W9-BOM-605

INTEGRATIVE NUTRITION

Feed Your Hunger for
Health & Happiness

Joshua Rosenthal

FOUNDER AND DIRECTOR, INSTITUTE FOR INTEGRATIVE NUTRITION

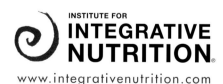

INSTITUTE FOR
**INTEGRATIVE
NUTRITION**®

www.integrativenutrition.com

Integrative Nutrition
3 East 28th St., Floor 12
New York, NY 10016
http://www.integrativenutrition.com

Distributed by Greenleaf Book Group LLC

For ordering information or special discounts for bulk purchases, please contact Greenleaf Book Group LLC at PO Box 91869, Austin, TX 78709, (512) 891-6100.

Page design, cover, and composition by Greenleaf Book Group LLC

Publisher's Cataloging-In-Publication Data
Rosenthal, Joshua.
    Integrative nutrition : feed your hunger for health and happiness / Joshua Rosenthal. -- 3rd ed.

    p. : ill., charts ; cm.

    Issued also as an ebook.
    Includes bibliographical references and index.
    ISBN: 978-0-9795264-5-9

    1. Nutrition. 2. Diet. 3. Health. 4. Holistic medicine. I. Title.

RA784 .R67 2014
613.2   2013952642

Printed in China on acid free paper

15 16 17 18 19 20   10 9 8 7 6 5 4 3

Third Edition

This book is dedicated to the health and happiness of people throughout the world and to the future of nutrition, which will offer new possibilities for everyone.

Contents

Acknowledgments

I am truly blessed to do the work I do everyday and to interact with so many incredible people who share a vision to change the world. Thank you to everyone who has been a part of my journey thus far.

I would especially like to thank:

The staff of Integrative Nutrition—you all contribute to the mission of the school. Your visions, creativity, intelligence, love and support consistently take the school to new levels.

The guest speakers who continue to inspire my students and offer new perspectives on the health and nutrition puzzle,

All of the students, alumni and their clients who have helped shape my view of things,

My dear parents for their unconditional love and support,

All of my friends who add love, laughter and support to my life,

Anyone who has ever purchased my books, joined the school's community, and everyone I've met along the way. You've all helped me get to where I am today.

Foreword

Life is a delicate balance between doing good and avoiding harm. The earliest single-cell organisms explored their environment looking for food, evading poisons and trying to avoid becoming food themselves. As life expanded into a multi-cellular animal kingdom, a kind of "inner knowing" developed. Animals have a sense of what to eat or avoid and instinctively know how to eat when sick, when breeding or in different seasons of the year. Our earliest human ancestors also had this inner knowing, as they ate local roots and greens and benefited from successful hunts and seasonal harvests.

Life has certainly become more complex. Our ability to process and transport foods has expanded beyond anything previously experienced in human culture. We fill supermarkets the size of football fields with more than 45,000 items, many of which are processed, packaged items wrapped in bright shiny packages and filled with sugar, fat and additives. Amidst all of this abundance, our compass of inner knowing has gone awry. It's become blocked by the magnetic attraction of foods that are engineered to tempt our taste buds but to neglect our health. We no longer instinctively know what to eat.

Adding to our confusion is an overwhelming glut of information about nutrition. A stampede of new diets on the market each claim to be the best and each have developed their own small following: High protein, low carbohydrate versus complex carbohydrate, low protein versus all raw foods versus vegan versus only grapefruit and on and on it goes. What each of these approaches misses is that we're all different. Our biological individuality allows one person to thrive on a diet that is a terrible for someone else. Following a diet plan designed by someone whose genetic makeup and nutritional needs are different from our own cannot restore our inner knowing. For real answers, we must look deeper.

In actuality, all of life is nutrition. Understanding this truth requires that we adopt a new perspective on food—one that integrates nutritional science, biological individuality and relearning our inner knowing. In this book, my friend and colleague, Joshua Rosenthal, presents an integrative holistic framework that will help readers see nutrition in an extraordinary light. His approach to nutrition offers a clear path to healthy living. I've watched his school, the Institute for Integrative Nutrition, grow from a small group to class sizes reaching more than 1,000 students. The word is out, because people are literally getting sick and tired of eating food that doesn't truly nourish them. With a simple, unique theory, Joshua's program addresses the full framework of nutrition. It focuses on truth rather than dogma, on real experiences rather than concepts and on a nutritional spectrum beyond food groups.

I know firsthand that a holistic, integrative approach like Joshua's really works. For decades I've seen how people who have lost touch with knowing what was good for them can recover health and balance. As a young physician in the 1970s, I began to practice a more natural method of patient care that included nutrition, vitamins, herbs, stress reduction, lifestyle changes and exercise. It became clear to me that people needed more education about how to be well. Like, Joshua, I created a school. When I started Omega Institute over 30 years ago, it was simply an adventurous experiment to create a space where people could learn and directly experience how to live in greater balance with themselves, others and our environment. I had no idea then that the holistic industry would become so large and in demand. People who come to Omega even for just a few days awe me with their capacity for transformation. I witness dramatic changes in their lives from eating whole foods, taking in lectures from inspiring teachers and experiencing nature.

Our society desperately needs more people who can help others to deeply nourish their health and inner beauty. Joshua and his students are part of a growing revolution to awaken and change society for the positive by recognizing the interdependence of all life. They represent a great opportunity for healing on many levels of our society and our planet.

This book encapsulates this different approach and new path. It offers you simple tools to help take control of your life by changing the way you view your health. Each of us can unlearn destructive habits and start living to our fullest potential. As we learn to tune into our inner knowing, we begin to listen to our bodies and fill them with whole, natural foods that nourish us.

We live in an era of "time poverty," where we're caught in a constant state of "hurry sickness." We consume massive amounts of caffeine to speed us up, eat fast foods to save time, work while eating to stay productive, but we never catch up. It is possible to shift these behaviors. Start by slowing down here and now: enjoy this book. Savor it like a good meal. Then start your meal with a few moments of silent breathing, chew slowly and enjoy the taste. Health and happiness begin with slowing down to enjoy every moment of your life.

Stephan Rechtschaffen, M.D., is cofounder of Omega Institute for Holistic Studies and chairman of Omega's board of directors. He is a holistic physician who uses concepts of time and healing as the focus for developing optimal health.

How to Use This Book

Set an Intention

To help you prepare for the journey ahead, please take a moment now to clarify your personal goals around health and well-being. What are your main health concerns? What is it you wish to learn or accomplish by reading this book? Devoting a small amount of time now to understand your optimal personal nutrition will result in a healthier, happier future later.

Experiment

In this book, you will find discussion of major dietary theories. But the food that is best for you is not going to be found in the pages of a nutrition book. No one diet is perfect for everyone. To best determine what is appropriate for your unique body and lifestyle, this book will guide you through experimenting with new foods and learning to listen to your body's responses.

Be Open to Discovery

A permanent shift in health may seem like a big challenge requiring a lot of dedication, but our approach is not about acquiring more self-discipline or willpower. It's about personally discovering what feeds you, what nourishes you and ultimately what makes your life extraordinary.

Climb One Rung of the Ladder at a Time

With this book you will unlearn old habits and absorb new information. Give yourself permission to go slowly. Big changes do not require big leaps. As far as your body is concerned, permanent change is more likely to happen gradually rather than through severe, austere diets. Proceed with care for yourself. Have fun.

Introduction

We all eat, all day every day, and we all know the saying, "we are what we eat." But for some reason, no one knows what to eat. Should we eat more grapes or drink more red wine? Are eggs a good source of protein or a source of bad cholesterol? Do dairy foods help us gain weight or lose weight?

Nutrition is a funny science. It's the only field where people can scientifically prove opposing theories and still be right. In science, we stick to facts. The earth rotates on an axis around the sun. The freezing point of water is 32 degrees. But we are yet to discover the same definitive truths about nutrition. We are only beginning to understand the relationship between our diet and our health. Despite all the nutritional research that's been done and all the diet books that have been published, most Americans are increasingly confused about food.

I have been working in the field of nutrition for more than 30 years and what I've learned is that there is probably no one right way of eating. I keep an open mind about new ideas that are published and respect others who are bravely working in this still-emerging field. My own background is in macrobiotics, an approach to healthy eating and balanced living developed in Japan that emphasizes the importance of whole foods and a plant-based diet. I've always been fascinated by food and health, and spent years experimenting with different ways of eating, noticing their effects and looking for the best ones for me and for my clients. I studied with the top macrobiotics experts and appreciated the simplicity and balance of their system. I spent years counseling and teaching others to follow the principles of macrobiotics to improve their health.

As I went along, I began to realize that macrobiotics was getting some people well, but not everyone. I started thinking there was more to health than simply eating healthy food. What was the missing ingredient? As I began to work with more and more clients, I found some interesting results. Some of my clients got better if they ate more raw foods, while others got better if they ate less raw foods. I had one client who didn't get better until she started eating some high-quality dairy products, even though macrobiotics advises against eating dairy. For other clients, it didn't matter what they ate. They got well by leaving a dysfunctional career or falling in love.

The more I observed human behavior, the more convinced I became that the key to health is understanding each person's individual needs, rather than following a set of predetermined rules. I saw plenty of evidence that having happy relationships, a fulfilling career, an exercise routine and a spiritual practice are even more important to health than daily diet. From these ideas I developed the concepts of Integrative Nutrition.

As I began evolving this new approach with clients, their results improved dramatically. I found many people were hungry for information about how to create a happy, healthy life and relieved to discover an approach that was flexible, fun and free of dogma and discipline. Drawing on my background in education, I started my own school to help individuals discover the foods and lifestyle choices that work best for them and to empower them to change the world.

Integrative Nutrition is a thriving school and community dedicated to helping evolve the future of nutrition, so that all beings can live healthier, happier and more fulfilling lives. For almost 20 years, people traveled far and wide to study at Integrative Nutrition in New York City. We now offer a life-changing online course, allowing students from all over the world to experience our unique program. As we spread our message to a global audience, the Integrative Nutrition community has grown exponentially. We are now 30,000 strong, with students and graduates in all 50 states and 100 countries.

We are the only school in the world integrating all of the different dietary theories—combining the knowledge of traditional philosophies like Ayurveda, macrobiotics and Chinese medicine with modern concepts like the USDA food guides, the glycemic index, The Zone, the South Beach Diet and raw foods. We teach more than 100 different dietary theories and address the fundamental concepts, issues and ethics of eating in a modern world.

We combine this information with simple steps for living a more balanced life full of laughter, joy and abundance. My intention is for you to uncover this process for yourself and share it with others.

I have noticed that as people improve their health, they become empowered to pursue the life of their dreams—the life they came here to live. If this book found its way to you or you found your way to this book, I trust it means you are a highly intelligent, highly sensitive human being with an appreciation for the benefits of whole foods and holistic living. Let this book empower you to stand up, speak up and act up for what you believe to be true. May your aliveness create a ripple effect in the world, and may all your hopes and dreams come true.

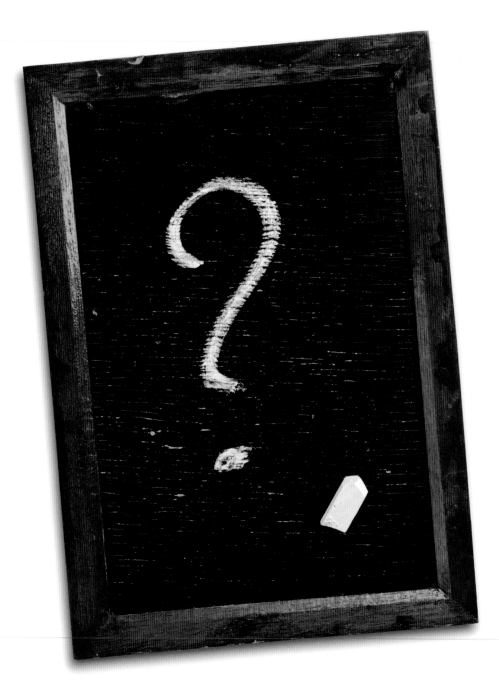

Question
What
You're Told

The Global Health Crisis

When I started Integrative Nutrition, I was just one person who felt that if I could improve what people eat, I would play a role in making the world a better place. I started in New York City because it's a place that sets trends for the world. The United States has the security, freedom and lifestyle desired by many people around the world. But Americans have become increasingly overweight, unhappy and unhealthy. Every year healthcare costs increase while overall health decreases; people continue to eat poorly, gain weight and depend on medications and operations to maintain their health.

Still, people around the world are hungry for American products—movies, television shows and cigarettes—and they love our food and drinks. American fast-food restaurants are sprouting up worldwide. McDonald's plans to open 700 new restaurants in China in 2013. Sales for Coca-Cola products slowed in developed countries, but the company announced in 2012 plans to invest $5 billion in India during the next 8 years.[1]

As our drinking and eating habits become fashionable throughout the world, so do our health concerns. More than half of the European Union's population is now overweight or obese.[2] In China, the World Health Organization (WHO) predicts that 50 to 57 percent of the population (mostly city dwellers) will be overweight or obese by 2015. They are rapidly catching up to America where 69 percent of Americans 20 years of age and older are overweight or obese.[3]

Overweight people now outnumber undernourished people in the world.[4] The WHO's estimates agree: globally, there are about 1.5 billion overweight adults, and 500 million of them are obese; in contrast, about 800 million do not have enough to eat. Even Africa, a continent previously thought of as being synonymous with hunger and food scarcity, is seeing a drastic rise in obesity and diabetes. More than one-third of African women are now overweight.

I saw firsthand the spreading of American food and health concerns when I visited Japan in 2005, after having been there twelve years prior. On my first trip, I traveled throughout Japan with Michio and Aveline Kushi, founders of the macrobiotic movement. During this time, I was overcome with the health of the Japanese people and spoke with many of them about their traditional ways of eating. The people talked about the value of their diet, which was rich in organic whole grains, vegetables, sea vegetables, fish and miso. They had perfect skin, clear eyes, slim bodies and a strong sense of peace and tranquility. However, on my last trip, I was shocked by the extent to which people's health had declined. Fast-food restaurants were everywhere. Many of the young Japanese people I saw were overweight, had acne and were missing that healthy glow I remembered so fondly from years before.

We are now witnessing a global health crisis. Today, more than one-third of American adults are overweight or obese. Worldwide, 347 million people have diabetes.[5] Every day, 2,500 Americans die from cardiovascular disease, such as coronary heart disease, heart attacks and stroke. By 2030, almost 25 million people will die from heart disease, which is predicted to remain the single leading cause of death.[6] Why are we so unhealthy and overweight?

Originally, the medical establishment's aim was to promote healing, but it increasingly relies on a pro-business model instead of a pro-health model at the expense of patients. The goal has become to increase profit, decrease expenses and let the chips fall where they may. This healthcare system is failing. In the U.S. Americans pay more for health insurance and have less time with doctors. Americans get more prescriptions and less guidance on how to create long-term health. U.S. health insurance today is really just prepaid medical expenses. Paying our monthly fees to insurance companies does not promise health; it just ensures that when you get sick you won't have to pay in full for your treatment.

The United States has the world's most expensive healthcare system. Yet, despite massive spending, Americans die earlier and experience higher rates of disease than people in other countries.[7] We suffer in increasing numbers from chronic health concerns, such as heart disease, obesity, diabetes, reproductive issues and depression.

An exorbitant amount of money is spent on medications and operations, while virtually nothing is spent on prevention, education and holistic health. The medical experts are basically saying, "Live it up, do what you want and when you get sick, we'll give you a magic pill that will make it all go away. If that pill doesn't work, we'll give you a different one, or a combination of a few, and if that doesn't work, we'll perform a quick operation, remove the problem and you'll be as good as new." What kind of system is this? Instead of asking citizens to pay for more pills and doctor's bills, wouldn't it be better to spend money on answering the question: *What would it take to have a country full of healthy, happy people?*

But it is not just American's suffering. Healthcare costs are straining governments and individuals around the world. About 100 million people a year are pushed into poverty by their medical bills, according to WHO.[8] Aging populations, the growing burden of chronic diseases and more expensive treatments are the main challenges governments face in funding healthcare.

In 2000, the World Health Organization completed the first ever assessment and comparison of the world's different healthcare systems. Examining various data including patient satisfaction, overall national health, medical responsiveness and distribution of services amongst the population, they rated the healthcare systems of 191 countries. The United States ranked 37th, despite the fact that we spend the highest proportion (over 16%) of our gross domestic product on healthcare. The United States spends more than $8,000 per capita on medical care compared with the average of more than $3,000 spent by other industrialized countries and twice as much as European countries like the United Kingdom, Sweden and France.[9] Our expenditure is significantly higher, yet we are the only industrialized nation that fails to offer universal healthcare to all our citizens. In fact, uninsured Americans reached an all-time high in 2010 at almost 50 million people.[10] Many of these Americans forego treatment because of prohibitive costs. Bankruptcy from lack of coverage and the excessive subsequent medical bills is commonplace. Job-based insurance premiums continue to rise, resulting in higher co-pays, deductibles and out-of-pocket expenses, according to the 2012 Employer Health Benefits Survey by the Kaiser Family Foundation and the Health Research & Educational Trust. Family coverage annual premiums have increased nearly 100 percent in the last decade, while costs for individual coverage are up 82 percent.[11]

The Affordable Healthcare Act, known as Obamacare, took effect in 2010, but it is not expected to make an impact on premiums until 2014 when its main provision—helping more uninsured gain access to medical care—kicks in. But two small provisions have already created positive ripples. Adults under the age of 26 can now remain on their parents' plan—this has insured 600,000 more young people than last year. Another provision requires new plans to cover preventative medical services with no patient cost-sharing, which is an overdue step toward prevention and education.

But even those with health insurance struggle to find an available, high-quality doctor in network. In addition, American patients report the greatest number of medical errors, including getting the wrong medication or dosage, incorrect test results, a mistake in treatment or late notification about abnormal test results. After carefully examining numerous indicators of performance, the Commonwealth Fund, a nonpartisan health policy think tank, gave the United States healthcare system a score of 64 out of a possible 100.[12] If we were in high school, this grade would be equivalent to a big, fat D.

If you were shopping in a store that had high-priced and low-quality products along with poor customer service, chances are you would not go back to that store. Why do we continue to tolerate this archaic, ineffective form of healthcare? Before blood pressure units and stethoscopes, doctors in Asia went from village to village caring for their patients. Using their ancient, traditional and so-called primitive skills of diagnosis, they would ask a few questions, look into a patient's eyes, check the tongue, take a pulse and then make recommendations. The next year, when the doctor returned, he was paid only if the patient was still healthy. If the patient had been sick, the doctor was not paid. Now that's a healthy healthcare system!

My passionate prayer is that people will become increasingly vocal about the exceptionally high cost of healthcare and demand answers from government officials at the local, state and federal levels. As Americans recognize the fundamental relationship between poor nutrition, expensive healthcare and the lamentable state of the public's health, my hope is that we can begin to set new trends for the world. What we eat makes a huge difference; yet very few doctors, corporations or politicians stand up for this truth.

The USDA

Good nutrition is straightforward and simple, but in America pressure from the food industry makes it almost impossible for any public official to state the plain truth. Public nutrition policy is dictated by the political process, which is now heavily dictated by a corporate agenda to maximize profits.

The primary agency responsible for American food policy is the U.S. Department of Agriculture, which was created in 1862 as a regulatory agency to ensure an adequate and safe food supply for the American public. The agency also took on the role of providing dietary advice to the public. From the start, the government had conflicting priorities. How can you protect public health on one hand and protect the interests of the food industry on the other? This opposition alone has led to decades of confusing and economically charged dietary advice.

As far back as 1917, when the USDA released its first dietary recommendations and launched the food-group format, it ignored research that Americans were eating too much, especially too much fat and sugar, because food manufacturers wanted to encourage the public to eat more.[13] It wasn't until the 1970s, when senators like George McGovern started to speak about the connection between overeating—especially fats, sugar, salt and cholesterol—and chronic disease that the USDA began advising people to restrict these foods in their diets with the *Dietary Goals* of 1977. With this new advice came strong objections from the meat, dairy and sugar industries.

The food industry's greatest allies are in Congress. It's the job of these politicians to protect the interests of their states, which includes not only the citizens but also the corporations and industries that live there. So, a senator from Texas will support the cattle industry. A senator from Wisconsin is going to fight for dairy by not allowing any wording into government guidelines that will negatively affect the dairy industry. Politicians, together with skilled, well-paid lobbyists, control legislation and nutritional information put out by the government. In 1977 when senators from meat-producing states such as Texas, Nebraska and Kansas saw the new dietary guidelines, they worked quickly—with the help of lobbyists for the National Cattlemen's Beef Association, among others—to amend the national dietary recommendations, removing any mention of decreasing the amount of meat in one's diet for optimal health.

This back and forth between the USDA, politicians and corporations continues to shape the public's awareness about what to eat. In 1991, the USDA and the Department of Health and Human Services created the first ever Food Guide Pyramid in an attempt to provide accurate guidelines about what to eat for optimal nutrition. Immediately, the meat and dairy industries blocked publication because they claimed it stigmatized their products. Marion Nestle, professor and former chair of the Department of Nutrition at New York University, chronicled the saga in her pioneering book, *Food Politics: How the Food Industry Influences Nutrition and Health*. The meat and dairy industries were upset because the Food Guide Pyramid placed their products in a category labeled "eat less." The USDA then withdrew the guide. It took more than a year to create a pyramid that was acceptable to the two industries. And that, my friends, is how our "politically correct" Food Guide Pyramid was created.

Let's take a moment to examine the pyramid that shaped American attitudes about health, diet and nutrition for more than 20 years. The USDA designed the pyramid in hierarchical form to indicate the importance and recommended quantity of each food group. The broad foundation is carbohydrates, including bread, cereal, rice and pasta. Next up is a slightly narrower band of fruits and vegetables, then a smaller layer of protein-rich foods, including meat and dairy. The very top has a small section of fats, oils and sweets.

Do you find anything odd about this picture? Anything you might question or disagree with? Almost everyone I meet has numerous issues with this pyramid. Even the experts who put it together must have known something

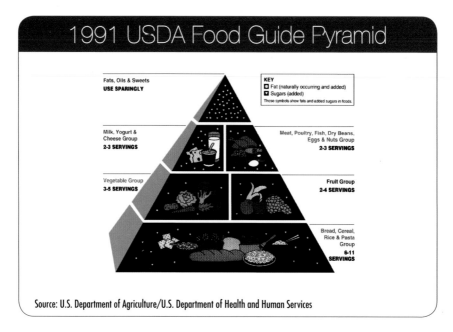

Source: U.S. Department of Agriculture/U.S. Department of Health and Human Services

was wrong here. Let's face it; the 1991 USDA Food Pyramid is a political document, not a scientific one. It encourages people to eat a lot of everything. This advice certainly helps the food industry and the senators protecting their financial interests.

The medical profession, registered dietitians, insurance companies, politicians and bureaucrats all advocated this Food Guide Pyramid from 1991 to 2005. The guidelines influenced government nutrition programs, food labeling and food promotion. Nutrition professionals used this as their foundation for working with clients, as did the makers of school lunch programs. These recommendations were the foundation of America's outlook on health, diet and nutrition for a time period that had a substantial increase in obesity and diet-related health concerns.

In 2001, the Physicians Committee for Responsible Medicine won a lawsuit, on the topic of the USDA's ties to the food industry. PCRM objected to the over-promotion of meat and dairy products by the government because of the prevalence of diet-related diseases such as heart disease, diabetes and hypertension. PCRM showed that the majority of the committee that reviews and updates the federal dietary guidelines had strong financial ties to the meat, dairy or egg industries.

"Having advisors tied to the meat or dairy industries is as inappropriate as letting tobacco companies decide our standards for air quality," Dr. Neal Barnard, president of PCRM, said.

The verdict found that the USDA had violated federal law by withholding documents that revealed a strong bias by the committee. PCRM's victory was a huge embarrassment to the USDA, especially because the government ruled against itself, which very rarely happens. Four years after the PCRM verdict, the Dietary Guidelines Advisory Committee reviewed and updated the dietary guidelines again. This time, they had the task of responding to recent statistics showing skyrocketing rates of obesity across the nation. The 2005 Dietary Guidelines were described as "the most health-oriented ever."

The report recommended that Americans eat more vegetables and whole-grain products, cut down on certain fats, such as butter, margarine and lard, and consume less sugar. The report strongly recommended that people "engage in regular physical activity and reduce sedentary activities to promote health, psychological well-being and a healthy body weight." In other words: Get off your butt, America, and start exercising.

Despite the improvements, the 2005 Dietary Guidelines still had many limitations. First, the guidelines were supposed to be about diet, and emphasizing weight loss through exercise shifts the responsibility for dietary change to the individual and away from the food industry's multibillion-dollar budget for marketing and promoting unhealthy foods. In addition, the guidelines didn't speak a language easily understood by the people who most needed the advice. Imagine if the guidelines said, "Stop eating Oreos, Jiffy peanut butter and Hostess cupcakes; Stop eating McDonald's, Burger King and Taco Bell." Now that's something we would understand!

MyPyramid

Following the release of the Dietary Guidelines in April 2005, the USDA redesigned the food pyramid, which stood more or less unchanged since its first appearance in 1992, and renamed it "MyPyramid." MyPyramid showed some improvements from the previous pyramid. It drew attention to both leafy green vegetables and whole grains, two groups the old pyramid was

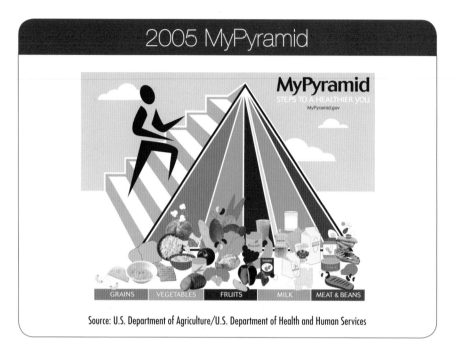

2005 MyPyramid

Source: U.S. Department of Agriculture/U.S. Department of Health and Human Services

missing. It also addressed the concept of healthy fats with advice to get most of your fat from fish, nuts and vegetable oils. For the first time, beans, seeds and nuts were recognized as legitimate sources of protein, and the pyramid even recommended to "vary your protein routine" and "choose more fish, beans, peas, nuts and seeds." The milk section included a comment for people who "don't or can't consume milk," marking the first time the USDA has acknowledged that not everyone can digest dairy. Even with these advances, MyPyramid was still far from an easily understood, legitimate and accurate presentation of what foods are necessary for health. The vegetable section was about the same size as the milk section, which seemed to imply you should consume the same amount of milk and vegetables.

MyPyramid promoted the idea that we can eat as much as we want, as long as we exercise every day. Calories in, calories out is a concept that benefits both the food and the exercise industries. The pyramid was constructed for people who exercise 30 to 60 minutes a day. A better plan would have been to create a pyramid for people who do not exercise at all, since most Americans are not active.

2010 Dietary Guidelines

The USDA released the updated 2010 Dietary Guidelines for Americans in January 2011. Like the 2005 report, the 2010 guidelines point out that Americans don't eat enough vegetables or whole grains and, instead, eat too much fat and sugar. Unfortunately, the guidelines continued to miss the mark and use vague terminology. "SoFAS" is used to describe added sugars and solid fats. To even a well-educated person, the word "sofa" is generally used to describe a small couch.

It's the use of these misleading words that led the Physician's Committee for Responsible Medicine (PCRM) to file yet another lawsuit against the federal government on February 15, 2011. PCRM states that using biochemical terms instead of naming actual foods like "meat and cheese" keeps Americans eating these unhealthy foods. "What Americans really should be told is we need to eat less red meat, less cheese, less ice cream, and less refined grains," Dr. Walter Willett said in a National Public Radio interview. Why is it so hard for the government to call out the main culprits?

Although the potential for conflict of interest still exists among committee members, these guidelines seem to be significantly more transparent than in years past. The guidelines committee recommended more action stating that the USDA and HHS convene separate committees to develop strategies for implementing these recommendations. They even admitted, "the actions needed to implement key recommendations likely differ by goal."

MyPlate

In response to the updated 2010 Dietary Guidelines, the USDA replaced MyPyramid with MyPlate. The icon was revealed by Agriculture Secretary Tom Vilsack and First Lady Michelle Obama. The goal was to simplify nutritional information to make it more useful to the average family. I commend the plate, as most people can understand that image.

Unlike the pyramids of the past, which attempted to convey how much you should eat based on the colors and relative sizes of sections on the pyramid,

MyPlate focuses on the portion sizes at each meal through simple divisions of a plate. It makes it visually obvious that half of your plate should be filled with fruits and vegetables. The MyPlate icon also features selected messages, like "avoid oversized portions" and "enjoy your food, but eat less." However, as with the pyramid, you must visit the MyPlate website for specific instructions on what to eat.

While MyPlate is a huge step toward instilling healthy changes in Americans, it still has many shortcomings. Why does dairy continue to be an essential part of the meal? Let's define grains more clearly, as we know there's a big difference between white bread and brown rice.

The Integrative Nutrition® Plate solves many of these issues. Adapted from the USDA MyPlate, this version also emphasizes the importance of vegetables, fruits and protein, but I swapped dairy with water and I've added fats and oils, which are essential to the diet. To complete the full picture of health, the plate is surrounded with lifestyle factors—primary foods—that create optimal health. The four types of primary foods are: relationships, physical activity, career, and spirituality. I encourage people to look at these aspects of life as a form of nutrition—a way to feed themselves at a much deeper level than food. The food you eat plays a critical role in your health and happiness, and discovering the right foods for you is very important. But the four forms of primary food truly nourish you and make your life extraordinary. We will explore these areas in depth later in the book.

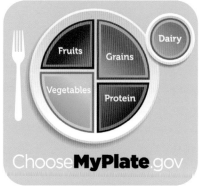

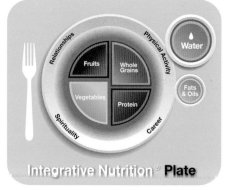

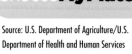

Source: U.S. Department of Agriculture/U.S. Department of Health and Human Services

Food Corporations

Food corporations are more or less free to deceive the public about the nature of their products, often using the guidelines—like the Food Guide Pyramid, MyPyramid and now MyPlate—as vehicles for their own agendas. The U.S. government even contributes to many food-marketing campaigns. Just think of the popular campaigns like "Got Milk?" "Beef. It's What's for Dinner" and "Pork. The Other White Meat." These campaigns, aimed at increasing Americans' consumption of dairy, beef and pork products, are part of the federal government's commodity promotion programs, called "checkoff" programs. Checkoff programs demonstrate the dual role of the federal government to both educate the public about nutrition and health, while still promoting its food. The question is, where are all the ads for vegetables or whole grains?

When the pyramid was released in 2005, General Mills announced that about 100 million boxes of its Big G cereal brands would carry MyPyramid on them, citing that the cereal box is one of the most-read items in the home.[14] The company also announced that they would reformulate their products to include whole grains, which was in line with the recommendation of the 2005 pyramid to eat more whole grains, thereby implying their cereals, including Lucky Charms, Trix and Golden Grahams, are healthy. Now that's savvy marketing.

Also in 2005, Frito-Lay, the potato chip manufacturer, devised its own food pyramid, showing packets of chips with happy, smiling faces filling the bottom section, implying that chips provide the carbohydrate foundation needed for good health. This is nonsense. The carbohydrates in chips are covered in fat, drenched in artificial flavoring and so highly refined that they immediately break down into simple sugars in the body. The supermarket shelf is a free-for-all in which companies can make many claims about their products, and public health authorities rarely interfere.

Of course, if people consumed junk foods only occasionally we would not have a global health crisis. But food and beverage corporations are big business. In 2012, PepsiCo had more than $60 billion in profits, Kraft $54 billion, Kellogg $13 billion—the list goes on and on.[15] The fast food and restaurant industries also generate billions in annual sales. McDonalds raked in over $27 billion in 2012, and it continues to open new franchises all the time.[16] These corporations put a big hunk of this money back into advertising.

It seems like every food corporation is trying to create a healthy image and pass off its products as being good for you. No one regulates the word "health" or "natural." No standards exist for the phrase "good for your health." So these food corporations are using their millions and billions of dollars to trick the public into thinking their products are healthy, simply because one of the ingredients is derived from a whole grain.

You may be wondering, how can food corporations get away with these tactics? Let me explain. The food industry spends a tremendous amount of money on lobbyists in Washington. In fact, in 2012, $26 million was spent on specific food and beverage lobbying. These big bucks pay off, giving these corporations major unfair advantages when it comes to food policy and regulations. Lobbying expenditures spiked from nearly $22.1 million in 2008 to nearly $56.8 million in 2009. Most of this increase came from the American Beverage Association. The ABA spent less than $700,000 in 2008 but spent almost $19 million in lobbying expenditures the next year.[17] The cause of such sudden massive spending? Congressional talk of a "soda tax" to help combat obesity.

That same year, Coke introduced 90-calorie mini cans to help fight concerns about obesity. How about reducing the amount of sugar and artificial ingredients in your products?

Soda company tactics have aggressively worked to deceive the public. In 2013 Coca-Cola released a new commercial touting their efforts to fight obesity saying, "All calories count, no matter where they come from, including Coca-Cola and everything else with calories." The American Beverage Association says its members have cut 88 percent of the calories shipped to schools since 2004 by offering less sugary drinks and emphasizing water, low-fat milk and juice in schools. But these are the same soda companies that made sure to solidify relationships with young customers through exclusive "pouring rights" contracts in public schools starting in the early '90s. In exchange for exclusive selling rights in school districts, Big Soda companies supplied schools all the beverages sold at snack bars, in vending machines and at sports events, offering the struggling school massive payments.[18]

Along with the drinks, the companies also filled the school with advertisements. But in response to growing pressure from parent groups and public health advocates, the ABA eventually announced voluntary restrictions on soft drink sales in elementary and middle schools, instead ramping up sales of bottled water and juices.[19]

Despite their efforts, U.S. soda revenues have plummeted by 40 percent in the last 10 years or so—due to the popularity of coffee and energy drinks, along with more nutrition education and even political bans. New York City Mayor Michael Bloomberg introduced legislation to ban supersized sodas (drinks larger than 16 ounces) in the city in 2013, causing a lot of uproar on both sides. The soda industry argues that the city is nagging consumers and imposing unfair burdens on businesses. But the mayor says the ban could help people drink fewer calories without even thinking about it.[20, 21] For someone who drinks soda every day, drinking a 16-ounce soda instead of a 20-ounce can could trim 14,600 calories in a year, or the equivalent of 70 Hershey bars.

Big Soda continues to market heavily overseas, trying to maintain that their products are healthy. In the U.K. Coca-Cola launched a Work-it-Out Calculator on their website, showing that you can still enjoy your soda; you just need to keep active. How about everyone keep moving and ditch the soda? In 2012, Pepsi launched a high-fiber, fat-burning soda in Japan called Pepsi Special. The drink contains a fiber-rich starch dextrin, which can be derived from arrowroot, potato or wheat. Japan's soda market is valued at almost $48 billion, but it's still a wonder why people would ever think getting fiber from empty, sugary calories could make them healthy.[22]

Not all food news is bad, though. The supersized soda ban in NYC has increased awareness about larger portion sizes, and as other cities consider similar measures it could just be the next big, successful health campaign. In 2011, McDonald's announced it would halve the amount of French fries and add fruit to children's Happy Meals in response to parental and consumer pressure.[23]

In January 2006, a big health victory came when the FDA required all packaged foods to list trans fat content on their Nutrition Facts labels. Trans fat is a compound created by chemically adding hydrogen to liquid vegetable oils. Food manufacturers have used trans fats for years to enhance flavor, extend the shelf life of packaged foods and give a more solid texture to baked and fried foods. In the early 1990s, studies began to link trans fats and heart disease. Research now shows that eating trans fats increases cholesterol and risks of developing heart disease, diabetes and cancer. Most corporations continued to use this substance until the law required them to list it as an ingredient. Companies had to choose between listing an unhealthy ingredient on their products and risking decreased sales, or finding an alternative ingredient. Now many products with bright lettering displaying "No Trans Fats" line shelves.

Government Policies

Ever notice that unhealthy foods are cheaper than healthy foods? You may think nothing of it, but our government policies and practices help lower the prices of unhealthful foods. Since the 1920s, American farmers have received government subsidies to help maximize production, reduce cost of raw materials, stabilize crop prices and keep the cost of food down for the American public, allowing farmers to stay in business. This originally well-intentioned government money has led to the overproduction of corn and soybeans, and consequently, lower prices for these crops and foods containing them as ingredients. This may seem harmless. Corn and soybeans are healthy, right?

In their natural states, these foods are not bad, but the outcome of the overproduction of these crops has led to their increased use as cheap, unhealthy ingredients found in processed foods on the grocery store aisles. High fructose corn syrup—an artificial ingredient found in most sodas and junk foods—is an inexpensive use of corn. Low corn prices have led to artificially low meat prices, because corn has become the number one feed for cattle—a major shift from a traditional grazing diet. The overproduction of soybeans and corn provides an inexpensive way to add flavor to packaged junk food, fast food, corn-fed beef and pork, and soft drinks. For consumers, these less nutritious foods are cheaper and particularly tempting to people living on a budget. These subsidies contribute to the obesity epidemic by making it cheaper to produce and purchase unhealthy packaged foods.[24]

As a result of the subsidies, growing fruits, vegetables and other grains is less lucrative for farmers. Less than ten percent of USDA subsidies are spent on fruits and vegetables. We should be asking why vegetables, fruits and whole grains aren't heavily subsidized so they can be cheaper and more accessible to everyone. Obviously, this change in policy would go a long way in helping

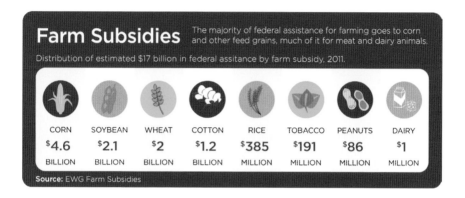

Farm Subsidies The majority of federal assistance for farming goes to corn and other feed grains, much of it for meat and dairy animals.

Distribution of estimated $17 billion in federal assitance by farm subsidy, 2011.

CORN	SOYBEAN	WHEAT	COTTON	RICE	TOBACCO	PEANUTS	DAIRY
$4.6	$2.1	$2	$1.2	$385	$191	$86	$1
BILLION	BILLION	BILLION	BILLION	MILLION	MILLION	MILLION	MILLION

Source: EWG Farm Subsidies

Americans follow their own government's nutritional guidelines. This disparity in government funding points out an awkward truth about the USDA: what it urges people to eat does not match what it pays farmers to grow.

Decades of food policy designed to benefit agribusiness and megafarms plays a big role in the American public health. Every five years, Congress must look at the national policies for agriculture, nutrition, conservation and forestry policy under a bundle of legislation, commonly known as the "Farm Bill."[25, 26] This legislation has the power to influence everything from the cost and availability of food to the protection of farmland throughout the country. The foods subsidized by the farm bill have an enormous impact on how the country eats. Some of the more promising aspects of the 2012 farm bill include expanding the Farmers Market and Local Food Promotion Program and $100 million of mandatory funding to encourage the purchase of fruits and vegetables in the Supplemental Nutrition Assistance Program, which serves the nation's low-income communities.

Another influential factor is political campaign contributions. Dependence on financial contributions from powerful lobbies prevents government agencies from stating the simple truths about nutrition. Politicians say the money they receive from corporate donors does not influence the policies they promote, but why would companies give money if this were true? Corporations are not known for their spontaneous generosity. Politicians need a lot of money to get elected, and food and drug companies are some of their biggest backers. McDonald's, Pepsi, General Mills, Kraft, Nestlé and Hershey depend on their friends in Washington, who make the food laws and guidelines. The top contributors to the former chairman of the Agricultural Committee, Frank D. Lucas (R-OK), were American Crystal Sugar, Dairy Farmers of America, National Beer Wholesalers Association, and National Cattlemen's Beef Association.[27] Of course, they want some return on their investment here.

Just Say No To Drugs

Something has gone terribly wrong in the pharmaceutical industry today. Medications in America are increasingly expensive. Every month a new magic pill emerges, and we are bombarded with commercials for drugs that cite side effects that sound worse than the original ailment. Does this sound familiar? "Warning: may cause nausea, headaches, constipation, dizziness, drowsiness or in extreme cases death."

Americans spent $307 billion on prescription drugs in 2010.[28] This boom of prescription drugs is partially due to advertising and doctors guiding the public to believe they need more medication. These advertisements, which usually feature attractive people—sometimes celebrities—smiling in the outdoors, send the message that what people need to be healthy is more prescription drugs. You name the health concern and a drug is out there for it. Drugs help us control cholesterol, lower blood pressure, regulate the menstrual cycle, prevent osteoporosis and end acid reflux. I frequently say that Americans are not prescription drug deficient. We are nutritionally deficient. The idea that prescription drugs cure diseases is a fallacy. They only work as a band-aid to a larger problem.

In addition to inundating the market with drugs and creating advanced marketing strategies, the pharmaceutical industry makes a killing, charging exorbitantly high prices for their products. In *The Truth About Drug*

Companies: How They Deceive Us and What to Do About It, Dr. Marcia Angell argues that drug companies must find a better, less expensive way of doing business. She says profits for pharmaceutical manufacturers really took off in 1980, when new legislation allowed university medical researchers and big drug companies to form an alliance. Before that time, taxpayers funded drug research, and findings were available to any pharmaceutical company that wanted to use them. With the new law, universities could patent their discoveries and grant exclusive licenses to drug companies. Suddenly, unbiased research disappeared. Then, Congress passed another series of laws extending monopoly rights for brand-name drugs to 14 years, another big win for the pharmaceutical industry. Under this law, pharmaceutical companies could market their drugs without competition for 14 years, charging whatever they liked. Only after the 14-year period could companies sell generic copies of the drug. This law allowed government-granted monopolies in the form of patents and FDA-approved exclusive marketing rights. As profits increased from these new policies, so did the political clout of drug companies.

Drug companies have one of the largest lobbying groups in Washington and give generously to political campaigns. By 1990, the industry had unprecedented control over its own fortunes. If it didn't like something that its regulatory body, the FDA, decreed, it could force change on the policy through direct pressure or friends in Congress.

The clout of the pharmaceutical industry led to a transformation in the ethos of medical school. Medical schools began searching for commercial opportunities and now welcome big sponsorships from drug companies. Pharmaceutical sales teams offer presentations to medical students, teaching them about the benefits of their products. Future doctors may have idealistic notions about preventing illness and making Americans healthier, but many of them graduate believing modern drugs are the quickest and most effective way to cure any symptom.

The FDA has the task of approving and regulating not only prescription drugs, but also food, supplements and other products that can be harmful to health. Their mission statement says:

> The FDA is responsible for protecting the public health by assuring the safety, efficacy, and security of human and veterinary drugs, biological products, medical devices, our nation's food supply, cosmetics, and products

that emit radiation. The FDA is also responsible for advancing the public health by helping to speed innovations that make medicines and foods more effective, safer, and more affordable; and helping the public get the accurate, science-based information they need to use medicines and foods to improve their health.

In 2008, poisoning became the leading cause of injury death in the U.S., and nearly 9 out of 10 poisoning deaths were caused by drugs.[29] This same year, these deaths exceeded the number of motor vehicle traffic deaths. Celebrities like Michael Jackson, Heath Ledger and Whitney Houston all died from overdoses and complications related to FDA-approved pharmaceutical drugs. These kinds of overdoses have tripled in the last decade and now have a larger toll than deaths from cocaine and heroin combined, according to a report from the CDC.[30]

Hello, where is the FDA? They appear to be overly focused on helping drug companies maximize profits rather than protecting consumer interests. Almost no one in the government is asking the right questions. People don't need more drugs. Maybe they need to understand disease prevention, the importance of exercise and how to eat a healthy, balanced diet. The fact that everyone is on medication should be questioned, discussed, and addressed.

The reason I share this information is not to blame the FDA or drug companies. I want the public to wake up to the fact that our system is broken. I want people to understand that even though a pill is out there claiming to help with a particular condition, there is another way—a healthy path that involves nutritious food, physical activity and a fulfilling life.

I want to tell you a little bit about my father. He is a fit, healthy, clever and humorous man who lives in Canada, and up until he was 82 years old was on no medication. My American friends and colleagues are surprised by this fact, but it is actually normal in other parts of the world for people to not take medication.

Scientists have even started studying certain regions around the world where people commonly live past the age of 100 years with little disease and no need for medication. These areas are called Blue Zones and are found in the mountain villages of Sardinia, Italy; the islands of Okinawa, Japan; the beach area of Nicoya Peninsula, Costa Rica and a community of Seventh-day

Adventists living in Loma Linda, California. What the people in these areas have in common is a healthy lifestyle including not smoking, staying active, engaging in social activities with people of all ages, putting family first and eating mostly plant-based diets, which is a far cry from lifestyles found in the Western world. I'll talk more about the Blue Zones later in the book.

Don't Trust the Experts

With nearly 74,000 members, the Academy of Nutrition and Dietetics (AND), formerly the American Dietetic Association (ADA), is the nation's largest organization of food and nutrition professionals. Founded in Cleveland, Ohio, in 1917 by a group of women dedicated to helping the government conserve food and improve the public's health and nutrition during World War I, the organization's mission is "leading the future of dietetics." AND members serve the public as "the most valued source" of good advice about food and nutrition, with a commitment "to helping people enjoy healthy lives."

Forty-six states currently have laws concerning professional regulation of dietitians and nutritionists, according to the AND's website. The group's rationale for protecting these titles is simple: the public deserves to know which individuals are qualified by education, experience and examination to provide nutrition care services.

The history of these laws began in 1987, when the Ohio state legislature passed a law, creating the Ohio Board of Dietetics, which prevented anyone from giving advice on nutrition except members of the AND. This law seems in line with public interest by restricting unqualified people from giving nutritional advice. However, the law was passed not to protect the public from poor nutrition advice, but to protect its own dietitians from competition. The Board asserts that only dietitians have permission to use the term "nutritionist" in their job title. Other professionals with master's degrees or Ph.Ds in nutrition, who are not members of the AND, are not allowed to use "nutrition" in their titles in Ohio. In addition, only dietitians are able to give advice, provide education and develop policies on nutrition. The Board put the issue into the national agenda, pushing for state-by-state

PROFILE

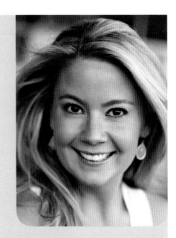

Elizabeth Rider, Billings, MT, USA

www.elizabethrider.com

"Consciously cultivating the ideal lifestyle is my religion."

Hi! I'm Elizabeth Rider. I help smart, savvy, successful women become even more successful by teaching them not just how to live well, but how to become the absolute BEST version of themselves.

My mantra in life is Happy, Healthy, Whole. It's about being in love with life, celebrating your unique talents, and living like you mean it.

I talk a lot about nutrition, but also about what it means to cultivate soul-shakingly good relationships, a heart-centered personal life, a healthy home environment, the importance of creativity (and fun!), kicking ass in your career, and making sure you show up as the sharpest, most giving, generous version of YOU that you can. Every. Single. Day.

And while my online business might look all sorts of fancy, I promise I'm really just a normal, down-to-earth girl. I grew up in Montana. I worked my way through college. I landed a spot at a Big 4 accounting firm. (I know—so different than what I do today.) I checked off all the boxes that society said would make me successful. And you know what? I wasn't happy. Something didn't feel right. And if I wasn't living the very best version of me, whose version was I living? And why?

So I decided to get serious about creating my ideal life. Or crazy, depending on who you asked at the time. Most people in my life thought I was insane to leave a highly successful corporate career (I had, after all, just won one of the firm's highest recognition awards). I took the leap to do something I absolutely loved and found the Institute for Integrative Nutrition—enrolling was one of the best decisions I've ever made.

I now run several nutrition-based businesses entirely online and enjoy an extremely comfortable lifestyle in which I can afford all of life's pleasures, work as much as I choose, and come and go as I please. I'm so extraordinarily blessed and grateful for everything I have in my life.

I'm completely determined to help others do what they were meant to do, and live the lives they were meant to live.

legislation to exclude everyone other than certified dietitians from giving nutritional advice.

Unfortunately, at the same time AND has been fighting against other nutrition educators, it has been taking money from Big Food. Michele Simon, a lawyer who specializes in legal issues with the food industry, released a report in 2013 detailing the number of food companies and trade groups that are paid sponsors of the academy. They more than tripled between 2001 and 2011, and more than 20 percent of about 300 speakers at its annual meeting had undisclosed financial ties to the food industry. Among some of the biggest sponsors? ConAgra, the National Cattlemen's Beef Association, Kellogg's, General Mills, Aramark, Mars and the National Dairy Council. How can an organization responsible for educating the public about nutrition educate its members using the same companies that are making people sick and obese? I attended a conference in 2012 and was shocked to see the likes of McDonald's, Kraft and Coca-Cola exhibiting and offering nutrition info at a meeting geared toward nutrition professionals.[31]

I'd like to point out that many dietitians are breaking away from conventional AND practices and do not support the corporate sponsorship of the organization. Many are making strides within the organization, like members of the Dietitians in Integrative and Functional Medicine, a group within AND that specializes in integrative, functional and holistic medicine, whole foods and natural healing modalities. This group is committed to inspiring more leaders in evidence-based practice for healing with whole foods, and I applaud their work. One of the fastest-growing AND practice groups is called Hunger and Environmental Nutrition (HEN), which looks at issues like antibiotics in animals, social justice and clean water issues. HEN's more than 1,400 members created their own listserv called Progressive Nutritionists. Others are working to create more awareness to expose AND's connection to junk food and big pharmaceuticals. At reallyeatright.org, RDs, nutritionists, AND members and citizens voice their concerns with AND's partnerships and its multi-state legislative effort to monopolize nutrition therapy.

Beginning in 1996, the board went after 795 people with lawsuits but made a serious tactical error when it turned its guns on Dr. Pamela Popper, a well-known nutritionist with two Ph.Ds who had designed an education program for an Ohio hospital but was not a member of the then ADA.

The Board came after Popper, threatening criminal prosecution. She not only fought the Board and the ADA but also vigorously campaigned to expose their practices, such as putting qualified professionals out of business, using heavy-handed investigation techniques, prohibiting the public to obtain unbiased nutrition information and failure to show that anyone had been harmed by nutrition advice given by someone who was not a member of the ADA. Popper made people aware that dietetics is only a small part of nutrition theory and publicized the fact that the ADA is heavily funded by the food industry, receiving millions of dollars a year from agricultural organizations and corporations that manufacture food and food additives.

The AND's positions on many health and nutrition subjects are, literally, bought and paid for. "With 15 percent of its budget—more than $3 million—coming from food companies and trade groups, it has learned not to bite the hand that feeds it," Sheldon Rampton and John Stauber wrote in *PR Watch*, the quarterly journal of the nonprofit Center for Media and Democracy.[32] "You can't take $50,000 a year from the sugar association and say bad things about sugar," Popper wrote. "This organization controls the educational programming and registration of the thousands of dietitians in the United States. It is my personal opinion that the influence of industry on the practice of dietitians is one of the reasons why nutrition in institutions such as hospitals, schools and nursing homes continues to be abominable."[33]

The story of the AND is just part of the long history of commerce in America. Each interest group tries to destroy the opposition in order to create a monopoly for itself, thereby acquiring more power, status and profit. If we cannot trust any of these groups to give us good advice about health and nutrition, whom can we trust?

The Turning Point

If we want to be healthy, we need to eat nutritious foods. It really isn't difficult. Unfortunately, billions of dollars are spent every day trying to seduce us not to do it. The food industry, drug companies, politicians, civil servants and even the medical profession all have strong vested interests in making money and not in protecting our health. In one way or another, almost all the sources of information we would expect to support our quest for overall health are contaminated for reasons of financial gain. If we face the facts, being sick and overweight keeps corporate profits healthy.

But the world is beginning to wake up to the reality that healthy food creates healthy people. We see it in the papers, on television commercials and hear all sorts of people talking about it. Sales of organic produce in the U.S. increased from $1 billion in 1990 to $28.6 billion in 2009.[34] Corporations are responding. The success of stores such as Whole Foods and Trader Joe's and the incorporation of organic sections at Walmart illustrate that consumers are concerned about their health and the quality of their food. When individuals like you and me stand up for improving our own health, things do change. If we buy our food from health-food stores, farmers' markets, and don't spend our money on unhealthful foods, corporations get the message loud and clear. Don't become a silent victim within the system. Think locally, act locally. Get involved with your local government, your school system, your office, your church or temple, and your family. With our dollars, our voices and our forks, we have the power to create change. If we all stand up and speak up for what we know to be true, we can dramatically improve the world's health and happiness. Margaret Mead said, "Never doubt a small group of thoughtful committed citizens can change the world; indeed, it's the only thing that ever has."

Exercises

1. Supermarket Field Trip

Go to your local supermarket with a friend or family member and walk around, looking into people's shopping carts. Ninety percent of Americans get their food from supermarkets. This should give you a good understanding of what people are eating in America today.

- Take out a piece of paper and write down the most common food items you see in people's carts.

- What is missing from people's carts?

- Imagine, how would you feel if you were eating these foods?

- What attracts you to the foods people have chosen (packaging, colors, etc.)?

2. Trustworthy Professionals

- Make a list of the "experts" in health and nutrition that you trust the most.

- Is there any expert you would trust with your life?

- Where has your most faithful, useful and solid health and nutrition information come from?

3. Get Involved

Contact your local government and find out where your local officials stand on food and health issues.

Here are some web resources to get you started:

- House of Representatives: www.house.gov

- Senate: www.senate.gov

- Project Vote Smart provides non-partisan information on each elected official and candidate for office: www.votesmart.org

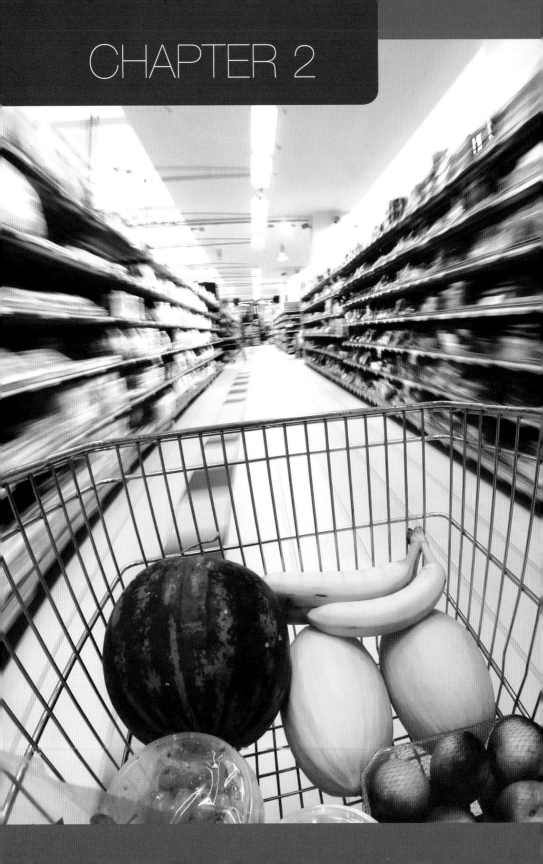

CHAPTER 2

Post-Modern Nutrition

Insanity: doing the same thing over and over
again and expecting different results.

—ALBERT EINSTEIN

We live in a world of modern nutrition. Almost everyone is on one diet or another. People dwell on calories, carbs, fats, proteins, restrictions and lists of good and bad foods. Each day we are hit with a new discovery, proclaiming the health benefits of a certain food or the best way to lose 10 pounds in a week. Diet books are best sellers. News programs feature stories about the global growing health crisis or the new wonder drug. Cooking shows are more popular than ever, while more and more families are eating out.

It wasn't too long ago that humans existed without this media blitz, without expensive medications and without diet gurus or celebrity chefs telling them what to eat. Instead they relied on intuition. People simply knew what to eat and how to prepare it. They didn't go to the gym to exercise; they just exercised. They didn't have a complicated career; they just worked. They didn't have such a cerebral interpretation of basic human needs. People naturally lived in harmony with the seasons and with their surroundings. They ate what was local and available and what gave them proper nutrients for their lives.

The world of nutrition has become incredibly complex. Nutrition is the only science in which two parties can comprehensively prove two different theories that are diametrically opposed to one another. Scientists unanimously agree, the speed of light is 670 million miles per hour; gravity is an attractive force between all matter; and water is made of two parts hydrogen and one part oxygen. How is it possible, then, that one expert can prove dairy is a necessary component of a healthy diet, while another expert can prove dairy is extremely detrimental to health; one expert can claim meat is essential to a healthy human body while another expert says meat is an unnecessary and unhealthy part of the human diet?

The publishing industry has largely shaped beliefs about food and health. Eager to earn money from the next best seller, they are the ones who "discover" and promote nutritional truths, not the medical industry. Think about it. Did you ever try *to Eat This, Not That!?* What about *The G.I Diet, The Sonoma Diet,* or *The Paleo Diet*? The *Dukan Diet* was a phenomenon in Europe. These are all popular diet books but they are not scrutinized for truth and scientific evidence about healthy eating; they simply aim to be best sellers. They grab attention by shocking, entertaining and providing quick ways to lose weight. But the dietary theories in these books are not usually sustainable for long periods of time. Once they stop working, the reader will try another diet book, and so on, and so on, consistently supporting the publishing industry. Remember the Atkins diet craze that hit the market in 2001? Sales of *Dr. Atkins' New Diet Revolution* exceeded 10 million copies, even though the book provided no medical evidence that the diet worked. In fact, it went against the standard nutritional advice to eat more vegetables and get more exercise.

My point is not to bash these diets. The Atkins diet was the beginning of public awareness about the glycemic index of certain foods and the unfavorable effects of simple carbohydrates. Each diet book exposes one more piece of the nutrition puzzle. Nutrition is still an emerging field in many ways, and we are only just beginning to understand all its facets.

Experts agree that we all need variety in our diets. But many disagree about other issues such as how much water to drink throughout the day or whether or not organic vegetables have more nutrient value than non-organic. Their theories are all missing a huge part of what nutrition is really about: the individual. Most nutrition books tell you what to eat without any reference to age, constitution, gender, size or lifestyle. We need to clarify that each person has very specific needs for his or her own health.

To avoid this perplexed, media-driven nonsense, I take what I like to call a post-modern approach to nutrition. One of the main concepts of this methodology is recognizing your bio-individuality. No perfect way of eating works for everybody. The food that is perfect for your unique body, age and lifestyle may make another person gain weight and feel lethargic. Similarly, no perfect way of eating will work for you all the time. You may notice you eat different foods on days when you are working eight hours than on a relaxing day spent reading. Foods you ate as a child may not agree with you as an adult. What you crave in the winter is completely different than what you crave in the summer.

Another critical part of post-modern nutrition is bridging the gap between nutrition and personal growth and development. These two entities are absolutely linked; you can't look at one without the other. People really want to be better. They crave growth. But very few experts in the realm of personal growth and development address the importance of nutrition. Likewise, traditionally trained nutritionists will give you a list of foods to eat and not to eat, but their advice will not work until you start to identify what in your life is keeping you from making healthy choices. Look at it this way: a person stuck in a bad relationship can eat all the broccoli in the world, but it won't change their relationship. This bad relationship will cause their health and well-being to suffer. Similarly, if your career is opposed to your spiritual values, you will have a hard time making big breakthroughs with a health concern. The energy spent at a draining job will ultimately outweigh the benefits of eating healthy food.

Being healthy is really not that complicated. The body knows what to eat. It's the brain that makes mistakes. Maybe you heard about a diet that sounded great in theory, but after a week of eating that way, you started to feel weak or bloated. You don't have to read nutrition books to know what to eat. Instead, you can foster a deep relationship with your body in which it naturally tells you what it needs to function at its highest potential. This post-modern approach will help you cultivate the ability to eat intuitively, trusting your body—not some book, chef or research study—to guide you to the foods that best support you and allow your body and mind to operate at their fullest potential.

Bio-Individuality

In 1956 Roger Williams published *Biochemical Individuality*, asserting that individuality permeates each part of the human body. This book explained how personal differences in anatomy, metabolism, composition of bodily fluids and cell structure influence your overall health. Each person, Williams wrote, has genetically determined and highly individualistic nutrition requirements. This theory influenced some independent-thinking minds in the nutrition world but is still largely ignored by mainstream medicine.

Watching fad diets sweep through the U.S., from high-carb diets in the '70s, to low fat in the '80s, to high protein at the dawn of the 21st century, I wondered how each of these nutrition experts could claim their diets worked for everyone. We are too individualistic to eat the same exact food. Ever notice that men eat very differently than women? Children, teens and adults all have very different preferences. People who work in an office eat differently than those who do physical labor. People eat according to their age, whether they are 25, 55 or 85.

Scientific research is starting to catch on to this concept. In a 2008 study, scientists found that men and women really do eat differently. The population survey of the Foodborne Disease Active Surveillance Network (FoodNet) looked at the eating habits of more than 14,000 American adults and found that generally men are more likely to report eating meat and poultry, and women are more likely to report eating fruits and vegetables.[1] I've noticed over the years that many times women try to get their male partners to eat more like a woman with more salads and vegetables. Years later, they wonder, where's my man? Now I know that both men and women enjoy a variety of foods, but isn't it interesting to tune in to these subtle differences?

One of the major factors shaping bio-individuality is ancestry. If your ancestors were Japanese, you will most likely thrive on a Japanese-type diet, high in rice, sea vegetables and fish. If your ancestors were from India, your digestive system will probably love basmati rice, cooked beans and curry. If many generations of your ancestors from Scandinavia were accustomed to eating dairy on a daily basis, it's natural that your body will be able to assimilate dairy foods. This theory also applies to foods that you have difficulty digesting. For example, many traditional African communities had an abundance of beans, grains, animal protein, sweet potatoes and green vegetables. Dairy was not easily accessible or easy to store in hot regions and, therefore, not a part of the traditional diet. So it makes sense that a lot of people of African descent are lactose intolerant.

My mother, who is now in her eighties, grew up in Hungary, where dairy was an important part of the daily diet. She drank warm, raw milk straight from the cow. When I first became involved with nutrition and health, I rejected dairy. I came to see that no other species naturally consumes dairy after infancy and that cow's milk is the perfect food to help a baby calf grow into a big, heavy cow but had no place in the adult human diet. I was eating brown rice and veggies, following my macrobiotic diet by the book. For years, I felt really good being off dairy. I stopped getting colds in the winter and stopped having mucus. Then I went on my first trip to India and visited many different Ayurvedic doctors, who all agreed I needed more dairy foods in my diet. They said I was lacking the calming, soothing, feminine energy that dairy holds. I remembered how strong my mom was and how much dairy she drank growing up. So, I gradually let go of my rigid attitude and began to experiment with milk, cheese and yogurt. Some people cannot tolerate any dairy; they get mucus, digestive trouble and allergies. Because my ancestors consumed dairy on a regular basis, it makes sense that I benefit from moderate amounts of high-quality dairy products in my diet.

Your blood type also influences your bio-individuality. Many people don't know their blood type, unless they have donated blood or received a blood transfusion, but the four blood types (A, B, AB, O) have evolved over thousands of years and offer insight into what foods work best in your body. Each type can be traced to a certain period of human history with distinct differences in diet, culture, and social conditions. Each blood type has developed particular strengths and limitations, and knowing them can influence your health. Many Type Os feel energized by eating meat, while Type Bs are better able to digest dairy. These preferences are based on a chemical reaction that occurs between the foods you eat and your blood. Some foods are capable of causing the cells of individuals with a certain blood type to clump together, while having no impact on the cells of individuals with another blood type. If you eat a food that is incompatible with your blood type, it could eventually lead to health problems, demonstrating how one person's food can be another person's poison.

Another aspect of bio-individuality is metabolism, or the rate at which you convert food into energy. Knowing your personal metabolic rate is useful when gauging the quantity of food your digestive system can process. Depending on your metabolic rate, your body may quickly convert calories to energy, or it may store the extra calories. You may recall that as a teenager you could wolf down a burger, fries, milkshake and ice cream all in one meal, without any indigestion or tightening of your jeans. That's because young people are still growing, have fast metabolic rates and burn calories more quickly than adults.

People can be divided into three general types of metabolic activity. Fast Burners, or Protein types, tend to be frequently hungry and crave fatty, salty foods and not do well on high carbohydrate or vegetarian-type diets. Their bodies burn through carbohydrates too quickly, and a higher protein intake helps slow down their metabolism. Slow Burners, or Carbo types, generally have relatively weak appetites, a high tolerance for sweets and problems with weight control. They require a higher percentage of carbohydrates to give them energy to speed up their metabolism. Mixed types generally have average appetites and moderate cravings for sweets and starchy foods. For them, the ideal diet is a balanced combination of protein and carbohydrates. You can determine your metabolic type by answering questionnaires or taking simple medical tests. Keep in mind that even your metabolic rate and sensitivity can shift as you age, or as stress levels or nutrient deficiencies shift in your diet or lifestyle. If this all seems too confusing and complicated, don't worry. Just observe how your own body responds to the food you give it. People are different, and getting to know your own body is an essential first step in discovering how to stay healthy.

Metabolic theory demonstrates that no one diet is right for all of us. You may know people who can eat processed carbohydrates, such as bread and pasta, and stay very thin while you gain weight on such a diet. It's not because

PROFILE

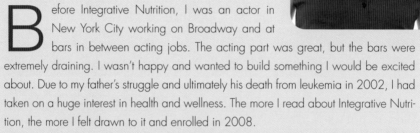

Heather Kenzie-Terry,
New York, NY, USA
www.nibmor.com

"Small changes are everything."

Before Integrative Nutrition, I was an actor in New York City working on Broadway and at bars in between acting jobs. The acting part was great, but the bars were extremely draining. I wasn't happy and wanted to build something I would be excited about. Due to my father's struggle and ultimately his death from leukemia in 2002, I had taken on a huge interest in health and wellness. The more I read about Integrative Nutrition, the more I felt drawn to it and enrolled in 2008.

The changes I've made since attending IIN are amazing. I was always stressed and struggled with emotional eating, sugar addiction, candida, as will as headaches, fatigue, and lack of focus. I started experimenting with every diet we learned about. Speakers inspired me with their voices and books. Today, I no longer work ridiculous hours, I have a fitness plan, I have conquered my ailments and I live a balanced life. It isn't always easy, but now I know how much I can take on and understand the art and power of saying "no."

Whenever I see individuals reaching out with new information, books or ideas on health and wellness, I applaud them. The more we reach out to the rest of the world, the more healing will happen. My personal mission is to educate and inspire anyone who will listen. If a person takes away one thing from something I say, or they pick up a NibMor product and are intrigued enough by a word or phrase to investigate it and make a change, then I've done my part in the world. Small changes are everything. Never minimize them. One small change leads to another and another and another. That is significant! And that is how happiness is achieved.

I never would have guessed I would own NibMor, an organic chocolate company. Talk about the surprises of life! We've been featured in all sorts of publications and on TV. Today, you can buy NibMor nationwide in over 3,500 stores, and we are growing fast. The plans we have reach for the stars with a mission of health and wellness for all. I am truly blessed and grateful. I followed the simple instructions at Integrative Nutrition and here I am. Oh how sweet it is!

carbohydrates are "evil" or your body isn't as healthy; it just shows that all people metabolize these foods differently. You might do better on a high-protein diet with lots of fresh vegetables and some whole grains. Knowing what foods you metabolize best will help you to choose foods that make you feel good and support your individual body.

Our personal tastes and preferences, natural shapes and sizes, blood types, metabolic rates and genetic backgrounds influence what foods will and won't nourish us. So, when the experts say "tomatoes are good for you" or "red meat is unhealthy," it's too much of a generalization. One person's food is another person's poison, and that's why fad diets don't work in the long run. They are not based on the reality that we all have different dietary needs.

Sometimes it takes millions of dollars in funding and years of research for scientists to prove what we already know. I am certain that science will soon discover diet needs to be based on bio-individuality.

The Laboratory of Your Body

Fortunately, you already have free, 24-hour access to the world's most sophisticated laboratory for testing how food affects your body and your health. Where is this lab? You're living in it. Your body is a sophisticated bio-computer. By learning to listen to your body and developing an understanding of what foods it needs and when it needs them, you will discover what is best for you.

If you doubt this connection to your body, begin by acknowledging that your body is highly intelligent. Your heart never misses a beat and your lungs are always breathing in and out. Even if you break up with a romantic partner, even if you receive traumatic news, your heart's four little chambers go right on pumping and your lungs continue to expand and contract. You can trust your body. It has evolved helpful instincts to keep you alive and well.

Just as a tree will always lean toward light, humans and animals know instinctively how and where to get food that is best for them. Animals don't read nutrition books. Their bodies tell them which plants to eat and which to avoid, or if they're predators, which animals to kill when they're hungry. They heal themselves when they are sick, usually by resting a lot and eating very little until the sickness passes.

We have the same instincts, but many of us ignore the messages our bodies are constantly sending. Dark circles under the eyes signal exhaustion—your body is telling you to slow down and get some rest. Constipation and bloating are signs that something you are eating, or the way you are eating it, is not appropriate. We ignore these messages until they become unbearable, and that's when we go to the doctor for medications and operations.

Give yourself time to explore the laboratory of your body and you will be surprised by its responsiveness, sophistication and intelligence.

Food-Mood Connection

Scientific research and personal experience both demonstrate that what we eat affects how we think and how we act. Still, most people don't acknowledge the connection between their food and their mood. Stop and think for a moment about how you feel throughout the day. Do you sometimes feel fuzzy and tired after lunch? Angry and irritable between meals? Energized by a great meal?

Food undoubtedly changes your mood. The most extreme examples are coffee or alcohol, which change your state of mind within minutes. For this reason, I don't even classify them as foods but as drugs. The standard American diet, high in processed carbohydrates and poor-quality animal meat while lacking in vegetables and water, leaves many people in a bad mood. It's hard to feel inspired and happy when you're living on chemical, artificial junk food. Julia Ross, author of *The Mood Cure* and a pioneer in the field of nutritional psychology, refers to this relationship as the law of malnutrition. The current epidemic of bad moods is definitely linked to an epidemic of deteriorating food quality and quantity: junk moods come from junk foods, she writes. Soda, chocolates, ice cream, potato chips and fries are all easily accessible foods that people turn to when they want to be lifted out of a bad mood, but the irony is that these foods are a big part of the problem. Salt can mess with your mood making you feel tense. Sugar can give you a high and make you feel energized. When your blood sugar goes up, you get that woo-hoo, good feeling. But as soon as it goes down, you feel like the world is coming to an end.

Think about the idea of comfort food. If you have a bowl of soup, you somehow feel all warm inside. It's soothing. The opposite of comfort food is focus food, which helps you work harder. Many people refer to protein, such as eggs, nuts or meat, as brain food. Ever notice how you crave more comfort food after work or more sharpening-type food to focus during a busy day at the office? We even crave more aphrodisiac food, such as chili peppers and spice, avocado and chocolate, when we are out on a date. What we are really doing with all this food is a form of self-medicating or seeking balance. We already understand the food-mood connection; we just don't have a language to discuss these habits with each other.

From a scientific perspective, the food-mood relationship is maintained by neurotransmitters—chemical messengers that relay thoughts and actions throughout the brain. Some neurotransmitters, such as serotonin, can make us feel relaxed. Others, such as dopamine, have a stimulating effect. The food we eat breaks down in our digestive tract, enters our bloodstream and creates changes in the behavior of these neurotransmitters, thus impacting our mood. Eating carbohydrates releases serotonin in the brain, which makes people feel more relaxed. Eating too many carbs or overly processed carbs like sugar and flour releases even more serotonin, causing drowsiness. You've probably experienced that sleepy feeling after eating too much pasta or heavy carbohydrates. Eating protein produces dopamine and norepinephrine in the brain which makes people feel more alert and full of energy, if protein is eaten in the appropriate portions. On the other hand, overeating protein can lead to tension and irritability.

Another experience of the food-mood connection comes from eating too much. Think of a big holiday dinner and how tired you become after indulging. Overeating often leads to drowsiness. To handle the excess food, blood flow is directed to the stomach, and away from the brain. The result is a feeling of lethargy.

It's surprising how deeply food affects us. In relationships, we often get irritated and blame our partner when actually it's our own mood swings that are causing the rift. Our moods go up and down like a yo-yo, and as soon as we come into a nutritional state of balance, suddenly our partner turns out to be a wonderful person.

Each person's food-mood sensitivity varies. Only you can determine the right amount of proteins, carbs and fats to keep yourself in balance. Once the correlation enters your consciousness, you will be more careful with your food choices. I simply encourage you to notice, explore, experiment and determine what works for you. I'm sure you've met people who are vibrantly healthy, despite the fact that they eat donuts and drink coffee for breakfast on a regular basis. You probably think to yourself, "If I ate that way, I'd be a mess." And you're probably right. There's nothing wrong with you or with the coffee and donut person, other than the fact that your food-mood sensitivity is different.

One of the best ways to discover how different foods affect your mood is to simply record what you eat and how you feel afterward. Try the exercises at the end of this chapter—both the **Breakfast Experiment** and the **Food-Mood Journal**—to explore how your body and mind respond to different foods.

Energy of Food

As you increase awareness about the foods you consume, consider that each food has its own unique energy, beyond vitamins, minerals, fats and carbohydrates. When we eat, we assimilate not only the nutrients, but also the energy of the food. Food has distinct qualities and energetic properties, depending on where, when and how it grows, as well as how it is prepared. By understanding the energy of food, we can choose meals that will create the energy we are seeking in our lives. Virtually no one in the field of health and nutrition speaks about the concept of food having energy, but if you stop and think about it, it intuitively makes sense. Vegetables have a lighter energy than proteins. Animal meat from tortured animals has a different energy than meat from animals that lived a peaceful existence.

If you practice yoga or have been to India, you may have heard the word *prana*, a Sanskrit word simply translated as "energy." This word is just one way to describe the vital life-force energy that exists around us and inside of us. Energy comes from the universe, from air and from food. Yogis believe that certain foods, such as fresh produce, have a greater amount of energy than foods that are heavily processed or that have been reused a day or two later. It makes sense: when you eat foods with more energy, you will have more energy.

Steve Gagné, author of *Energetics of Food: Encounters with Your Most Intimate Relationships*, says that all food has an essential character. He analyzes where foods come from to help identify their essence. Plants sprout from a seed; some animals are hatched from eggs, while others are birthed by their mothers and nurtured through infancy. Regarding plant food, consider where, when and in what direction it grows. Greens, such as kale, collards and bok choy, reach up toward the sun, soaking up the chlorophyll. Eating foods that are rich in chlorophyll provides our blood with oxygen. For this reason, greens are powerful mood enhancers, lifting the spirit. Squash and gourds grow level with the ground and help balance moods and energy levels. Root vegetables, such as carrots, parsnips, beets and burdock, grow into the ground and absorb the nutrients from the soil in which they grow. Therefore, they have a strong downward energy and are great for grounding us when we feel overstimulated.

In contrast to these vegetables, reflect for a moment on the character of a donut. It starts with dough, made of wheat and sugar; then it's deep-fried, probably in a less-than-desirable oil. Often it's filled with jam, cream or custard, or topped with a sweet glaze of icing. What kind of energy do you imagine you get from this donut? How would that differ from the energy you get from eating organic roasted root vegetables? As you cultivate awareness around the energy of your food, and how it is passed onto you, you will begin to make greater strides in recognizing your own mind-body connection.

Cross-Species Transference

Taking food energetics to the next level, I would like to introduce a theory I call Cross-Species Transference, which asserts that character traits can be passed from animals to humans. Essentially, you become more like the species you eat. Modern nutrition experts claim that a protein is a protein is a protein. The current dietary guidelines say that meat, poultry, fish, beans, eggs and nuts are basically the same. In The Zone diet, Barry Sears recommends that every meal have an adequate serving of low-fat protein. But he doesn't distinguish between the types of proteins. I have to disagree. Energetically, it makes an enormous difference if you are getting protein from any of the following sources: dahl or minestrone soup; soy milk or cow's milk; beef, chicken or fish; organic or non-organic protein.

The main American food is cow. It's either beef in the form of burgers, hot dogs or steak. Or it's dairy in the form of cow's milk, ice cream, cheese, yogurt and so on. These foods compose a large part of the daily diet and are available in almost every restaurant. Contemplate the effects of eating beef every day for more than 20 years, as many Americans do. Increasingly, I have noticed Americans developing big, beefy bodies and wide eyes. We are beginning to look like cows! We even have a herd mentality, in which many people are trying to keep up with the crowd.

This theory may seem esoteric and difficult to prove, but I became convinced during my years of working with clients that I could spot the influence of specific animal foods on individuals. When I would meet people with pronounced, beak-like noses and tense, nervous dispositions, I would ask, "Have you eaten a lot of chicken?" Nine times out of 10, they would answer "yes." Think about Frank Purdue in all those commercials for his chicken conglomerate. He looked like a chicken. When I'd bump into someone strong and muscular, with a red face and ask if they ate a lot of beef, they would invariably answer "yes."

One client had me stumped. At the time, I was deeply engrossed in studying facial diagnosis, which looks at how disorders, diseases and strengths are manifested on the face in the form of lines, wrinkles, colorations, moles, dimples, structure and so on. Using this method, I would accurately guess the animal diets of clients and friends, but this one client showed none of the familiar signs. He was a huge guy with very large ears, a big, round nose, thick arms and legs and small eyes. Yet he was not loud or aggressive and was actually very gentle and shy.

I continued to observe him throughout the consultation and finally asked, "What was the animal food you ate growing up?"

"Well, I grew up in South Africa and we used to eat a lot of elephant meat," he said, not missing a beat.

I practically fell off my chair. "Really? You're kidding!"

"No, I grew up with my family on a forest reserve. My father was a game-keeper. The elephant population had to be culled from time to time, so we had a lot of free meat. It's actually pretty good, you should try it sometime." He smiled at me playfully, and I could almost imagine him there for a minute, lumbering through the veld. After this experience, I became convinced of the strong correlation between animal foods and human development.

In addition to influencing facial structure, cross-species transference produces animal-like habits in humans. Chickens spend a lot of time and energy creating a pecking order to establish who is higher on the social scale. They are generally noisy, nervous, frenetic creatures and, when raised in factory farms, they are cooped up in small, overcrowded cages most of their lives. Chicken may be the perfect food for someone who is very quiet and lethargic and wants to be more social. But for a high-strung, stressed-out person, chicken is probably not a good food choice.

Our bodies absorb the energetic qualities of our foods, especially when we eat meat. Once you open your eyes to this information, it's amazing to discover how much it impacts us daily. What impresses me is how sensitive and adaptable the human body can be. We can change our moods, our bodies and our mindsets by making small changes in our daily diet. I hope understanding the flexible nature of your own biological organism will encourage you to explore and experiment with different foods. Your body will respond to the changes you make, and you will feel the difference. Just give it a try.

Weight Loss

Weight loss is a huge issue today. Our society idolizes people who are thin. But with an overabundance of snack foods, junk foods and fast foods, combined with a lack of daily exercise, many people struggle with their weight. One of the most popular New Year's resolutions is to lose a few pounds. People turn to modern nutrition's approach of counting calories and trying to get fit. When they have trouble following their own diet regimen, they look for help in the more than $66-billion diet and weight loss industry, which includes everything from commercial chains like Weight Watchers and Jenny Craig to diet pills, artificial sweeteners, diet books and magazines, meal replacement shakes and belly-stapling surgeries.[2] Year after year, many Americans realize that these fad diets don't work. In fact, about 90 percent of all dieters regain some or all of the weight originally lost. Diet and exercise theories like the 40-day, 20-day or even 8-minutes-a-day to a thinner you are aimed at quick results and book sales.

In recent years, the idea of eating more and weighing less has become popular. Why not? When given the choice, most of us would rather eat more. The trick is understanding caloric density or volumetrics, which means you can eat as much as you want of foods that are nutrient-rich and low in calories. I like to use the example of a package of Oreos. One package has 2,200 calories. For that same amount of calories, someone could consume 1 pound of carrots, 1 pound of papaya, 1 pound of apples, 1 pound

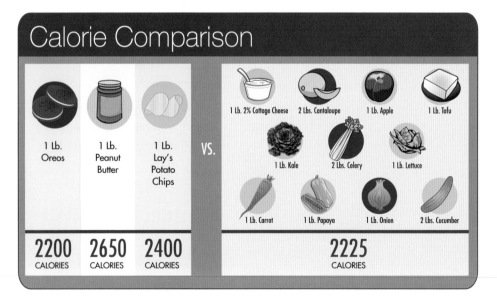

Calorie Comparison

| 1 Lb. Oreos | 1 Lb. Peanut Butter | 1 Lb. Lay's Potato Chips | VS. | 1 Lb. 2% Cottage Cheese | 2 Lbs. Cantaloupe | 1 Lb. Apple | 1 Lb. Tofu |

1 Lb. Kale   2 Lbs. Celery   1 Lb. Lettuce
1 Lb. Carrot   1 Lb. Papaya   1 Lb. Onion   2 Lbs. Cucumber

2200 CALORIES   2650 CALORIES   2400 CALORIES   2225 CALORIES of onions, 1 pound of lettuce, 1 pound of kale, 1 pound of tofu, 1 pound of 2% cottage cheese, 2 pounds of cantaloupe, 2 pounds of celery and 2 pounds of cucumber.

Another way to think about caloric density is that your body only needs a certain volume of food each day. If you're having a bowl of soup, your body doesn't know if the bowl of soup has 100 calories or 1,000 calories. By choosing foods that have a low caloric density, you can feel full without packing on the pounds.

Many people who have lost weight and kept it off have looked past the diet books and fads and found what works best for their own bodies. I encourage people who want to lose weight to experiment with different methods and see what works.

Weight Loss Suggestions

Always eat breakfast. People who eat breakfast are much more successful at keeping weight off. When you skip meals, you become calorie deficient and usually end up binging later in the day.

Snack throughout the day. You know the saying, "Don't go shopping when you're hungry?" Try it. Snacking can actually help some people eat less. By eating between meals, you can help reduce hunger pains and binging later in the day.

Drink more water. By replacing soda, alcohol or coffee with water, you can cut a significant amount of calories from your daily routine. Many people can effortlessly lose 10 pounds by simply replacing soda with water throughout the day. Be aware of alcoholic drinks as well—a jumbo margarita can have up to 700 calories. Also try drinking water before your meal. The water will help break down the food more effectively.

Make your own meals. Restaurant food generally has more salt, more fat and more calories and is served in larger portions than food cooked at home. When you make your own meals, you can control the amount of salt and oil, as well as the portion size. If you have to eat out, try splitting one dish between two people or ask for half the meal to be wrapped up before it comes to the table.

Reduce your stress levels. Many people eat more when they feel stress; the stuffed feeling makes them feel comfortable and helps them relax. Try other ways of relaxing, like a hot bath or a walk around the block. Also try slowing down, breathing and enjoying each meal. Say a prayer beforehand or take a moment to be grateful for the food you are eating.

Get enough sleep each night. Growing evidence supports that missing out on sleep can increase your appetite. Most people need about 7-8 hours of sleep each night.

Keep moving. Start with small changes like getting off one stop earlier on a train and walking the rest of the way or parking in the back of a parking lot. Take the stairs whenever possible. Instead of meeting a friend for coffee, meet for a walk, or a bike ride or take a dance class together.

Keep track. Whether you keep a food journal or use a free weight-loss app on your smart phone, find a method that will keep you motivated and help you track your progress.

Be a food detective. Read food labels and don't eat anything you can't pronounce. Stick to simple, whole foods that will nourish your body.

Identify your temptation foods. You know whether they are salty or sweet, fried or creamy, and you know that if they are within reach, you will want them. Do not keep these foods in your home or office and get support from your family and friends with these foods.

Take a multivitamin. Everyone can benefit from well-rounded nutrients. Some evidence suggests that by adding specific high-quality nutrients to a well-balanced diet, you can improve your metabolism and many enzyme processes for greater vitality and health.

If you want to lose weight fast, you don't have to go on a fad diet. Just switch from simple to complex carbohydrates and eat lots of vegetables. You'll lose weight and improve your health. Plant foods are so low in calories that they force the body to burn its own fat. Nobody gets fat on a diet that's made up largely of green vegetables, sweet vegetables, whole grains and small amounts of high-quality animal products. But throw in a bunch of cookies, white bread, French fries and a few quarter-pounders, and you've got yourself a serious weight problem. Many of the students that attend Integrative Nutrition end up losing weight when they start shifting some of their food choices. They usually report having more energy, more excitement about their food and, oh yeah, they lost 25 pounds. When people make the connection that healthy, whole foods really make you feel better, the weight becomes a secondary issue.

Exercises

1. The Breakfast Experiment[3]

As a way of tuning into your body and learning how to listen to its messages, explore eating a different breakfast every day for a week. Jot down what you eat and how you feel, both right after the meal and then again two hours later.

Day 1: scrambled eggs

Day 2: scrambled tofu

Day 3: oatmeal

Day 4: boxed breakfast cereal

Day 5: muffin and coffee

Day 6: fresh fruit

Day 7: fresh vegetables

Day 1 Breakfast:

    Right after eating I felt:

    Two hours after eating I felt:

Day 2 Breakfast:

    Right after eating I felt:

    Two hours after eating I felt:

Day 3 Breakfast:

    Right after eating I felt:

    Two hours after eating I felt:

Day 4 Breakfast:

    Right after eating I felt:

    Two hours after eating I felt:

Day 5 Breakfast:

    Right after eating I felt:

    Two hours after eating I felt:

Day 6 Breakfast:

    Right after eating I felt:

    Two hours after eating I felt:

Day 7 Breakfast:

    Right after eating I felt:

    Two hours after eating I felt:

Once you get the knack of this experiment, you can expand it to include your whole daily intake, exploring how different foods and liquids affect you. For example, for one week, make a point of drinking more water during the day, or eating more leafy greens or meat. Notice how your body feels and how each change of diet affects your mood.

2. Food-Mood Journal

Write what you eat at each meal or snack and how you feel afterwards. Be sure to record how you feel immediately after and then again a few hours later. You may feel great right after eating candy or drinking coffee, but two hours later it's often a different story. You may write, "I had tea first thing this morning, and I felt good. I had coffee at 11 a.m. and still felt okay, but the second cup of coffee after lunch put me over the top." Or you may notice, "I had too much animal meat today and felt lethargic." Or, perhaps, "Every time I eat bread, my stomach hurts." Or, "Yesterday I had a nice spinach and lentil soup, but wanted something more. I had a small piece of chocolate for dessert and felt satisfied." Soon you will know what energizes you and what drains you. Certain foods will give you gas; certain foods will prevent you from sleeping well; other foods will enhance your ability to concentrate at work.

3. Friend Food Inventory

List the three healthiest people you know and the three unhealthiest people you know. Write down what they eat. See how the foods correlate with their level of vibrancy.

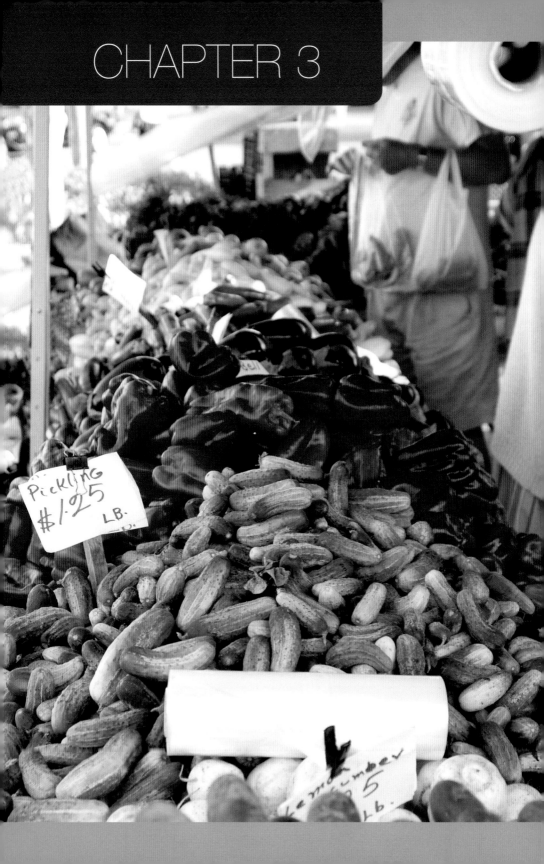

CHAPTER 3

What,
When
and How
We Eat

Peace begins in kitchens and pantries, gardens and backyards, where our food is grown and prepared. The energies of nature and the infinite universe are absorbed through the foods we eat and are transmuted into our thoughts and actions.

—MICHIO KUSHI, *ONE PEACEFUL WORLD*

Now that you know the fundamentals of post-modern nutrition, let's go a little deeper. Part of the modern experience of eating has to do with the quality of the food we eat and the quality of our eating experience. In just a few generations, humans have completely transformed what, when and how we eat. Supermarket food contains chemicals, additives and sweeteners wrapped in boxes with bright colors and catchy slogans. We eat this stuff, along with fried, fast foods, in our cars, in front of our TVs or at our desks, giving little thought to where our food comes from and how our food choices impact the world around us. We eat with all of our senses, but many of us never stop to enjoy the look, smell, sound, texture or even taste of our food. Most people don't really chew their food. They spend time at doctors' offices complaining of upset stomachs, constipation and a range of other digestive disorders without thinking about these larger issues.

The Integrative Nutrition approach to this problem is quite simple: eat and *enjoy* high-quality food. Take a look at what you're eating, when you're eating it and how you eat it. You may be surprised to find that by making a few adjustments, you can dramatically improve the quality of your life. Better food equals better health. It's really that simple.

What We Eat

The Food Our Ancestors Ate

Throughout history, people have eaten food essentially as nature produced it. People ate whole and unprocessed vegetables, fruit, grains and beans; and chicken, fish and other animal foods. Small amounts of sugar and honey or some wine and beer in the diet were balanced by regular physical labor, from sunrise to sunset, for every member of the family. They had no cars, planes, trains or bicycles for transportation. Life was active.

Our ancestors would not recognize the food in today's supermarket. In the last 100 years or so, large-scale food processing has become the norm. Breads and other baked goods that were once made of whole-grain flour are now made from processed, white, bleached flour that is far less nutritious. American consumers have developed a taste for processed foods like pastries, cookies, crackers, chips and other foods that are far removed from their origins. I think most people would agree that Doritos don't grow on trees.

Many people don't realize that processing food strips it of many nutrients. Think of the difference between white bread and wheat bread. Both come from wheat. But wheat bread uses the entire grain, while white bread is made by removing the bran and the germ (parts of the grain) during the milling process. Manufacturers remove these parts to create lighter, fluffier bread and to extend its shelf life. The germ, specifically, contains natural oils that could make bread go rancid. Wonder Bread can sit on the shelf for about 21 days before it loses its moisture and gets hard, while bakeries typically sell their fresh-baked bread within 24 hours.

In addition to leaving out or removing essential nutrients, processing foods generally involves adding sweeteners, colors, flavors and preservatives. Manufacturers now add sugar to everything from ketchup to toothpaste. Supermarket shelves are filled with highly chemicalized foods, including soft drinks, packaged snacks, frozen dinners, boxed desserts and condiments. Nearly all of these items contain artificial ingredients, rather than fresh, natural ingredients.

Sometimes manufacturers try to reintroduce nutrients to foods by a process called enrichment. But a laboratory can't possibly reintroduce all the vitamins, minerals, carotenoids and fiber that the original plant source contained. A single tomato contains more than 10,000 phytochemicals. Scientists have identified thousands of phytochemicals that can help boost immune function, prevent DNA damage and protect cells from the damaging effects of toxic substances that can result in cancer and heart disease.[1] When you see the word "enriched" on bread labels, such as "enriched white flour" or "enriched wheat flour," it means they took out the good stuff in the processing and tried to put some of it back at the end. A similar process occurs with fortified cereals, which typically feature highly processed grains and sweeteners doused with a few vitamins. A simple way to think about enriched foods is to imagine you have $100 in your wallet. If someone stole the $100 but then decided to put back $20, would you feel enriched? I think most people would feel like they're still missing $80.

The fact that we have to inject nutrients back into our food demonstrates how strange our eating habits have become. Not that long ago, we ate what was fresh and available. Now we eat foods that are cheap, fast and convenient with little thought about whether they give our bodies the nutrients we need to get us through our day. I wonder what our ancestors would think. My guess is that, if they could see us buying food from drive-thru windows and from automated vending machines, they would think we were from another planet. If they tasted all the chemicals, preservatives and added fats and sugars, the flavor of our modern foods would be so intense they would probably spit them out.

What we buy in the grocery store may look like food, and it may taste like food, but it's not the food our great-grandmothers ate. I encourage you to eat foods in their whole, natural states as much as possible. Before you put products in your cart at the store or before you place your order at a restaurant, think about the processing the food went through to get to you. If you're at a Mexican restaurant, the corn tortillas are probably made from processed corn flour and a mix of preservatives. If you're buying Twinkies from the store, think about how they were created—using highly processed flour and sugar and stuffed with a white filling made from cream, which comes from cow's milk and contains added sugar. Many different machines are involved in both the production and the packaging of processed foods like this one.

Many people are disconnected from real, whole foods and have lost touch with the reality that our food comes from the earth. Simple eating celebrates the richness of whole foods. Think of the juiciness of a ripe piece of fruit, the crunchiness of a whole carrot or the creaminess of mashing an avocado. I encourage you to find simple pleasures in the foods you eat.

Organics

One of the most profound ways to experience the energetic nature of food is to notice the properties of organic food. Have you noticed that eating organic food can make you feel more vital and that the taste is cleaner and more flavorful? It's not surprising that organic products continue to be one of the fastest-growing categories of food. Worldwide, 1.6 million producers farm organically, and about 80 percent of them are in developing countries—India, Uganda, Mexico and Ethiopia top the list. The global market for organic sales reached $59.1 billion in 2010, according to Organic Monitor. The countries with the largest markets include the U.S., Germany and France. In the U.S., organic fruit and vegetable sales were up almost 12 percent in 2010 from 2009.[2]

Originally, all foods were "organic"—grown without synthetic pesticides, herbicides, chemical fertilizers or hormones. Large-scale farming with chemicals began around World War II, around the same time that food processing exploded. Large-scale farming works against the natural cycles of the earth, relying on chemicals to produce big returns. This process has depleted much of the world's soil of its minerals and nutrients. The resulting vegetable and animal foods are not only deficient in nutrients, but they are also full of pollutants and agrochemicals.

The modern denaturing of foods through massive refining and chemical treatment degrades their original life force, making it difficult to foster equilibrium and health for the people eating them. Pesticides, which are present in most commercial produce, must be processed by our immune systems and have been shown to cause cancer as well as liver, kidney and blood diseases. In addition, as pesticides build up in our tissues, our immune system weakens, allowing other carcinogens and pathogens to affect our health.

In contrast, organic farming works with the land. Crops are rotated from year to year to allow the soil to retain its nutrients between growing cycles. Animals graze in different areas each season to let grasses recover and replenish between seasons. Farmers feed the soil with broken-down plant waste (compost), rather than using artificial fertilizing methods. Some farms even

Pesticide Residues in Produce

The produce ranking, developed by analysts at Environmental Working Group (EWG), is based on the results of nearly 60,700 sample tests for pesticide residues on produce collected by the U.S. Department of Agriculture and the U.S. Food and Drug Administration between 2000 and 2010. EWG is a not-for-profit environmental research organization dedicated to improving public health and protecting the environment.

Dirty Dozen™
Produce with the most residues
(in order from most contaminated)

1. Apples	7. Grapes (imported)
2. Celery	8. Spinach
3. Sweet Bell Peppers	9. Lettuce
4. Peaches	10. Cucumbers
5. Strawberries	11. Blueberries (domestic)
6. Nectarines (imported)	12. Potatoes

Clean 15™
Produce with the lowest levels of residues
(in order from least contaminated)

1. Onions	9. Eggplant
2. Sweet Corn	10. Kiwis
3. Pineapple	11. Cantaloupe (domestic)
4. Avocado	12. Sweet Potatoes
5. Cabbage	13. Grapefruit
6. Sweet Peas	14. Watermelon
7. Asparagus	15. Mushrooms
8. Mangos	

cultivate good pests to help rid the area of bad pests, and plant seeds in coordination with the cycles of the moon. All of these practices are long-term, sustainable methods of farming that work with the natural environment, instead of adding chemicals to it.

Fresh, organic produce contains more vitamins, minerals, enzymes and other micronutrients than intensively farmed produce. According to research published in the *Journal of Agricultural and Food Chemistry*, organic fruits and veggies have 50% to 60% higher levels of cancer-fighting antioxidants than non-organic fruits and veggies.[3] The average conventionally grown apple has 20 to 30 artificial chemicals on its skin, even after rinsing. Though organic food is usually more expensive, the extra money you pay may save you hundreds, if not thousands, of dollars in future doctors' bills.

Some people avoid organic produce because it looks less colorful and less perfectly shaped than conventionally grown produce. But have you ever bought a big, red juicy tomato from the store, only to find that when you bite into it at home, it has no flavor? Have you ever picked a small, funny-shaped tomato right off the vine and found it incredibly sweet? It hasn't spent weeks on a truck or been exposed to harsh chemicals, so its natural taste is preserved. Organic fruits and vegetables may not look as bright or "perfect" as some conventionally grown foods (which are sometimes dyed to look more appealing), but they certainly taste fresh off the vine. Another thing people notice when first buying organic produce is that the fruits seem smaller. Americans believe that bigger is better, but try to reverse this saying when you look at organic produce. It is actually grown to its natural size, resulting in a more flavorful, and often sweeter, taste than its larger, non-organic counterpart.

Another reason to eat organic is to avoid genetically modified organisms (GMOs), also known as genetically engineered foods. A GMO is any organism in which the genetic material has been altered or shuffled around in a way that does not occur naturally. This technology allows individual genes to be transferred from one organism to another. This science is used to cultivate GM plants, which are then used to grow GM food crops. GMOs on the market have been given genetic traits to provide protection from pests and diseases or resistance to pesticides, or to improve the quality of the crop. The most prevalent GM crops were created to resist harsh chemicals; these

Unlocking the Produce Code

One way to spot organic produce in the store is to check out each food's price look-up number or PLU. You'll find a PLU label on each piece of produce, attached as a sticker. The International Federation for Produce Coding standardizes PLU codes for every grocery store in the country. Conventionally grown fruits and vegetables have 4-digit numbers and generally begin with a 3 or a 4. Organically grown fruits and vegetables have 5 digits and begin with a 9. Genetically modified fruits and vegetables also have 5 digits and begin with an 8. For example, the PLU for a conventionally grown banana is 4011; for an organic banana it's 94011; and for a genetically modified banana it's 84011.

Source: Adapted from www.plucodes.com

crops have DNA traits from bacteria, fungi or other plants that create this resistance. Farmers who use GM crops can spray their fields to kill everything growing in the area except the food crop. Imagine what is being killed in our bodies when we eat these foods.

The most common genetically engineered crops in the United States, which is the largest grower of GM crops in the world, are canola, corn, soy and cotton. Genetically engineered soy, corn and canola are used in many processed foods, but the government does not require labeling of these foods and regards these foods as generally safe. Many experts estimate that about 70 percent of the foods in grocery stores in the U.S. and Canada contain genetically engineered ingredients.

During the past decade, food safety experts have identified several potential problems with genetically engineered food crops, according to reports from the Union of Concerned Scientists. These problems include the possibility of introducing new toxins or allergens into previously safe foods, increasing toxins to dangerous levels in foods that typically produce harmless amounts or diminishing foods' nutritional values. Many scientists have raised environmental concerns about these crops, as GM crops tend to dominate over wild plants and conventional crops, potentially disrupting natural ecosystems.

In the 2012 U.S. election, California introduced legislation aimed at labeling GMOs called Prop 37. Proponents argued that labeling would allow consumers to know which foods on supermarket shelves contain genetically engineered ingredients and prohibit these products from getting labeled as "natural." More than 40 other countries including most of Europe, Japan and India already require labeling. But big food companies like Monsanto, Dupont, PepsiCo, Coca-Cola, Kraft, General Mills and Kellogg donated millions of dollars to oppose the bill, saying that it could increase food costs by billions, forcing farmers and food companies to implement new operations and switch to more expensive, non-genetically engineered foods.[4]

But in early 2013, Whole Foods Market made headlines as the first national grocery chain to set a deadline for labeling all GMO products in their stores. By 2018, all products in their U.S. and Canadian stores must be labeled about whether they contain GMOs. Until then, if you want to avoid these foods, be a food detective. Look for organic or products labeled by the Non-GMO Project, a collaboration of manufacturers, retailers, farmers and consumers, who have developed North America's first independent third-party Non-GMO Product Verification Program.[5] Jeffery Smith, director of the Institute for Responsible Technology and a leading advocate for healthier, non-GMO choices, agrees that food labeling is crucial. He believes if a labeling law were passed, food companies would most likely remove GMOs from their products rather than label them.

Environmental Effects of Food Choices

Our personal food choices not only have an impact on our bodies but also on our environment. Each meal is made up of food that requires a significant amount of energy and resources to reach your plate. The journey of our food is a much longer process than many of us realize. Some people refer to this journey as food miles, which is the distance food travels from field to plate, and the higher the mileage, the larger the impact on the environment. Food travels further these days partly because of large corporate grocery stores, which have centralized methods for distributing food. In some cases, a crop of cherries may travel across the country to be packaged and then sent back close to where the cherries were originally grown. In other cases, stores fly in food from all over the world to ensure they have fresh produce, whatever the season. This practice causes us to have organic bananas from Peru, organic kiwis from New Zealand, organic avocados from Mexico, at any time of year. Locally produced, seasonal foods cut energy use and therefore leave a smaller impact on the environment.

The decision about whether or not to eat meat is also a big one, and it can have significant impacts on the environment. In John Robbins' book, *Diet for a New America*, he points to many areas that are impacted by factory-farmed beef consumption. Cattle require huge amounts of water every day. Giving up one pound of beef a year could save more water than if you stopped showering for six months, according to his book. Corn-fed cattle also impact the environment, because each bushel of corn they eat has been treated with about 1.2 gallons of oil-based fertilizers. Each cow consumes about 25 pounds of corn each day, which translates into a lot of fossil fuel energy. Cattle also need land for grazing. About 70 percent of the lands in western national forests are used for grazing, according to the book. And although the U.S. is the world's largest producer of beef, worldwide demand for beef has caused massive deforestation in other parts of the world. Between 2000 and 2006, Brazil lost about 150,000 square kilometers of forest—an area larger than Greece—and since 1970, about 600,000 square kilometers (232,000 square miles) of Amazon rainforest have been destroyed.[6] The leading cause of deforestation in the Brazilian Amazon is cattle ranching. The growth in Brazilian cattle production—80 percent of which was in the Amazon—was largely export driven. While deforestation has slowed since 2006, it still continues at a rate of 13 million hectares per year, or 36 football fields a minute. Environmental groups are working with scientists to help achieve zero net deforestation by 2020, according to the Living Planet Report.[7]

But you don't have to eat a strict vegan diet to eat in an environmentally friendly manner. Get to know where your meat comes from by making friends with your local farmers and ranchers or look online to find better sources than what's available at your local store. Look for meat that is grass-fed, certified organic and local, whenever possible. Think about reducing the amount of meat in your diet and therefore lessening your overall environmental footprint.

When We Eat

Seasonal Foods

One Christmas, I was visiting India and went to the market to buy fruit. It was still frigid in Massachusetts, where I live, and I hadn't had good, fresh fruit in several months. I filled bags with grapes, pomegranates, mangoes and limes, and, after feeling the ache in my arms on the walk home, realized I had overdone it. As I came to the gate of my apartment building, I offered some of the fruit to the guard outside the apartment where I was staying.

"No thank you, sir," he said, smiling politely. I knew he was a poor man and fruit was a relative luxury for him, so I was confused.

"Do you eat fruit?" I asked him with curiosity.

"Yes, sir, thank you, sir. You are very generous, sir. But I don't eat fruit in the wintertime because the weather gets cold at night."

Although he'd probably never read a diet book, the guard instinctively knew that fruit is a cooling food. He knew not to eat food that reduced his body temperature during a cold time of year because it would lead to sickness. Returning to my apartment, I realized it probably wasn't such a great idea for me to be eating all this fruit either. I had some anyway, but it was an "aha" moment. I learned more from this man than from all the diet experts' books. Our ancestors ate seasonally because they had no choice. Fresh greens grew in spring, fruit ripened in summer, root vegetables kept them going in the fall, and people relied on animal food to get them through the winter. But when California and Florida were settled and highway transportation and refrigerated trucks were invented, pretty soon Americans could eat more or less anything they wanted, anytime they wanted. But there are costs to this kind of convenience. When we have ice cream in the middle of January and hot barbecued foods on the 4th of July, it's likely to confuse the body. Eating

Seasonal Food Guide

Because produce is available year round, choosing what's in season can be confusing. Generally, look for ripe, fresh produce in abundance and check with your local farmers to get location-specific assistance for each season. For reference, here is a rough guide that links the harvesting season to many popular fruits and veggies.

Fall Foods

winter squash	figs
(acorn, butternut,	grapes
buttercup,	mushrooms
delicata,	parsnips
hubbard,	pears
kabocha)	pomegranates
apples	pumpkin
beets	quince
Belgian endive	sweet potatoes
Brussels sprouts	Swiss chard
cranberries	

Winter Foods

chestnuts
grapefruit
kale
leeks
lemons
oranges/tangerines
radicchio
radishes
rutabaga
turnips

Spring Foods

apricots	mangoes
artichokes	mustard greens
asparagus	new potatoes
avocados	peas
carrots	rhubarb
cherries	spinach
chicory	spring lettuces
chives	strawberries
collards	sugar snap and
dandelion greens	snow peas
fennel	watercress

Summer Foods

bell peppers	nectarines
blackberries	okra peaches
blueberries	pineapples
raspberries	plums
broccoli	summer squash
corn	tomatoes
cucumbers	watermelon
eggplant	zucchini
green beans	

locally grown food in accordance with the seasons will help you live in harmony with yourself, your body and the earth.

In the wintertime, it's natural to crave animal food because that's when the body needs to feel more solid and insulated from the cold. Look at how animals get ready for the winter. Squirrels gather nuts and fatten up to prepare for the cold season. Humans also need more fat in the winter. Allow yourself to eat heavier meals at this time and be sure to have plenty of oils, protein and nuts. If you want to remain on a vegetarian diet through these cold months, it may be an interesting experiment to grill your vegetables, giving them more heat and density, and to avoid raw vegetables and salads. Thick soups—such as pumpkin, pea or potato—will help to keep your body feeling sturdy.

Daily Eating Habits

Pay attention to the times of the day that you eat. Most of us eat habitually at regular, clocked times: before work, during the lunch break and in the evening. We may take a couple of coffee or snack breaks during the day or make a late-night visit to the fridge. Few of us pause to check whether we are really hungry when we eat. We use food as entertainment and comfort whether we are socializing or alone, passing time or feeling bored.

Time of day determines how well our bodies assimilate food. Ayurvedic philosophy advocates for people to eat their biggest meal in the middle of the day, because it's the best time for our bodies to take in and digest a large meal. If you look at many cultures in Europe, this practice is very common. People close shop, go home and eat a large meal with their families and friends. In our country it's harder to find this time during the day, but you can find creative ways to have your largest meal at lunch hour. You may find that this works best for your body, or you might find you feel best when you have a large meal at breakfast or at dinner instead. Some people eat a large breakfast and lunch and then have a small snack for dinner; others do best with five small meals throughout the day. Experiment with the sizes and timing of your meals; only you can determine what is best for your body. Each meal is an experiment. Take the time to listen to your body and notice what it needs.

PROFILE

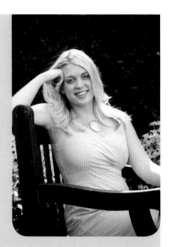

Lindsey Smith, Pittsburgh, PA, USA
www.FoodMoodGirl.com

*"I went from stressed out to blissed out,
and from purpose-less to purpose-full."*

Before attending the Institute for Integrative Nutrition, I was struggling to figure out my purpose, passion and how I could make a single dent in the world. I always knew I was meant to help others, but I struggled to figure out "the how to."

As a pre-teen, I suffered from general anxiety disorder which left me hospitalized at age 11 as the result of severe panic attacks. Despite my young age, I had this inner voice telling me, "There has to be a better way to live your life." After I exhausted all the traditional therapies for anxiety, my family sent me to a local holistic wellness center. In six short months, I was a completely different person. I was anxiety free, loving life and emotionally stable. I was super passionate about my changes and loved talking to people about it, but I never once thought of it as a career option. I thought, "Could I really get paid to share my story? To have a career that is an extension of who I am?"

Then, IIN showed up. After one phone call with the admissions department, I said, "SIGN ME UP!" I KNEW this was where I was meant to be.

Since graduating, I have successfully built my brand called the Food Mood Girl and travel the country speaking to groups and organizations about the food and mood connection. I have also authored two books: *Junk Foods & Junk Moods: Stop Craving and Start Living* and *Bliss Cleanse: Your Two-Week Mind, Body, Spirit Guide to Greater Health and Happiness.*

I have been featured on local and national TV shows and news outlets, have my own TV show called, "Healthy Inspirations," and at 24 years-old, I know this is only the beginning.

I am still in awe that one school could not only be so supportive, but also help guide me to a life of happiness—physically, mentally, emotionally and spiritually. I went from stressed out to blissed out, from fearful to free, and from purpose-less to purpose-full and I have my education at IIN to thank for that!

Many health experts emphasize that we should not eat after 7 p.m. or 8 p.m. I agree that it's a good idea to avoid eating three hours before bed, because when we sleep, digestion slows and food tends to stay in our stomachs the whole night. Strange dreams and restless sleep can result from late-night eating and affect the next day's energy. Some experts say we gain more weight from food we eat at night. I don't know if this is scientifically true, but I do know that I don't sleep well on a full stomach, a strong indication that it's not working well for my system. But, again, it's something for you to explore, using your own body as your laboratory.

How We Eat

Drive-thru Eating

People dine in odd ways and places: standing up, driving a car, on the subway, discussing business deals, watching television, reading a book and playing video games. Eating is no longer viewed as an activity in and of itself, worthy of exclusive quality time. What most people don't realize is that while we eat food, we are also assimilating energetically whatever else is going on around us. During eating, the body is in an open and receiving mode, and we take in more than just the vitamins and nutrients in our meal. We also absorb what is happening in the environment around us. If we eat in an ugly, noisy, neon-lit room, the energy of that space is going to penetrate us. If we eat quietly in a beautiful park or by the ocean, we will also absorb the positive qualities of those surroundings. When eating with other people, we absorb their moods, their laughter, their complaints and their busy minds.

Many people suffer from a range of digestive disorders, from acid reflux to irritable bowel syndrome and more. These conditions are connected not just to what we eat, but how we eat it. Our bodies have sensors that connect our guts to our brains and our five senses. When these sensors are triggered, they get our digestive juices flowing, helping us to properly process our food. They tell us when we have had enough to eat, so we don't overload our systems. When we eat too fast, on the run or under stress, these sensors don't have enough time to go off. Our bodies are unable to rev up and prepare for digestion. By the time our brains get the message that we are getting full, we've already scarfed down a huge meal and moved on to our next activity. As a result, our bodies barely recognize that we have eaten, even though there is plenty of food in our stomachs. I'm sure you've had this experience. For example, many of us eat while driving and then wonder why we feel hungry a few hours later, and some of us will eat more. This overeating can overwhelm the body and eventually lead to chronic conditions.

Because the nature of our bodies is to "rest and digest," the body likes to be relaxed, inactive and in a peaceful environment when assimilating food. The body doesn't want to be in tense "fight or flight" mode, alert for danger and unexpected events. In this state, the eyes tighten, the heart beats faster and blood goes to the center of the body. Proper assimilation of the nutrients in food is essential to health, and if we want this assimilation to take place, we need to be calmer when we sit down to meals.

Healthy eating means eating with all of our senses. We need to see our food, smell it and spend time enjoying it. People used to enjoy food by eating dinner together. This traditional daily ritual had a binding effect on the family as an organic unit. As the saying goes, "A family that eats together stays together." Sharing meals made the family more cohesive and, in turn, kept them interwoven within a much bigger collective fabric, a whole mindset about the kind of society we all wanted. This mindset is rapidly changing. Now kids eat prepackaged microwave dinners because both parents are working and have no time to prepare home-cooked meals. If Dad eats a burger for dinner, Mom has a large salad and the kids eat pizza on the run, it's natural that the family will have difficulty relating to one another later in the evening. Each member of the family will have different energy, thoughts and feelings depending on his or her individual meal.

Whether you are a single person or part of a family unit, experiment with ways to eat in a calmer, quieter, more loving way. Maybe you can organize your family to eat a home-cooked meal together once a week. Notice the difference this makes in your energy and connection. Try simple rituals to make mealtime special, like eating off of your good plates, lighting a candle or saying a blessing before your meal. If you tend to eat at your desk at work, try to change this habit. Simply going into a different room to eat, or better yet, eating outside, may make a big difference. Be creative and discover what you can do to bring your body into a more relaxed state during your meals. It could make a big difference to your overall health.

The Importance of Chewing

Many of us inhale our food. We use our fork as a shovel, putting the next bite in before we've finished the previous one. It's part of our fast-paced culture. Aside from missing the enjoyment of a long, relaxing meal, eating quickly can be detrimental to our health. Digestion actually begins with the chewing process. If you think about your stomach working to break down every little bit of food you put into your mouth, it makes sense that the more you break it down in the chewing process, the easier the digestion process will be. If your food is not properly broken down before entering the esophagus, it can remain undigested and cause bacteria overgrowth in the intestines. In addition, the action of chewing and the resulting production of saliva both, send a message to the stomach, intestines and entire gastrointestinal system that the digestion process has begun. These organs can then prepare for their digestion tasks and keep the body in balance.

Chewing also makes food more enjoyable. The sweet flavor of plant foods is released only after they have been chewed thoroughly. Complex carbohydrates start breaking down in the mouth by an enzyme in saliva known as amylase. It is only by chewing the carbs thoroughly and mixing them with amylase that we can taste all of their sweetness. This sweet flavor becomes a reward for chewing. Do you see the brilliance of the natural food system involved in this process? Leveraging our inherent craving for sweetness, our body works with nature to ensure we get the nutrients we need.

I do not have a recommended amount of time people should take to chew each bite, although some of my students experiment with chewing each bite 20 to 50 times. In general, I recommend putting down your fork or utensils in between each bite to help you focus on the food in your mouth. Once you are done chewing, then you can take your next bite. It can be difficult to focus on chewing when eating with others, so try eating on your own and focus on fully chewing each bite. Turn off the TV, resist the urge to text or surf the web and really focus on your eating experience. You'll see that it takes you longer to eat your meal but that you get full faster. Another useful tip to help people slow down is to try eating with chopsticks. They can only pick up a limited amount of food at a time, and it can be a fun eating adventure.

Exercises:

1. Organic Apple Taste Test

Go to the supermarket and pick out your favorite apple variety. See if you can find one conventionally grown and one organically grown and see if you can see differences in the look, texture and smell of the apples. Take each one home and do a taste test for yourself.

2. Visit Your Local Farmers' Market

Find a farmers' market in your area. Walk around the market and notice all the fresh vegetables. Talk to the farmers about where they come from and ask about the journey the vegetables took to get there. If they are local and organic, they are most likely in season. Filling your bag with local produce is a way to ensure that you are cooking and eating in season. Share some of your favorites finds with your friends and family.

3. Chew Your Food

At your next meal, count how many times you chew each mouthful of food. See if you can chew 100 times per bite. Or try 50. Become more aware of each bite and practice chewing slowly and with intention. Notice how you feel at the end of your meal. Share your experience with your friends and family and encourage them to chew as well.

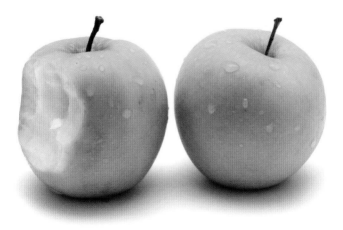

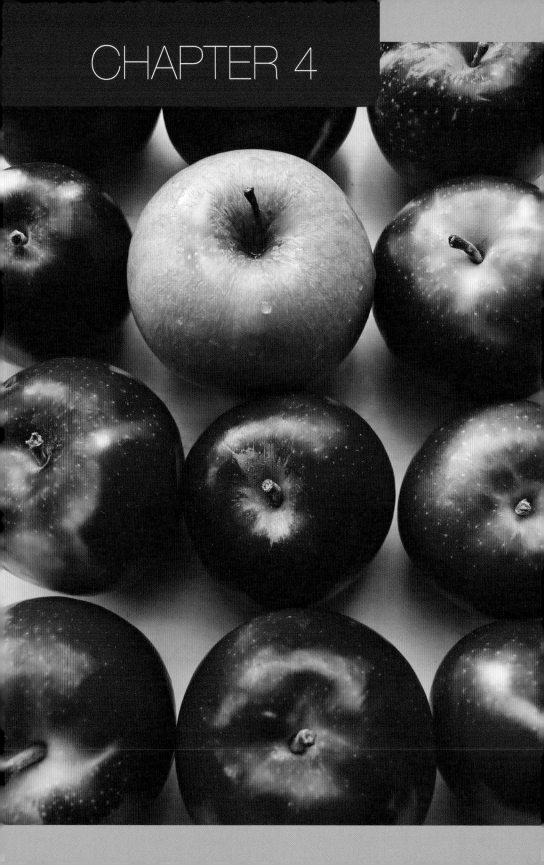

CHAPTER 4

Dietary
Theory

When it comes to diet, one size definitely doesn't fit all.
—Christiane Northrup, MD

have always been interested in food. As a child, I was excited to go shopping with my mother. I was enthralled by the enormous supermarket filled with shopping carts and aisles upon aisles of food. I wondered how my mother knew what foods to choose and what to leave on the shelf. At home, I would help put the food away in cupboards or in the fridge and the food would come out again in some order that my mom knew was the right order. The whole process—how food transformed from packages on shelves to warm, delicious meals on a plate—fascinated me.

As I grew up, my passion for food continued. In my 20s, while getting my master's in education with a specialization in counseling, I noticed that there was no overlap between the sciences of psychology and nutrition, but I knew a connection existed. At that time, I encountered someone on a vegetarian diet. With that friendship, I became much more conscious of my eating habits, which led to a further understanding of the food-mood connection. I realized that to best support my clients emotionally, I would have to incorporate dialogue about food. The clients who upgraded the quality of their food became more clear, optimistic and healthy. In turn, I became clear that emotional counseling had to be preceded by counseling on food and diet.

At the age of 25, my interest in natural foods led me to macrobiotics. I read every book on the topic that I could find (about 50 at the time), went to macrobiotics conferences, studied at the macrobiotics center in Toronto and eventually studied extensively with Michio and Aveline Kushi, two of the chief students of George Ohsawa, the man who created macrobiotics as it is known today. Then, when I was director of the macrobiotics center in

Toronto, I increased my frequency of visits to the Kushi Institute, learning as much I possibly could. Considering that my nutrition philosophy evolved out of this Japanese-based theory, I'd like to share a few stories to illustrate why macrobiotics initially attracted me.

Michio invited me to go with him to Japan, where I met people whose families had grown traditional macrobiotic foods for centuries, such as umeboshi plums and high-quality brown rice. I met miso masters and even someone who made sake from brown rice. On this trip, I gained a deep under-standing of Michio, Aveline and traditional macrobiotics. Upon our return, I enrolled in their intensive 10-day macrobiotic educator course, which boasts such esteemed alumni as Paul Pitchford, Dr. Dean Ornish and Dr. Christiane Northrup, to become an official, expert macrobiotic teacher. We studied medicinal cooking, visual diagnosis, shiatsu massage and performing consul-tations to gain an in-depth understanding of macrobiotic theory and prac-tice. Students would take turns cooking and eat three meals a day together. Michio and Aveline were known for their finely tuned taste buds and skills in judging how food was prepared by its taste alone. At mealtimes, they would intuitively know who at the table had prepared each dish and what his or her thoughts and feelings had been as they cooked. They could tell a lot about a person by just tasting his or her food.

Macrobiotics follows the premise that every action on the food affects the quality and nutritional value of the meal. Every single slice, chop and shake, the speed of the stirring, the mood the cook is in, as well as the cleanliness and order of the kitchen, is consumed with the food. One day my friend Vince decided to challenge the precision of Michio and Aveline's intuition, as well as test the legitimacy of this theory. He cooked the meal in a messy kitchen and went wild running around the kitchen singing, shouting and dancing. He also manipulated the food much more than was necessary, but all along maintained the integrity of the ingredients for a proper macrobiotic meal. As Michio tasted the food, he commented, with studied Japanese politeness, "This is good, but very strange." At the end of the meal, he turned to my col-league and said calmly, "Maybe you need a doctor."

Another time, I was preparing a meal for 10 people as part of my certi-fication exam, when, thirty minutes before mealtime, someone announced that Michio had returned from a visit to Japan and would be joining us for dinner. He had an entourage of 10 students with him. Since I had no time to prepare extra of my carrot-burdock sauté or roasted root vegetables, I decided to quickly add more soba noodles to the soba dish and more water to the miso soup, and cross my fingers that it would all still taste okay. When Michio and Aveline arrived, they inspected the food, admired its appearance and offered a prayer. Everyone sat down and began to eat. Utter silence filled the room as Michio and Aveline tasted the food.

After a few bites, Michio looked up and said, simply, "Noodles are good. But why did you add water to the soup at the end of its cooking?" He looked at me steadily, waiting for an answer. With his wise eyes on me, I suddenly felt like I was the only person in the room.

"Uh, no I didn't," I stammered.

Michio continued watching me, but I could see a smile playing on the corners of his lips. Everyone else at the table had looked up from their plates and was watching me too.

"Okay, I did, I did," I admitted, blushing. "I didn't know how to make the meal feed everyone." He just smiled in a non-egotistical way without needing to say another word.

During the time I spent training at the Kushi Institute, I was repeatedly awed by the depth of Michio's awareness of the subtle aspects of cooking and consuming food. He inspired me to commit my life to the development of this kind of understanding, and, eventually, to help my students develop this understanding as well. Studying with him, I learned how to use my body as a walking, talking laboratory to conduct a vast array of experiments in my search for optimum health.

For a while, macrobiotics supplied all the answers for me. Like many dietary theories, it promised longevity, peace of mind and extreme wellness to those who followed its complex rules. But I also encountered some issues that wouldn't go away. Many macrobiotic teachers smoke cigarettes, drink alcohol and indulge in quite a few donuts on a regular basis. These habits always seemed odd to me since the macrobiotic diet is so rigid in its prohibition of tomatoes, potatoes, oranges and garlic, as well as other restrictions, yet the teachers were regularly consuming much more harmful foods. Over time, noticing these contradictions was helpful for me; they freed me from becoming a "true believer" about nutrition. My growing awareness of the limitations of macrobiotics spurred my quest to gather a broader base of knowledge and information about food and health.

Moving to Kripalu, the largest residential yoga center in the United States, was another formative step in the evolution of my thinking on nutrition. Part of Kripalu's philosophy is to expose students to many different types of yoga, from Iyengar to Anusara to Kundalini. Watching the skillful teachers move seamlessly between yogic styles, I began to see the beauty and wisdom of assimilating different learning styles from a variety of traditions, instead of having to decide on one alone. By applying the same principle to nutrition, I realized I could relieve a lot of needless suffering and release people from the notion of one "perfect diet." I decided to create a new kind of nutrition school, one that would cover the best of every diet system and support people in their own quest for nutritional knowledge.

Most nutrition people believe their theory is the right one and everyone else's theory is wrong. They see the emergence of new information as competition and attempt to dismiss all other diet plans as "fad diets." My approach is just the opposite. I am thrilled when new dietary theories emerge because it shows that people are continuing to uncover what will help us all live happier, healthier lives. When a new theory appears, I read about it, research it, try to understand where its creators are coming from and then add their wisdom to my teaching.

I like to discuss all the different dietary theories, covering the pros and cons of each, because the interesting thing is that they all work. When people decide to go on a diet, they have already become conscious of their self-destructive eating habits and realize it's time for a change. Whatever diet they choose is going to work because they are shifting from a chaotic, disordered way of eating to an ordered way of eating. They are going to stop eating chemicalized, artificial junk food and get better. The general rule is that any attention to diet is better than none. Diet theorists miss this fact because they want to attribute success to their unique approach.

All diet programs contain elements of truth. When I talk about various diets to my students, including programs ranging from raw foods to Paleo, some students always swear that a particular diet really helped them. The extent to which people can benefit from specific diets is amazing. This fact reminds me to appreciate how we as a species are so diverse and unique. I believe that when a diet is successful, a placebo effect may be responsible for at least some of the benefits. Experts in the field of nutrition rarely discuss this phenomenon because experts like to take credit for discovering the latest weight-loss method. Many studies illustrate the power of the placebo effect. A group of patients all suffering from the same ailment take sugar pills and are told they contain a breakthrough medicine that will help cure them. With no active ingredients in the pills, a significant percentage of the patients will recover simply because they believe they are being treated. It's the same with diets. Many of them work because of this mind-over-matter factor.

Most people will lose weight on any given diet program for a limited period of time, and then revert to a less disciplined way of eating. Why? Because most diet books instruct people to eat a limited spectrum of recommended foods. People follow the program with all good intentions, slowly narrowing their list of acceptable foods, squeezing their eyes shut while scurrying past a Dunkin' Donuts or Starbucks, determined not to stray from the chosen path. Sooner or later, though, the cravings become too intense, their determination fades and they fall off the wagon. These people are not weak, ignorant or lacking in willpower. Their cravings occur because humans are omnivorous creatures with roving appetites. We all have unique bodies, cravings and lifestyles, and a list of "acceptable" foods is not always going to align with our individual needs or satisfy our cravings. So, just as all diets work, they all also don't work.

I've learned this fact as much from my own personal experience as from that of my students. Late one evening, after I had been more or less vegetarian for a few years, my craving for meat grew so strong I found my car pulling into a fast food drive-thru window. I saw myself ordering a burger with extra, extra vegetables and parking on a deserted street to wolf down the forbidden food. I had never experienced such exhilaration. The thrill of giving my body exactly what it needed, even though it went directly against my beliefs at the time, was undeniable. It felt so good and so bad at the same time! For years, I kept these clandestine moments of what I thought were weakness to myself, hiding them from my friends, family and colleagues. They only stopped when I was able to come to a deeper, clearer understanding of balanced eating. This understanding came from listening to my own body and studying every dietary theory I could.

The following is a description of many of the theories that I have found the most useful, interesting and applicable throughout the years.

Macrobiotics

Central Philosophy: Translated literally, macrobiotics means "great life." The philosophy is based on eating only natural foods, and balancing yin and yang in the body. The idea is to live within the natural order of life.

Foods Encouraged: Whole grains comprise about 40–60% of the diet, followed by fresh vegetables, which are about 25–30%, beans about 5–0%, soups 5–10% and sea vegetables about 3–5% of the diet. Fish is allowed about 1–3 times a week.

Foods Restricted: dairy, meat, eggs, refined sugar products, chocolate, tropical fruits, coffee, hot spices, nightshade vegetables

····· **SAMPLE DAILY MENU** ·····

Breakfast: miso soup with daikon radish and shiitake mushrooms, brown rice porridge, steamed leeks and Chinese cabbage

Lunch: millet with toasted pumpkin seeds and tamari, blanched broccoli and cauliflower, aduki beans with carrot, ginger and sea salt

Snack: bancha tea, brown rice syrup–sweetened ginger cookie

Dinner: arame seaweed with toasted almonds, sweet and sour beets, chilled soba noodles with watercress, roasted kabocha squash

The modern macrobiotic movement began in the early 1900s with George Ohsawa, a Japanese dietary innovator, who combined theories of Eastern philosophy with food and medicine. Macrobiotics is a modified version of the ancient concept of yin-yang, which points to an underlying order in the universe based on a dynamic, ever-changing balance between two apparently opposite yet complementary principles. Yang embodies the masculine qualities of hard, strong, active, tight and contractive. Yin embodies the feminine qualities of soft, yielding, passive, receptive, loose and expansive. The dance between these two universal energies includes not only men and women, but sweet and salty; day and night; winter and summer; dark and light. The list goes on and on. Regarding food, the yin-yang theory of balance asserts that we should avoid foods that are too yin, or too yang, to avoid imbalance which eventually leads to illness.

It wasn't the dietary aspect of macrobiotics that interested me initially, but the simple, ancient wisdom of the yin-yang philosophy, the dance of opposites. How could Western theorists and dietitians overlook such a simple and self-evident system of universal dynamics? On further study, I learned that Ohsawa's key to good health is to maintain yin-yang balance by following a traditional, grain-based diet. He taught that there is only one basic human disease: living out of balance. Macrobiotics is based on the age-old concept that grains are the principle food in the diet, sacred in virtually every traditional society. Ohsawa reintroduced this idea to the West, helping to establish brown rice and soy products as staple foods in Europe and America. Macrobiotics originated in an enclosed Japanese island culture with limited food resources, where people were obliged to eat the same foods—rice, local vegetables, fish and seaweed—over and over again. They did not have dairy or much animal meat. To keep their meals appetizing and healthy, they developed different ways to cook the same foods, often based on the season of year.

When I first encountered macrobiotics in the 1970s, eating seasonal, locally grown, organic produce and traditional foods made me feel vibrant and energized. I was also intrigued by some of the lifestyle suggestions, including singing a happy song every day. The recommendation to sing really surprised me. A singing diet? Unbelievable! But when I did it, I noticed I felt better, happier and more relaxed. This opened my mind to the concept of being nourished on different levels, not only physically, but also mentally, emotionally and spiritually.

Other macrobiotic suggestions include keeping your home simple, neat and clean, wearing more cotton clothes and fewer synthetic fibers, keeping a sense of humor, allowing time for prayer and meditation, avoiding excessive jewelry or chemical perfumes and growing green plants in the home. Another recommendation is to be on good terms with all people, creating more balance in your personal life.

Understanding the Yin-Yang Qualities of Food

MORE YANG	MORE YIN
sea salt	alcohol & chemicals
	sugar & coffee
eggs	honey & spices
miso & tamari	dairy
	oil
red meat	tropical fruits
	local fruits, nuts & seeds
cheese	tofu
poultry	leafy green vegetables
	roots & winter squash
fish	beans
grains	sea vegetables
LESS YANG	LESS YIN

For several years I followed a vegan macrobiotic diet—eating no dairy, meat, honey or eggs. I did eat fish about once a month. I became very healthy and strong and any time I went for a checkup all my blood tests were normal. Gradually, however, I began to notice the downside of this way of eating. Although macrobiotic theory advises people to eat the traditional diet of their ancestors, most macrobiotic teachers, books and sections in natural food stores strongly emphasize Japanese foods. This issue wasn't too problematic when I started my nutrition school in Toronto, but when I moved to New York I was dealing with a much more diverse clientele—students who went home to feed Puerto Rican, African American and Jewish families. Imposing a Japanese diet on these people can practically pose a threat to break up their families. Moreover, for New York's singles and working moms, preparing complex macrobiotic recipes added unnecessary stress to their already crowded daily lives.

The drawbacks of macrobiotics are largely due to the reliance of salt in the traditional Japanese diet. The diet rarely incorporates herbs and spices, and sugar is never recommended, so salt is the main flavoring for everything. Miso soup, for example, is very salty, as are soy sauce and umeboshi plums. Unfortunately, as a result of this overabundance of salt in the diet, stomach cancer is a significant problem among the Japanese. Every medical student and health practitioner knows that too much salt can lead to hypertension, accompanied by rising blood pressure. If a patient has high blood pressure, a macrobiotic diet is probably not appropriate for them.

One of the most difficult aspects of the macrobiotic diet to follow is the suggestion to drink only when thirsty. The body doesn't normally feel the urge to drink until it is already dehydrated, a kind of neurological time lag. Our body needs water, but our brain doesn't get the message in time. I spent years on a macrobiotic diet, and I never thought I was thirsty because my body was accustomed to a very low level of water. Too much salt and not enough water are both independently problematic for the body, but to combine the two is a recipe for disaster.

Even though your head can convince your body to obey a diet for a while, your body will reach a certain point and reassert itself, sometimes with tragic results. It's amazing how people get carried away with their beliefs, confusing food with religious fervor. Macrobiotics certainly has its share of fanatics. To such people I want to say, "It's just a diet. It doesn't matter that much. You are not going to heaven for eating so many vegetables, and you will not go to hell for drinking too much water."

Ayurveda

Central philosophy: Ayurveda is an ancient healing system from India that emphasizes eating in accordance with your individual body type and the seasons. The system promotes health and disease prevention through balancing the doshas, or mind-body types.

Foods Encouraged: A basic meal should have something warm, something with protein, a salad and/or vegetables with good oil, spices and flavorings, a small sweet for dessert, walk and rest. Each meal aims to cover all six tastes: sweet, sour, salty, pungent, astringent and bitter. Examples of sweet foods are fruits like figs, grapes and oranges, and cooked starchy vegetables like sweet potatoes, carrots and beet roots. Sour foods include sour milk products, such as yogurt, cheese and whey, sour fruits, like lemons, and fermented substances like soy sauce, vinegar and sour cabbage. Salty foods include sea salt, rock salt and pickles. Pungent foods include radishes, onions and spices, such as ginger, cumin and mustard seeds. Bitter foods are olives, grapefruits, eggplant, chicory, spinach and zucchini, along with fenugreek and turmeric spices. Astringent foods are honey, walnuts, lentils, sprouts, rhubarb and green leafy vegetables.

Foods Restricted: heavily processed foods, excess sugar and caffeine, large amounts of animal protein

····· SAMPLE DAILY MENU ·····

Breakfast: hot cereal with walnuts, honey and spices

Lunch: portobello mushroom curry with basmati rice, mung bean dahl and sautéed spinach

Snack: almonds, Eater's Digest tea

Dinner: tandoori salmon with yogurt, turmeric and pineapple chutney, broccoli salad with sesame oil and sesame seeds

Dessert: rice pudding with cardamom, cinnamon, honey and almond milk

The ancient Indian healing system of Ayurveda, which translates as "the science of life" in Sanskrit, was developed at least 3,000 years ago. In recent times, Ayurvedic medicine and its accompanying herbal remedies have become increasingly popular in the United States and Europe. Ayurveda recognizes that all life—human, plant and animal—must live in harmony with nature in order to survive. Creating optimal health and balance begins by adopting the concept of "food as medicine."

In Ayurveda, proper diet is determined by the three harvesting seasons: late fall, spring and summer. The late fall harvest is rich in nuts and grains— all warming and insulating to combat the cold, dry extremes of the coming winter. Meat is not typically recommended in an Ayurvedic diet, but it is more accepted during cold times of year. In the wet, rainy and congested spring, the naturally occurring harvest is rich in low-fat and astringent roots, sprouts, grapefruits and berries. These foods help to decrease the seasonal tendency to make mucus, and fight against allergies, colds and weight gain. In the summer months, the naturally occurring harvest is rich in cooling fruits and vegetables, and eating these foods moderates the accumulated heat of the season. Cultures that still rely on food from local farmers practice these universal principles of Ayurveda by naturally changing their diets with the rhythm of the seasons.

In Ayurvedic theory, the five elements of nature are space, air, fire, water and earth. These elements materialize and combine to create the three basic fundamental principles in nature, called doshas. Space and air combine to form the principle called vata. Fire and water combine to form the principle called pitta. And earth and water combine to form kapha. These principles are used to categorize mind-body types, also called doshas. Thus, Ayurveda has three seasons, three primary harvests and three doshas.

Vata

The qualities of vata as seen in nature are cold, dry, rough and constantly moving. Winter is the season in which vata predominates. During this time of year it is cold, our skin gets dry, precipitation becomes cold and dry in the form of snow, and the wind blows without restrictions as the trees are without leaves.

The vata body type is what we imagine when we think of our contemporary notion of beauty: thin-boned, tall and skinny, or short, slim and petite.

Vatas have sharp minds and a tendency to worry; they are light sleepers and have nervous dispositions. These people usually have a fast metabolism, experience difficulty gaining weight, and are characteristically weak in their intestines, suffering from poor absorption of nutrients. As the squirrel needs nuts in the winter and as the natural harvest is rich in warm, heavy foods, so the wintry vata requires highly nutritious food, with an abundance of cooked vegetables and whole grains to promote healthy assimilation and bowel function. Vatas benefit from eating small amounts of animal food, but must be careful not to overdo it. Fish and low-fat meats are usually best. Vatas need regular exercise to release nervous tension. They do best with more meditative, gentle and calming practices such as yoga.

Pitta

During the summer months the environment accumulates heat. The property of fire or heat is called pitta.

The pitta body type embodies the qualities of fire. This body type is physically oriented, with more muscle and a fiery temperament. Pitta people usually have yellow or reddish colored skin that is sensitive to rashes. They often sweat profusely and are easily irritated. Their bodies and temperaments both tend to be hot. For the most part, they have a very strong and athletic constitution.

Pittas tend to be leaders and are well-organized, intelligent and charismatic. They are usually emotional, competitive and passionate, and in need of a good eight hours' sleep per night to rest and cool off. They have enormous appetites for food and life experience, and can become gluttons if not careful. Pittas benefit from seeking balance in eating, avoiding hot spices and too much animal food, emphasizing sweet vegetables like squash and pumpkin, and whole grains like barley and oats. Most importantly, pittas must avoid excess and include regular exercise in their daily schedules.

Kapha

Spring, which is the kapha season, is a very wet and heavy time of year. It is allergy season, the rainy season, full of heavy mud and potential congestion.

Influenced by the qualities of springtime, those with kapha body types are big-boned, full-bodied, and physically strong and tend toward weight gain. Their solid skeletons protect them from osteoporosis. Skin color is pale and cool, and eyes are large and often dark. They are frequently easygoing, slow, methodical types, with balanced, peaceful temperaments. Kapha types radiate competence, even when they are quiet or shy.

Kaphas have slow metabolisms and strong intestines, and the ease with which they assimilate nutrients means that they don't have to eat much to stay in good health. In fact, they should avoid overeating because their main health concern is danger of obesity. The heart is their weakest organ.

Kaphas should eat lots of vegetables and light foods, including a wide range of grains. Their primary animal food should be eggs. All spices are good for kaphas, but they need to restrict intake of oil as much as possible. Regular, non-strenuous physical exercise, like taking a stroll in the park, suits them best.

If this system intrigues you, I encourage you study it further. In India, Ayurvedic doctors usually do not tell a patient his or her body type. Instead, they look at a patient's susceptibility to imbalance. With this information, they can employ preventative techniques to avoid disease and maintain good health.

Our greatest lesson from Ayurveda is to learn from nature, eat in harmony with the seasons and live a life of balance.

5 Element Theory

Central Philosophy: An ancient Chinese belief system that says we are surrounded by five energy fields: wood, fire, earth, metal and water. Keeping all the elements in balance promotes harmony in our surroundings and in ourselves.

Foods Encouraged: Eat foods from each of the five phases including grains, tubers, beans, vegetables and fruits.

Foods Restricted: meat, sugar, overly processed chemical foods, deep-fried foods, liquor, beer, wine

····· **SAMPLE DAILY MENU** ·····

Breakfast: steel-cut oats topped with walnuts and blueberries

Lunch: grilled shrimp with corn and black bean salad

Snack: air-popped popcorn

Dinner: broccoli and tofu stir-fry with brown rice

Dessert: watermelon slices

Based on ancient Chinese philosophy, the 5 Element Theory relates all energy and substances to the elements—fire, earth, metal (or air), water and wood. Each element is associated with a direction of the compass and a season of the year with late summer as the fifth season. In the creation cycle, one element gives birth to the next and nourishes it through the flow of energy. Wood creates fire, which creates earth, which creates metal, which creates water, which creates wood. In the destruction cycle, wood injures earth, fire destroys metal, earth controls water, metal attacks wood and water injures fire.

Wood is associated with the morning and the spring season. It is associated with the liver and the gallbladder organs and the emotions of impatience and anger. Wood vegetables are artichokes, broccoli, carrots, string beans, zucchini, sprouts, parsley and leafy greens. The effect of wood on the body is purification.

Fire is associated with twelve noon and the summer season. The related organs are the heart and small intestine. The related emotion is joy. Fire vegetables are asparagus, Brussels sprouts, chives, dandelion, scallions and tomatoes. Coffee and tobacco are also fiery. Fire creates circulation in the body.

Earth is associated with the afternoon and the late summer season. The stomach and pancreas are the active organs, and sympathy and worry are the correlated emotions. Chard, collards, parsnips, spinach, squash and sweet potato are the earth vegetables. The taste of earth is sweet, and other earth substances are carob, honey, maple syrup and sugar. The related bodily function of earth is digestion.

Metal is associated with the evening and the autumn season. The lungs are the active organs. The emotion is grief. Cabbage, cauliflower, celery,

5 Element Chart

	TREE/WOOD	FIRE	SOIL/EARTH	METAL	WATER
TIME	morning	noon	afternoon	evening	night
SEASON	spring	summer	Indian summer	autumn	winter
ORGANS	liver gall bladder	heart small intestine	stomach, spleen, pancreas	lungs large intestine	kidneys bladder
GRAINS	barley, oats, rye, wheat	amaranth popcorn	millet	rice sweet rice	buckwheat
VEGETABLES	artichoke broccoli carrot string bean romaine lettuce parsley zucchini	asparagus Brussels sprouts chive dandelion endive scallion tomato	chard collards eggplant parsnip pumpkin spinach squash sweet potato	cabbage cauliflower celery cucumber daikon radish onion	beet burdock hijiki kale kombu wakame water chestnut
FRUIT	avocado grapefruit lemon lime plum pomegranate	apricot raspberry strawberry	banana apple (sweet) cantaloupe coconut date fig raisin	peach pear	blackberry blueberry cranberry watermelon
LEGUMES	black-eyed peas green lentil	red lentil	chickpea	navy soybean	adzuki kidney
NUTS	brazil cashew	pistachio	almond pecan pine nut	walnut hickory	chestnut
ANIMAL MEAT	chicken chicken (liver) beef (liver) lamb (liver)	shrimp squab beef (heart)	salmon swordfish tuna pheasant rabbit	cod flounder halibut turkey beef	crab lobster mussel duck ham pork
OTHER	lard nut butters vinegar olives pickles	beer coffee chocolate ketchup liquor tobacco	carob honey maple syrup rice honey sugar - brown sugar - white	mint mochi peppermint spirulina tofu tempeh	decaf coffee miso salt tamari bancha tea
COLOR	green	red	yellow orange	white	gray black deep blue
EMOTION	anger	joy	sympathy worrying	grief	fear
TASTE	sour	bitter	sweet	hot pungent	salty
SOUND	shouting	laughing	singing	weeping	groaning
ENERGY	planning decision-making	commanding to action	imagining	establishing rhythmic order	preserving by will power
BODY	purification	circulation	digestion	respiration	elimination

cucumber, daikon and radish are the metal vegetables. Peppermint, spirulina, tofu and tempeh also belong to the metal family. Respiration is the related bodily function.

Water is associated with night and the winter season. The active organs are the kidneys and the bladder. The emotion is fear. Beets, burdock, sea vegetables and kale are water vegetables. Miso, salt and tamari are also water foods. Elimination is the bodily function.

By eating foods associated with each of the elements, you can promote balance in the body. Knowing which foods, seasons, emotions and bodily functions are associated with which element can make you a master of balance. Say, for example, it's the middle of winter and you are feeling constipated and tight. It's the water time of year, so increasing sea vegetables with water energy and drinking more water could help. Or say you are craving coffee and cigarettes, which both belong to the fire element. You could deconstruct those cravings and ask yourself, "Where else can I add fire, passion and joy into my life?" You might also increase the fire vegetables, like green leafy vegetables, in your diet. Chances are your craving for coffee and cigarettes would subside.

According to 5 Element Theory, the way you cook changes the energy of your food. Stir-frying and deep frying give food a wood energy, grilling and barbecuing give food a fire energy, boiling gives food a water energy, baking gives food a metal energy and steaming gives food an earth energy.

If you are interested in exploring this theory further, use the chart with the elements and components of each element clearly listed. In your food journal, you can record what you eat from each element every day for breakfast, lunch and dinner. This will help you see your natural tendencies and find balance. If you notice that you are eating mostly earth foods, it may help to increase wood foods because wood holds down the earth.

High-Carbohydrate Diets

Central Philosophy: High-carbohydrate diets are a modern take on traditional diets that relied on whole grains, beans and vegetables.

Foods Encouraged: About 80% carbohydrates, 10–15% protein and 5–10% fat. Foods encouraged include whole, unprocessed grains including brown rice, millet, barley and oats; a variety of vegetables and fruits, and beans, such as black, chickpea, lentils, lima and pinto.

Foods Restricted: Generally, avoid meats, oils, high-fat dairy products, sugar, alcohol and caffeine. Some high-carb diets are also low-fat diets and restrict commercial products with more than 2 grams of fat per serving, such as Dr. Dean Ornish's diet.

····· **SAMPLE DAILY MENU** ·····

Breakfast: oat-wheat-rice pancakes topped with sliced bananas and served with a side of orange slices

Lunch: tabbouleh salad with broiled red and yellow bell peppers and a scoop of hummus

Dinner: lentil tacos, with garnish of shredded lettuce, diced tomatoes, chopped green onions, shredded carrots and low-fat cheese with a side of wild rice

Dessert: fruit meringue

Snack: vegetable juice made with carrots, apples and celery and rye crispbreads topped with peanut butter

I pinpoint 1972 and the publication of *Diet for a Small Planet* by Frances Moore Lappé, as the beginning of a trend toward high-carbohydrate diets in America. This book eventually sold more than three million copies worldwide. Lappé postulated that human practices, not natural disasters, cause worldwide hunger. Food scarcity results when grain, rich in nutrients and able to support vast populations, is fed to livestock to produce meat, which yields only a fraction of those nutrients to many fewer people. Lappé theorized that traditional cultures stay healthy by mixing vegetable proteins together, such as the pairing of beans and grains. Her book's publication coincided with an American hippie subculture that was turning its back on fast food and embracing natural foods, macrobiotics, Indian-style vegetarianism and a grain-based diet as part of a general "back to the land" movement.

Then came Nathan Pritikin, a medical doctor who studied indigenous cultures around the world, and noted they did not have the types of chronic disease suffered by people in developed countries. He attributed their health to a low-fat diet with lots of carbohydrates. Based on these insights, he created the Pritikin Longevity Center in 1976. In 1980 he co-authored a best-selling book, *The Pritikin Program for Diet and Exercise*, in which he advocated a low-fat, low-protein diet, with most nutrients coming from complex carbohydrates. Recommended foods included fresh and cooked fruits and vegetables, whole grains, breads, pasta, and small amounts of lean meat, fish and poultry. He also encouraged a daily regimen of aerobic exercise.

In 1977, George McGovern, former director of the "Food for Peace" program under President Kennedy, headed the U.S. Senate Select Committee on Nutrition and Human Needs. After years of discussion, scientific review and debate, the committee encouraged the movement toward vegetable and grain-based diets in America—unwelcome news for the meat and dairy industries. Six years later, in 1983, Dr. John McDougall attracted public attention by designing a vegan diet of high-carbohydrate, low-protein foods. In 1993, Dr. Dean Ornish published the best-selling *Eat More, Weigh Less*, shattering the commonly held notion that losing weight requires starvation. To actually eat more and still shed pounds was a truly revolutionary idea. Ornish embraced macrobiotics but had the foresight to realize that the Japanese foods, like seaweed and miso, and yin-yang philosophy were too foreign for most Americans. He incorporated the system's basic dietary principles into his new diet and used more familiar American foods and concepts.

In 1988, the U.S. Surgeon General, in conjunction with the American Medical Association, conducted a study of various weight-loss plans. The study showed that two-thirds of people on these plans gained all their weight back in one year, and 97% regained all their weight within five years. A few years later, Ornish showed that under his plan, patients lost 24 pounds in the first year and kept more than half the weight off for five years. He attributed much of his success to the fact that his patients could eat more food, thereby avoiding hunger pangs and cravings normally associated with dieting.

Ornish then approached insurance companies like Blue Cross Blue Shield, pointing out how much money they could save on payouts for heart bypass surgery if they instead enrolled their clients in his program. In response, the insurance companies put 300 people on his program and saved millions of dollars. The Ornish program for reversing heart disease is now commonly accepted by insurance companies as a deductible expense, a huge break-through for the nutrition world. His program recommends a diet largely com-posed of grains and vegetables, with a formula of 10% fat, 20% protein and 70% carbohydrates. He also recommends yoga, meditation and developing a loving heart—"hugging is healthy!"—to keep the arteries clean and clear.

Boredom is one of the biggest challenges for people on a high-carbo-hydrate diet. Eating meals consisting largely of grains and veggies may be great for some people's health, but it can be very frustrating for the palate. One thing you must learn if a high-carbohydrate diet is going to work for you is how to make simple food taste delicious.

Vegan Diet

Central Philosophy: Veganism is the practice of abstaining from all ani-mal products, rejecting the commodity status of sentient animals. Followers often extend the ethical principles of veganism into other areas of their lives and oppose the use of animals or animal products for any purpose.

Foods Encouraged: fruits, vegetables, plenty of leafy greens, whole grains, nuts, seeds, legumes

Foods Restricted: all animal products and by-products including eggs, dairy and honey

····· **SAMPLE DAILY MENU** ·····

Breakfast: sriracha-infused scrambled tofu, sliced avocado, sweet potato home fries

Lunch: three bean burrito with salsa, vegan cheese, romaine lettuce in Ezekiel wrap

Dinner: mushroom, pea and asparagus risotto with broccoli rabe

Dessert: almond, date and banana bites

Snack: kale chips, cacao nibs, spicy baked chickpeas

The vegan lifestyle is becoming increasingly popular these days with help from famous figures like former president Bill Clinton, television host and comedian Ellen DeGeneres and actress Alicia Silverstone that make it seem more acceptable and doable. Also known as a plant-based diet, vegans do not eat any food from animal sources including red meat, chicken, eggs, dairy or honey. They avoid wearing shoes, belts or any other clothing made from an animal source, as well. A 2012 study by the Vegetarian Resource Group in the U.S. found that 2.5 percent of the country now identifies as vegan, up from 1 percent in 2009, showing that the numbers have more than doubled recently.

While vegan eating probably began in India or Asia, the first known vegan cookbook, *No Animal Food: Two Essays and 100 Recipes* by Rupert H. Wheldon, was published in 1910 in London.[1] The Vegan Society started in 1944 and created World Vegan Day, which is an annual celebration held on November.[2] The Physicians Committee for Responsible Medicine (PCRM) has recommended a no-cholesterol, low-fat vegan diet since 1991 and they have even created their own food groups: legumes, grains, fruits and vegetables, to replace the old USDA food groups: meat, dairy, grains, fruits and vegetables.

Today, people go vegan for many reasons including health, animal rights and the environment. From a health perspective, a well-balanced vegan diet greatly increases your intake of fruits and vegetables and reducing foods like cheese can be helpful for weight loss. Many people choose to be vegan to live a more activist lifestyle. By choosing to not support the way farmed animals are raised and treated or to eat any animal products, they take a strong stance on living a compassionate life. For some, it's all about helping our environment. Plant-based diets require about one third of the land and water needed to produce a typical Western diet, according to the Vegan Society.

Many athletes choose to adopt a vegan diet to help their performance. World famous track star Carl Lewis went vegan to prepare for the World Championships in 1991, running what he called the best meet of his life. He earned 10 Olympic medals over his career, nine of them gold. At age 40 Rich Roll was 50 pounds overweight and completely out of shape. He made some major changes to his diet and lifestyle and became the first vegan to complete an Ultraman competition finishing in the top 10 males. After tennis star Venus Williams was diagnosed with a rare autoimmune disease she drastically changed her diet and is now a raw vegan. She continues to dominate in her sport.

High-Protein Diets

Central Philosophy: High-protein diets restrict carbohydrates, causing the body to burn its own fat for fuel, instead of carbohydrates. When the body is in this state, many people tend to feel less hungry, and as a result, lose weight.

Foods Encouraged: foods that are high in protein, including eggs, seafood, beef, poultry, dairy products and nuts

Foods Restricted: foods that are high in carbohydrates, such as breads, pastas, grains, and some vegetables and fruits

····· **SAMPLE DAILY MENU** ·····

Breakfast: egg omelette with cubed ham and red pepper

Lunch: ½-pound browned ground beef, shredded lettuce, tomato, cheddar cheese and salsa; two cups salad greens

Snack: sugar-free Jello or two ounces of cheddar cheese

Dinner: chicken and vegetable stir-fry with onion, garlic, tomato, basil, broccoli and zucchini

Beverages: water, decaf coffee or tea

People love eating protein. It makes us feel stronger, more alert and more aggressive. It increases our sense of power and confidence—two of the most highly prized qualities in our contemporary culture and part of the reason high-protein diets are so popular today. High-protein diets can also lead to significant weight loss, important to many in this time of rising obesity rates.

Anne Louise Gittleman, Ph.D., C.N.S., former head nutritionist at the Pritikin Center, and the first to see the downside of a low-fat, high-carbo-hydrate diet, began to distinguish between "good" and "bad" fats. Saturated fats in dairy products and trans fats in processed foods like potato chips and margarine clog the arteries and contribute to inflammation in the body. Olive oil, avocado oil, omega-3, omega-6 and oils from seeds and nuts nour-ish the body and prevent the accumulation of cholesterol and triglycerides in our arteries. Ironically, a lack of good fats can actually lead to just the kind of heart disease dangers that low-fat diets are trying to avoid! Omega-3 fatty acids, found mainly in fish oil, are especially effective at clearing the arteries.

Gittleman also pointed out that the average American does not know the difference between healthy and unhealthy carbohydrates. The experts might be talking about the need to eat brown rice, millet, quinoa, whole-grain breads, vegetables and beans, but most Americans have no idea what these foods are or where to find them. Thinking that all carbohydrates are the same, they eat more refined wheat products, such as bread, pasta and pizza. In addition, Gittleman warned about the dangers caused by gluten in wheat, which acts like a kind of glue in the body and can cause aller-gies, brain fog, candida and mineral deficiencies. Gittleman's contribution to understanding the subtleties and implications of high-carbohydrate diets is significant.

Many people who embrace high-protein diets follow the program pre-scribed by Dr. Robert Atkins. Atkins began his work in 1972 with the pub-lication of Dr. Atkins' Diet Revolution and died in 2003, at the age of 73. The title of a recently released biography about Atkins, *The True Story of the Man Behind the War on Carbohydrates*, describes his life's mission well. Atkins' supporters claim that, under his plan, you can "eat delicious meals you love, never count calories, enjoy a cheeseburger when you're hungry, see amazing results in 14 days, reach your ideal weight and stay there." Dieters can also supposedly eat all the meat and all the fat they want, and still lose weight. With such a generous range of permitted foods, how could anyone not want to go on such a program?

Atkins encourages weight loss by depriving the body of the carbohydrates that our digestive system routinely converts into sugar. Once the body recognizes that it's not getting carbohydrates, its preferred fuel, it will burn protein for a few days instead. But hundreds of thousands of years of evolution from hunter-gatherers has taught us that burning protein is not a great idea. Protein is our primary muscle constituent, and without muscles we will have no strength to hunt for food. Burning protein is counterproductive to survival, so the body won't do it for very long.

Once the carbohydrate stores are burned and we've burned protein for a few days, our bodies will say, "Okay, it's time to start burning fat." At this point, the brain protests, because it prefers only carbohydrates as a fuel source, so our liver performs a little chemical magic and converts fat into ketones, a substance that the brain can burn. Now our body is in a state of ketosis, burning fat and losing weight. During the first few days on a high-protein diet, the body loses a lot of water, which accounts for much of the initial, encouraging weight loss. High-protein diets also reduce hunger, so we are satisfied with our meals and not tempted to eat more.

The Atkins approach could benefit many vegetarian-type people. Vegetarians often suffer from extreme ups and downs in their blood sugar levels. This simply doesn't happen to people following the Atkins program. When a vegetarian goes on Atkins, the pancreas gets to rest because sugar consumption decreases while protein intake increases. People who suffer from candida or diabetes, both of which are aggravated by too much sugar consumption, can sometimes benefit from this way of eating for a short time.

The downside to Atkins and other high-protein diets is that too much animal protein may lead to illness, especially heart disease and cancer. Animal meat is full of saturated fats that can spike blood cholesterol levels, has no fiber to aid digestion and is low in many essential plant-based nutrients, such as antioxidants, carotenoids and phytochemicals. In addition, there is increasing concern about tainted meat, hormones and antibiotics in factory-farmed meat. If you decide to go on the Atkins diet, you should eat organic animal food as much as possible.

Another problem is that this program doesn't distinguish between animal proteins. In Atkins, eating beef, fish, chicken or eggs is the same: a protein is a protein is a protein. In reality, each of these has a completely different quality and impact on the body. Further, the body is always trying to maintain an acid and alkaline balance. Protein is a very acidic substance. If you eat a lot of protein, your body will try to create a more alkaline environment in your stomach by leaching calcium from your bones and teeth, which can contribute to bone loss and osteoporosis.

People also say these diets lead to constipation, depression, bad breath and body odors.

The Zone Diet and Glycemic Load

Central Philosophy: The Zone Diet is based on a theory that excess insulin, a hormone that helps control blood sugar levels, makes us gain weight and keep it on. By regulating blood sugar levels with a perfect balance of carbohydrates, fats and proteins at every meal, the body burns fat more efficiently and has more energy.

Foods Encouraged: A ratio of 40 percent carbohydrates, 30 percent fat and 30 percent protein, found in foods such as fresh vegetables, fruits and nuts, leafy green vegetables and sufficient protein; fats from olive oil, avocados, almonds, fish and fish oils. The diet also encourages drinking eight glasses of water a day.

Foods Restricted: processed carbohydrates, found in bread, pasta and white grains and saturated fats

····· SAMPLE DAILY MENU ·····

Breakfast: buckwheat blintz with ricotta and apples

Lunch: grilled chicken BLT club sandwich, side salad of mixed greens with balsamic vinaigrette

Dinner: grilled pork loin with barley pilaf and sautéed green beans with garlic and sliced almonds in white wine sauce

Snack: banana mini muffin, crab cake or low-carb pretzels

The Zone Diet was developed by Dr. Barry Sears in the '90s. He is the author of the bestseller *Enter the Zone*, which is based on more than 15 years of his research in the field of bio-nutrition and the role of diet in hormonal response, gene expression and inflammation. The Zone is sometimes called a high-protein diet, but it's less extreme than Atkins. The diet's primary aim is to keep you in "The Zone," a sports term, describing an almost mystical state of heightened awareness and relaxed intensity in which athletes perform at their best and without effort. The goal is to become balanced, relaxed and well-fed, so your energy level is optimal for normal day-to-day living.

The Zone offers a specific meal plan based on each person's gender, activity level and amount of body fat. It's called "the 40-30-30 diet" because for all the Zone snacks and meals, you get 40% of your calories from carbohydrates, 30% from protein and 30% from fat. This proportion contrasts sharply with the accepted nutritional standard of 65-15-20. The theory is that the more you give your body 40-30-30, the faster it will get accustomed to processing this food combination, and settle into a specific metabolic state, leading to weight loss.

One of the goals of the Zone is to avoid peaks and valleys in blood sugar levels. A recommendation that I find effective is to eat a meal within one hour of waking up in the morning because that's when your blood sugar is lowest. The Zone encourages people to eat more fruits and vegetables, and reduce bread, pasta and white grains. The diet is big on drinking water, which I agree with wholeheartedly. I also like the Zone's relaxed attitude about mistakes: no big deal if you fall off the diet, since you are only one meal away from getting back on track. People on the diet tell me, "Yes, it's great. I'm never hungry, and my energy is great!"

A downside to the Zone is that, unless you're a scientist, it's very hard to design each meal to be a perfectly balanced 40-30-30. It's also difficult to be on a Zone diet and be a vegetarian because of the diet's strong emphasis on eating protein. In response, the Zone has a plan called "Soy Zone," which recommends eating more soy products. However, many people are allergic to soy or have difficulty digesting it in large quantities, so this is not a viable option for all vegetarians.

Critics of the Zone often argue that weight loss on this program comes from restricting calories and not from any biochemical magic induced by the

40-30-30 formula. They also assert that, contrary to Sears' claims, athletic performance may be impaired by reducing carbohydrates.

South Beach Diet

Central Philosophy: The South Beach diet is similar to other low-carb diets but offers a unique approach by distinguishing the right kinds of carbohydrates and fats and puts emphasis on lean proteins.

Foods Encouraged: fresh vegetables, lean proteins, such as eggs, poultry, pork and fish, cheese and nuts

Foods Restricted: bread, rice, potatoes, pasta, baked goods, fruit, candy, ice cream, sugar, beer and alcohol (the latter two, mostly, in the strictest phase of the diet)

····· **SAMPLE DAILY MENU** ·····

Breakfast: two scrambled eggs with Monterey Jack cheese and salsa, a slice of whole-grain toast and half a grapefruit

Mid-morning snack: one hard-boiled egg

Lunch: roast beef wrap with reduced-fat cream cheese, spinach and red onion

Mid-afternoon snack: four ounces of yogurt

Dinner: lemon couscous chicken with steamed broccoli

Dessert: lemon peel ricotta creme

When South Beach's own Dr. Arthur Agatston, a cardiologist, developed a diet for his heart patients and saw the dramatic weight-loss results, he published it in the early 2000s so beachgoers and others could reap the benefits.

At first glance, this diet may not seem very different from other high-protein, low-carbohydrate weight-loss plans. But South Beach focuses more on the type and quality of carbohydrates consumed, using the glycemic index to differentiate. The glycemic index indicates how quickly a particular food makes your blood sugar rise; it's a system of measurement used in the nutritional management of diabetes.

Like the Zone, South Beach encourages people to eat three normal-size meals and two snacks each day with no need to count calories, weigh food portions or deprive themselves of tasty food. The diet works in three phases. The first two are restricted periods, and the third is offered as an ongoing lifestyle. Phase one is very similar to Atkins, restricting all carbohydrates, with dietary emphasis on lean meats, low-sugar veggies, low-fat cheeses, nuts and eggs in order to maximize the rate of weight loss. In phase two, some of the banned foods are slowly reintroduced, while weight loss continues. Phase three is a maintenance diet.

Other diet authorities have challenged many of the medical statements made in Agatston's book, *The South Beach Diet*. For example, his alluring invitation to "lose belly fat first"—obviously something every dieter would love—seems implausible given the fact that the areas where we lose and gain weight on our bodies are largely determined by our genetic predispositions. Agatston's diet is offered as a repeat formula. Whenever you gain weight, just jump back from phase three to phase one and start again. It sounds easy, but temporary weight loss and repeated dieting can be more damaging to the body than not losing weight at all.

Another controversy with South Beach doctrine concerns Agatston's recommendation not to drink beer at any stage of his diet because of its high glycemic rating. Anheuser-Busch brewing company took out full-page ads refuting Agatston's claim that beer is loaded with maltose, a sugar derived from malted barley, explaining that although it is present in the early brewing stages, the sugar disappears during the fermentation process. One of the leading researchers in the field, Jennie Brand-Miller, author of *The Glucose Revolution*, has written that beer has too few carbohydrates to assess its glycemic index, giving it essentially an index of zero. Agatston has since changed his stance on the subject, saying that beer in moderation is acceptable in the later phases of the diet.

Agatston's book has sold millions of copies, and in a multi-million-dollar deal, Kraft, the largest U.S. food company, tied more than 200 of its products to the diet. Oreos, Kool-Aid and Cheez Whiz carried the "South Beach seal of approval" as foods lower in carbs and fats. The goal? Naturally, to lure shoppers back into buying Kraft products as consumers slowly become more health conscious.

While the South Beach Diet could have come and gone like many fads, Dr. Agatston works to remain relevant. In 2011, Agatston released *The South Beach Wake-Up Call*, which he described as not a diet book but instead more of a lifestyle book to offer inspiration and tools for breaking unhealthy habits. In it, he addresses how inflammation is at the core of many of today's health problems, the importance of cooking more meals at home and gluten intolerance and its role in many health problems from GI issues to autoimmune disorders. Not surprisingly, he published another book in 2013 called *The South Beach Diet Gluten Solution*, tackling the question of gluten confusion. As more and more gluten-free products hit the market, he created a 3-Phase diet plan to help people determine their own level of gluten sensitivity and how to make the right choices around gluten overload. I'm happy to see this topic getting a more bio-individual approach.

Blood Type Diet

Central Philosophy: The Blood Type Diet is an individualized approach to eating that combines anthropology, medical history and genetics. Each blood type (O, A, B and AB) is derived from a different time in human evolution, and thus affects how people of each type react to food and disease.

Foods Encouraged/Restricted: Each blood type has its own set of good and bad foods.

····· **SAMPLE DAILY MENU** ·····

Type O

Breakfast: fried eggs with black-eyed peas, one strip of bacon and rice toast

Lunch: cream of kale soup made by substituting yams or sweet potatoes for cream, served with 100% rye bread

Dinner: beef roast with mushroom stuffing

Type A

Breakfast: carob buckwheat pancakes topped with almond butter and puréed pears

Lunch: curried peanut tempeh with carrots and broccoli served over rice

Dinner: salmon teriyaki served with grilled asparagus

Type B

Breakfast: apple-walnut spelt scones

Lunch: turkey lettuce roll-ups with carrots, scallions and sprouts

Dinner: poached catfish in apple cider vinegar served with veggie slaw salad

Type AB

Breakfast: mung bean porridge

Lunch: tuna salad with rice crackers

Dinner: butternut squash and tofu mash with mixed vegetables

One of the keys to finding your own healing diet is to figure out how much protein is right for your body, and the Blood Type Diet is an excellent guide to determining protein needs. The best-selling book on the subject, *Eat Right for Your Type*, was written by Dr. Peter D'Adamo and published in 1996, but the work was pioneered by his father, Dr. James D'Adamo.

The Blood Type Diet is based on the theory that each major stage in human social evolution is associated with new environmental conditions and a different blood type. Human beings began as hunter-gatherers, chasing herds of wild animals. Our diet was primarily meat and a combination of wild plants and roots, and we adapted genetically to maximize the nutrition from these sources. D'Adamo maintains that modern people with this common O blood type function best on a meat-centered diet. Wheat and dairy had not been cultivated at the hunter-gatherer stage, and so O types find them difficult to metabolize.

When humans stopped hunting and started farming the land about 15,000 years ago, our diet changed dramatically from meat to a plant-based diet centered on grains, vegetables and beans, as well as milk from domesticated cows. The genes of these agrarian peoples gradually adapted to a new way of eating and produced blood type A. People with this blood type function best on a plant-based diet and, of all the blood types, are the most suited to vegetarianism.

Nomadic people emerged later and consumed a diet that was a combination of cultivated plants and animal foods. This led to the development of a third blood type, B, as people needed flexibility in their diet so they could absorb nutrition from both plant and animal foods. According to D'Adamo, B types are better able to consume dairy products than O and A types. Nine hundred to 1,000 years ago, the AB blood type evolved. AB blood types tend to be highly sensitive, rare and mysterious. They are destined for modern life and have the combined attributes A and B blood types. AB's can usually tolerate a mixed diet in moderation.

I've seen a great deal of truth in the Blood Type categories. Type O's tend to be more physically oriented, as hunter-gatherers once were, and have greater demands for protein. Also, type O people often have difficulty metabolizing and digesting wheat. People with type A blood are frequently attracted to vegetarianism. B types do a little better than others with dairy foods.

However, like most other dietary programs, this one takes its basic premise to the extreme. People with type O blood do not require the large amounts of animal foods that D'Adamo recommends. Beyond a certain point, protein is injurious to everyone's health, regardless of blood type, and is one of the reasons why we suffer from high rates of osteoporosis, digestive disorders, heart disease, and breast, colon and prostate cancers. Most Americans already eat six times the amount of protein their bodies actually need, so encouraging O types to eat more can lead to health problems.

In addition, humans evolved to become dependent on grains, including O types, though they typically do better eating brown rice, millet, quinoa and amaranth than they do with wheat and barley (the two high-gluten grains).

Following this diet in a family situation can be very challenging, as it might demand cooking for two or three different blood types at the same time.

Traditional Diet

Central Philosophy: Traditional diets are just what they sound like, following the ancient traditions of our ancestors with food in their most pure, unprocessed form. These unrefined, natural foods are revered for their nutrient density and should be prepared just as your great-great-great grandmother did.

Foods Encouraged: pastured, grass-fed and free range animal products: whole, raw dairy milk, eggs, meats, organ meats, fish eggs, fish and cod liver oil; butter; sprouted grains and mostly cooked vegetables

Foods Restricted: refined sugars, low-fat or no-fat dairy products, non-organic meats and vegetables

····· **SAMPLE DAILY MENU** ·····

Breakfast: scrambled eggs with toasted sprouted bread, butter. A glass of whole milk (or raw milk, if desired)

Lunch: minestrone soup, made with bone broth and fresh, seasonal vegetables

Snack: chopped pear served with drizzled raw honey and soaked sunflower seeds

Dinner: grilled swordfish served with artichokes in a lemon butter sauce with baby potatoes, collard greens

Dessert: ginger snaps made with ground ginger and bulgur flour

Many foods have a long history of supporting good health. For centuries humans existed without the need to read books about their diet. They ate from the land and grazed what was around them, and the traditional diet looks to reclaim these ways.

Nina Planck, author of *Real Food* and *Real Food for Mother and Baby* explains that traditional means a food has been farmed or raised and processed pretty much the way it used to be. Foods like grass-fed beef and wild salmon are two to three million years old. In contrast, modern foods like corn syrup were developed in the 1970s. In her books, she explains how ancient foods like beef and butter have been falsely accused of causing health problems, while industrial foods like corn syrup and soybean oil have created a triple epidemic of obesity, diabetes and heart disease. She writes that real food is never an imitation of something else.

The real food movement can be traced back to the early 1900s, when Dr. Weston Price, a dentist who believed nutrition was the foundation for well-being, studied the diets of many ancient societies and decided that by eating nourishing, traditional foods and farm produce, we could achieve optimal health. He traveled the world studying indigenous people's dental and physical health. He found that the further away people lived from civilization, the healthier they were. They ate from local food sources. They had fewer cavities, and some cultures never experienced any cancer or heart disease.

Sally Fallon Morell brought Price's work to a larger audience in her books *Nourishing Traditions: The Cookbook That Challenges Politically Correct Nutrition and the Diet Dictocrats*. I really appreciate that her work and other traditional diet followers ignores the current fads and politics around food, and instead looks to our heritage to determine what foods are ideal for human consumption. Perhaps one of the most controversial parts of traditional diets is that raw dairy products are considered an important part of a healthy diet. Followers argue that for the past 9,000 years, humans have relied on milk to meet their needs for protein and fat and that the problem is not milk, but the modern methods used to make dairy cows produce milk. Selective breeding and genetically engineered hormones, along with pasteurization, which makes the proteins in milk difficult to absorb, interfere with the benefits from milk.

The traditional diet also asserts that it is impossible to obtain adequate protein on a vegetarian diet. Fallon Morrell cites studies of primitive cultures that relied on animal meat and had healthy bones and claims that certain health problems, such as bone loss and tuberculosis, developed when agriculture was introduced and people began depending on grains and beans for sustenance. Fallon Morrell says animal food is the only source of complete protein, with all 22 amino acids necessary for the human body to thrive. She acknowledges that abstaining from commercial meats is a good practice, and that avoiding meat for a certain period of time can be cleansing and healing. But she cautions that strict vegetarianism can be dangerous, causing mineral deficiencies and health problems.

Fallon Morrell stresses the benefits of the natural fats in meat, eggs and dairy, and encourages people to avoid the no-fat or low-fat alternatives to these products. In addition to high-quality animal meat, she recommends eating other quality fats, such as virgin olive oil, unrefined flax oil, coconut oil and palm oil. Carbohydrates from organic whole grains are another essential element of her diet. She also recommends high-quality water, meat stocks, vegetable broths, unrefined sea salt, raw vinegar, fresh herbs and naturally fermented soy sauce.

In modern, whole-food nutrition, it's difficult to find people who recognize that high-quality dairy can be beneficial for us. On the other hand, her diet is so rich in protein and fat, it's not what most people need right now. The average diet is mainly lacking in vegetables and fruits, a fact she does not address adequately. Fallon Morrell's suggestions may prove beneficial for some but will not work for everyone.

Paleo Diet

Central Philosophy: Our bodies are designed to thrive on foods that were available to our early paleolithic ancestors from 10,000 years ago.

Foods Encouraged: grass-fed, pasture-raised meats, fish, eggs, vegetables, fruit, roots and nuts

Foods Restricted: grains (flour), beans, dairy products, potatoes, refined sugar, salt and processed oils

····· **SAMPLE DAILY MENU** ·····

Breakfast: shrimp and scrambled eggs with basil and steamed kale, handful of blueberries

Lunch: portabella mushroom "sandwich"—grilled organic chicken, sliced tomato, guacamole and fresh spinach leaves

Snack: handful of almonds or macadamia nuts

Dinner: grass-fed ground beef marinara over baked spaghetti squash

Dessert: grilled banana and apricots with cinnamon and walnuts

Similar to the traditional ways of eating, the paleo diet, also known as the paleolithic or caveman diet, harkens back to the eating ways of our ancestors. This diet first came on the scene in the 1970s thanks to Walter L. Voegtlin, a gastroenterologist who wrote *The Stone Age Diet*. In it, he argues that humans are carnivorous animals needing mostly fats and proteins and that our jaws and teeth resemble other carnivorous animals like dogs rather than plant-eating animals like sheep. Loren Cordain, author of *The Paleo Diet*, links the movement to a 1985 article in the New England Journal of Medicine that claimed the diet could be a reference standard for modern human nutrition.

In 2009, Mark Sisson said you could reprogram your genes in the direction of weight loss, health and longevity by following 10 laws in his book *The Primal Blueprint*, which is a stricter variation of paleo, allowing more healthy fats and cracking down on the use of artificial sweeteners that other paleo diet books allow. By 2010, *The New York Times* ran a piece about new-age cavemen, or urban dwellers who follow the paleo path. The article chronicled a modern-day renaissance of the diet, following a few New Yorkers who kept large amounts of meat in their freezers and said the diet had helped them clear up health issues. The article also publicized CrossFit, an intense fitness program that combines weightlifting and gymnastics, stating that many paleo dieters also enjoy these rigorous workouts.

Again, I think any diet with a focus on protein will become popular in the Western world. I do like that this diet focuses on eating whole foods rather than processed foods, and I think many people benefit from this diet simply by removing flour and dairy from their diet, as many people are allergic or have sensitivities to these foods. The downside of this plan, like many other diets, is that a strict eating plan can be impractical for most people. While it may feel good for a time, many people have a hard time keeping up with such intense food rules.

Mediterranean Diet

Central Philosophy: By adopting the eating style of the people who live in the Mediterranean region of the world, particularly Southern European countries like Greece, Italy, France, Portugal and Spain, people can enjoy longer lifespans and less risk of developing chronic disease.

Foods Encouraged: vegetables, fruits, beans, nuts, seeds, olive oil, yogurt, cheese, moderate amounts of fish, poultry, eggs, small amounts of red meat and red wine

Foods Restricted: refined sugars and carbohydrates, processed oils, animal protein, especially red meat

····· **SAMPLE DAILY MENU** ·····

Breakfast: low-fat Greek yogurt, granola, strawberries and a drizzle of honey

Lunch: grilled chicken served with green salad, balsamic vinaigrette and feta cheese

Snack: wholegrain crackers with hummus dip

Dinner: grilled wild salmon served with quinoa, infused with rosemary and pine nuts, grilled cauliflower, broccoli and carrots drizzled with olive oil; a glass of red wine, if desired

Dessert: baked apple with cherries and almonds

The Mediterranean diet is less of a diet and more of a lifestyle. People who live in the southern, coastal regions of Europe and the Middle East dine leisurely, engage in regular physical activity, spend time with family and, of course, eat a heart-healthy diet with lots of vegetables, healthy fats and beans. The region emphasizes fresh, regional cuisine, simply prepared with very little fried foods.

Interestingly, a Minnesota physiologist named Ancel Keys was the first scientist to talk about the health value of a Mediterranean-style diet. He was also one of the first people to talk about the role of saturated fats in contributing to heart disease. His work began in the 1940s, but he became known for his landmark epidemiological research that he called the Seven Countries study starting in the late '50s. He studied 12,000 healthy middle-aged men living in Europe, Japan and the U.S. and revealed that the Mediterranean diet was protective against heart disease even though about 35 percent of the calories come from fat. Yet, most of those fats are monounsaturated fats from plant sources. Even more interestingly, Keys lived to be 100 years old.

In the last decade or so, scientists have continued to study this region extensively, mostly looking at how residents enjoy such good health. In 2011, researchers examined 50 studies linking the Mediterranean diet to reduced risk of developing metabolic syndrome, which leads to heart disease, diabetes and stroke. But even more striking was the first major clinical trial to measure the diet's impact on heart risks. The study ended early after only about five years because the results were so staggering: about 30 percent of heart attacks, strokes and deaths from heart disease could be prevented in high-risk people simply by switching to the diet. The results were published in a 2013 *New England Journal of Medicine* article, and mark the first time a diet was shown to be a powerful means to reduce disease risk in a clinical setting. In the study, a low-fat diet went head to head with the Mediterranean diet, which allows for healthy fats and a more balanced way of eating. Not only did the Mediterranean diet have better results, but the study participants were able to stick with it and feel satisfied. Other studies have shown that the diet can help maintain a healthy body weight and lower risk for diabetes.

I like this diet's traditional roots and agree that a balance of good food and lifestyle factors can help you live longer and enjoy your life. Of course, many people wonder if this diet can really be recreated around the world and if it makes sense to advise, say, people in China to eat more like people in Italy. Again, I think people benefit more from adopting the more traditional diet of their own regions.

Raw Food Diet

Central Philosophy: Raw or living food diets are based on unprocessed and uncooked plant foods. Raw foodists believe that eating food above 116 degrees will destroy vital enzymes in the food and disrupt your body's ability to absorb nutrients from the food.

Foods Encouraged: Fresh fruits and vegetables, nuts, seeds, beans, grains, dried fruit, seaweed and coconut milk. About 75% of the diet must be raw.

Foods Restricted: foods cooked above 116 degrees and meat and dairy products

····· SAMPLE DAILY MENU ·····

Breakfast: fruit smoothie with soaked flax seeds, banana, fresh fruit and dates

Lunch: almond avocado stew with apple cider vinegar and sunflower sprouts

Dinner: green curry pasta: zucchini and mango slices topped with a Thai nut curry cream and coconut noodles

Snacks: carrots served with raw hummus made from sprouted garbanzo beans and fresh garlic

Many people are moving toward a raw food diet, choosing to eat food that is not cooked or heated. The basic premise of raw food theory is that we are the only species that cooks our food, which destroys its natural enzymes. In its raw state, food is composed of living cells. Raw foodists view cooked or heated food as dead and lifeless. Heating food changes its basic molecular structure, making it toxic. According to this theory, cooked food stresses the body because the liver, heart and kidneys all have to work overtime to eliminate the toxins ingested with the food, ultimately leading to disease. Raw food theory also states that cooked foods are addictive and extremely difficult to give up, but once people shift to eating primarily raw foods, they will experience clarity of mind, body and spirit. Raw foodists believe raw plant food is the only food humans should eat.

Raw food is very cleansing, healing and refreshing to the body, and is especially good for people who have eaten a lot of meat and processed food. Eating raw food may improve digestion and increase vitality. It is an environmentally supportive and ecologically friendly way of eating that can lead to a feeling of deep spiritual connection to nature. Going on a raw food diet can feel like fasting, as it helps remove toxins quickly and effectively from the body and can lead to weight loss. One of the biggest benefits of going on a raw food diet is that it gets people off sugary, processed junk foods.

On the other hand, this diet can be too cleansing for people whose systems are weak and need building. People with a sensitive digestive track may find the nutrients in raw food too intense, and the cell walls of the vegetables may be too thick to break down and assimilate. The cooling effect of raw foods on the body makes this diet difficult to sustain during the winter months. People who are, to use a macrobiotic term, very yin—tall, thin and/or spacey—may need a more grounding diet as raw foods are also very yin. Getting adequate protein can be a challenge while following a raw foods diet. Some people can also experience sweet cravings from eating too much sugar from raw fruits.

Some raw foodists are very adamant in their belief that cooked food is unfit for human consumption. Some eat 100% raw, some 75% raw and some eat 15% raw. I encourage people to experiment with the percentage of raw food in their diet and notice how it affects them, especially in the summer months, when raw foods are easier for the body to process.

Cleansing Diets

Central Philosophy: You can detoxify the body with a restricted plan of simple, whole foods or through fresh fruit and vegetable juicing or even a master cleanse mixture of water fasting to boost health. Results from a cleanse include increased energy, better digestion, understanding food allergies sensitivities and/or greater mental clarity.

Foods Encouraged/Sample Daily Menu: It depends on the plan you are following.

One of the most well-known cleanses today is the Master Cleanser, or Lemonade Diet, a liquid mono-diet, consisting of water with fresh lime or lemon juice, maple syrup and cayenne pepper. Stanley Burroughs, the creator of Master Cleanser, recommends drinking the mixture 6 to 12 times a day, for a minimum of 10 days, and a maximum of 40 days, depending on a person's physical health. A laxative herbal tea, taken twice a day, and saltwater bathing are also recommended, but no other food is consumed during the cleanse. Directions for coming off the diet include a slow re-incorporation of raw fruit, fruit juice, nuts and vegetables. Burroughs suggests doing the cleanse four times a year for optimum health. The goal of Master Cleanser is to correct all health disorders. This lemonade drink was first shown to help aid stomach ulcers, and then Burroughs began to recommend it for other conditions. He believes that when we cure one disease, we help cure them all and create vibrant overall health.

Improper diet causes the accumulation of waste, toxins and poison in the colon. These filter into the bloodstream and circulate throughout the body, inhabiting tissues and cells. The settling of these toxins weakens the cells and the entire immune system, exposing the body to disease. Cleansing the body of this built-up waste rejuvenates its innate healing mechanisms. It then functions at optimal capacity, reducing toxicity, restoring health and vitality, and increasing our life force.

Other people try less extreme forms of cleansing either with fresh fruit and vegetable juices or simply eating unrefined, whole foods for a time. Joe Cross helped bring attention to the power of juicing in his documentary, Fat, Sick & Nearly Dead, which tracked his progress on a 60-day juice fast. He lost nearly 100 pounds and got off his prescription medication for an autoimmune disease, simply by increasing his consumption of fruits and vegetables. In 2008, Oprah and her staff embarked on a 21-day vegan cleanse and found amazing results from adopting this diet that is free of all animal products. Even in cleansing, we can see how some people thrive and others struggle with certain ways of eating or eliminating food from their diet even for a relatively short period of time.

Doing a cleanse or simply eliminating coffee, tea, sugar and comfort foods for a set period of time is a freeing experience. Many people report that cleanses help them lose weight and feel healthier.

It's common for people to decide they are going to fast in the springtime, especially if they've put on weight during the winter months. I've seen this pattern many times. People overeat during the holiday season and then, when the weather gets warmer and the days get lighter, they announce to everyone they know, "Okay, now I'm going to clean it all up by going on a fast."

Being healthy is a daily practice. I do not believe that long-term fasting is an effective weight-loss method. Just follow the simple instructions in this book and you will lose weight in a healthy, gradual way. Sudden fasts are a bit like going to pray once a week, instead of integrating spirituality into your everyday lifestyle. The way I see it, I fast half my life. Pretty much every day, I fast from 8:30 p.m. to 8:30 a.m. I break my fast with my morning meal, called breakfast. This process has improved my digestion and my sleeping and allows me to wake up in the morning with a greater appetite for food and for life.

If you are unable to practice this simple form of daily fasting, there is no point in going on an extreme fast. Long-term fasting is a sophisticated art practiced by people who have already developed an ascetic habit and choose not to eat as part of a spiritual discipline. They begin with shorter fasts, and then gradually extend to longer periods without eating.

If you really want to fast, the best way is to cut out a specific, selected food, rather than reducing the overall quantity of food you eat. Just eliminating one food from your diet can be a major undertaking. For example, you might decide not to eat sugar for a week. This is a very big deal. Just try it and see. Or, if you know you eat too much chocolate, just cut out this one item, and create a fast this way. You can also fast by adding food such as freshly cooked vegetables every day. This will crowd out other, less healthy foods. If you have success with adding and subtracting things on your menu, you can begin to cut more undesirable foods, one by one, and add more healthy foods, one by one.

PROFILE

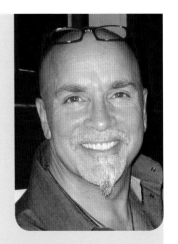

Nick Oddo, Briarcliff Manor, NY, USA
www.tenstudiohill.com

"We must listen to our bodies and teach others to do the same."

For almost 20 years I worked as a banker and banking consultant. At age 47, I started worrying about my health, suffering from depression and brain fog. It scared me because my father and grandfather suffered from the same symptoms and both committed suicide at a young age. I wanted to get this under control for my two children and me. I would never want them to suffer with this nasty disease. I cried out to the Universe and the magic started to happen.

I was led to a nutritionist who taught me about the blood type diet and how the food I was eating was responsible for my depression! I made some necessary dietary changes and my depression started to ease. I also started feeling more energetic, lost 40 pounds, my allergies disappeared and all those little arthritis aches and pains that I thought were natural aging vanished. I was amazed by this healing, and started talking about nutrition and food to whoever came into my path. I wanted to learn more and more.

In 2007, I was introduced to Integrative Nutrition through a friend and enrolled immediately. I didn't know that this could become a career; I simply wanted to learn more about health and nutrition. Since I never completed college, I decided this was going to be my college experience. At 40, I discovered I was living with learning disabilities my entire life. I had no retention memory and barely made it through high school! But now I know that my learning disabilities were actually food disabilities. I was eating all the wrong foods my whole life.

When I started classes at Integrative Nutrition, I instantly knew my entire future! I was going to be a motivational speaker and spread the word about the importance of food, health and nutrition. Joshua and IIN have taught me the most invaluable lesson I have ever learned—we must listen to our own bodies and teach others to do the same. We were all born with the tools necessary to understand what is right for our own unique self.

I am a Positive Life Health Coach, Motivational Speaker and Energy Therapist, I now know my mission for this lifetime—to teach people the importance of working on themselves as a whole—mind, body and soul. I have finally found my passion and immensely enjoy working with those who are ready to awaken to happiness, health and wealth.

When it comes to fasting and cleansing, remember that heroic activities may appeal to your mind but can wreak havoc on your body. I suggest taking a middle path, doing things in moderation and realizing that your body doesn't necessarily know what your mind is thinking.

Calorie Restriction/Longevity Diets

Central Philosophy: Calorie-restriction diets aim to expand life expectancy through minimal caloric intake. This restriction sets your body at an ideal weight to achieve maximum metabolic efficiency, slow the aging process and reach a maximum life span.

Foods Encouraged: nutrient-dense foods with few calories, such as vegetables, fruits, lean meats, egg whites and quorn (a high-protein, low-calorie meat substitute made from a cultured strain of the soil mold *Fusarium venenatum*); good fats found in avocados, nuts and olive oil; low-fat dairy products

Foods Restricted: foods with empty calories, such as highly processed cookies, crackers and other snack foods and sweets

····· **SAMPLE DAILY MENU** ·····

Breakfast: scrambled tofu with one slice of mixed-grain bread and half a grapefruit

Lunch: one bowl of vegetable salad, which has dried chickpeas, brown rice, wild rice, carrots, broccoli, sweet potato, mushrooms, tomatoes, romaine lettuce, bell peppers, zucchini and cabbage with a dressing of non-fat yogurt, buttermilk and balsamic vinegar served with a slice of rye toast

Dinner: ½-cup of millet with ¼-cup of peas, 3 ounces of oysters cooked with ¼-cup of onions, 2 stalks of steamed broccoli and 1 cup of steamed collard greens

Snack: ½-cup nonfat yogurt with ½-teaspoon of cinnamon

The calorie-restriction diet, also known as a longevity diet or simply CR (for calorie restriction) diet was pioneered by Dr. Roy Walford, who spent more than 35 years studying anti-aging diets in his laboratory at the UCLA Medical School. He was a top expert in the field of gerontology—the study of aging—and a physician for two years inside Biosphere 2, a 3-acre structure built as an artificial closed, ecological system in Arizona. He practiced the CR diet on the people who lived in Biosphere 2. The principles of the diet are based on laboratory research into the relationship of diet and aging. It's one of the few diets around based on scientific evidence. In his book, *Beyond the 120 Year Diet*, he describes the CR diet as a means to create food combinations and menus with all the recommended nutrients but with minimal caloric intake. The program calls for gradual weight loss until you reach an ideal weight point, which will slow down aging, preserve mental and physical function and substantially reduce your risk of degenerative diseases, such as heart disease, cancer and diabetes.

In the last few years, this research has made it to the mainstream but has been mixed. The National Cancer Institute, the American Diabetes Association and the National Institutes on Aging have all committed to funding long-term studies of calorie restriction in humans. In 2004, researchers at Washington University in St. Louis published a study that presented evidence of the long-term results of the CR diet in humans. The study indicates positive shifts in the biomarkers associated with disease risk, including decreased total cholesterol levels and blood pressure. But a 23-year study published in 2012 found that the CR did not extend life or reduce age-related deaths in monkeys. It did, however, offer other health benefits like a reduction in cancer.[3]

The CR diet is a radical departure from typical Western perception of "more is better." We are accustomed to super-sized portions and access to a wide array of snack foods 24 hours a day. For most people, cutting down calories may really help them lose weight. Artificial, chemicalized junk foods are high in calories, while whole, unprocessed foods are generally lower in calories. Therefore, watching caloric intake usually leads to a natural reduction in unhealthy foods and an increase in vitamins and nutrients. But the question of whether most people can sustain long-term calorie restriction remains to be seen. Yes, it works well in the lab, but can it work with real people who have real cravings? Another disadvantage of the diet is that it may cause your body's temperature to go down, which is a consequence of the body's increased efficiency. This drop may feel great to people living in warm environments but not so great to people living in colder climates.

The diet also does not address people's relationships to food. While it may be beneficial for people to reduce their calories, eating less is not always that simple. People have deep-rooted attachments to food. Giving up certain comfort foods may pose a great challenge to them. This diet is also not intended for people with a history of eating disorders, since calorie restriction may cause a lapse in their issues with food and body image.

DNA Diet/Nutrigenomics

Central Philosophy: The DNA diet is a customized approach to health and diet, which offers specific recommendations for food based on the results of genetic testing.

Foods Encouraged/Restricted: Foods encouraged or restricted are based on your unique biochemical makeup.

The DNA diet or nutrigenomics is a personalized way of eating based on your genetic blueprint. The idea spun out of the Human Genome Project—the government project that identified nearly 25,000 genes in the human body. Many studies have evaluated nutrigenomics and the correlation between diet and genes. Scientists have started using this information to research cures for dozens of genetic disorders, such as diabetes. Testing an individual's personal variations in the genes can provide many answers to health issues, such as heart and bone health, detoxification, and antioxidant capacity, insulin sensitivity and tissue repair. Small differences can influence how your body metabolizes food, utilizes nutrients and excretes damaging toxins. The idea here is that genetic makeup is the reason why one person can handle a diet rich in sugar, while that same diet will give another person hypoglycemia or even diabetes.

Many biotech labs now offer do-it-yourself testing kits, which look at 19 genes to determine a person's future health. You can purchase these kits at a clinic, online or even at some supermarkets. The kits come with sterile cotton swabs, used inside each cheek to collect cells for the DNA sample. They also come with a lifestyle questionnaire that asks about eating habits and family history. Once all the information is submitted, it takes about three weeks to get a printed report with details about each of the 19 genes.

Dr. Mark Hyman says that food is not just calories, but it's information. We generally think of food as a means to get energy and fuel our bodies, but he says that food can literally talk to our genes, giving your body instructions on things like how to control metabolism or turning on cancer protective genes. Nutrigenomics is literally food as medicine—working to turn off certain genes when you eat well or turn on certain genes if you go for foods that are unhealthy to the body, like chemicalized, artificial junk foods.

Critics of the diet call it generic advice and that analyzing 19 of the 25,000 human genes can't provide enough information to identify risk factors, much less specific foods you should eat. They say the advice is nothing more than common sense information about eating habits that would help anyone lose weight and be healthier, regardless of their genes. The nutrigenomics industry came under further attack when four of the leading companies came out with a line of supplements called "nutraceuticals" that were being sold for close to $2,000 per year and were supposedly tailored to the customer's unique DNA, but upon further examination were shown to be remarkably similar to the multivitamins sold at any local drugstore.

Still, this kind of diet is closer to a bio-individual approach than many of the fad diets out there. It may prove to be effective simply for offering a personal approach, which can help motivate people. Research in this field has only just begun.

Joshua's 90-10 Diet

I've noticed that when many people try to eat totally clean and pure diets, they can only do it for a limited period of time. Sometimes it's a day, a week, a month or even a year. But at a certain point, no matter how strong our idealism or willpower, certain foods we're avoiding become increasingly appealing. This realization inspired me to create my own dietary theory. Since so many other diets work on recommended proportions, 40-30-30, 40-40-20, or 50-25-25, I decided to express my diet in the same way, as the "90-10 diet."

Since I'm not very much into rules, this diet has only one rule. And even that rule is flexible. The rule is that 90% of the time you eat what is healthy for you, and 10% of the time you eat whatever you feel like eating. A lot of people try to stay 100% on their chosen diet program, which is bound to cause stress and likely to result in failure. Why turn dietary "mistakes" into sins? Having fear and guilt around food is not healthy. Cravings are an opportunity to listen to the body and fine-tune eating habits. Instead of creeping guiltily to the fridge at 2 a.m. for a pint of ice cream, publicly enjoy an ice cream with friends at a pleasurable social occasion, or get a delicious ice cream cone and eat it outside on a nice day. By giving yourself a 10% range of flexibility, you can indulge yourself without guilt and maintain a basically healthy diet.

Finding the Right Diet for You

All of these diet programs, and many more, are covered in greater depth in the curriculum at Integrative Nutrition. Students tend to get enthusiastic when we discuss the pros, then disappointed and confused when we reveal the cons. "Which dietary theory is right for me?" is a question I frequently hear.

But it's not about choosing the right theory. It's about finding what works best for you, then creating your own nutrition theory based on your individual desires and needs. I want you to find what's right for you. This task is far more challenging than getting swept away by the latest media-hyped fad and jumping on an already-rolling bandwagon. In the end, however, it will be far more rewarding because you will have come to understand your own nutritional needs, and you will arrive at a place of lasting health and physical well-being. It is a very empowering experience to realize you don't need to follow someone else's guidance but can control your own destiny and trust your own intuition and intelligence. The result is worth the extra effort.

Exercise

Create Your Own Diet

This is an invitation to create your own diet. It will help clarify your understanding of how diets work and what works best for you.

1. Get out a piece of paper and list three major diet programs that appeal to you.

2. Write down five aspects of these diets that seem the most essential to you.

   Example:

   I like_____ because_____.

3. Use these five qualities to create your own diet.

   Give your diet a name:

   The _____Diet.

   Be creative! Try finding a name that will catch the public's imagination.

4. Make up your own rules.

   The five most important points of The_____ Diet are:

   a.
   b.
   c.
   d.
   e.

5. How long should your diet be followed?

6. What results might someone expect from following your diet?

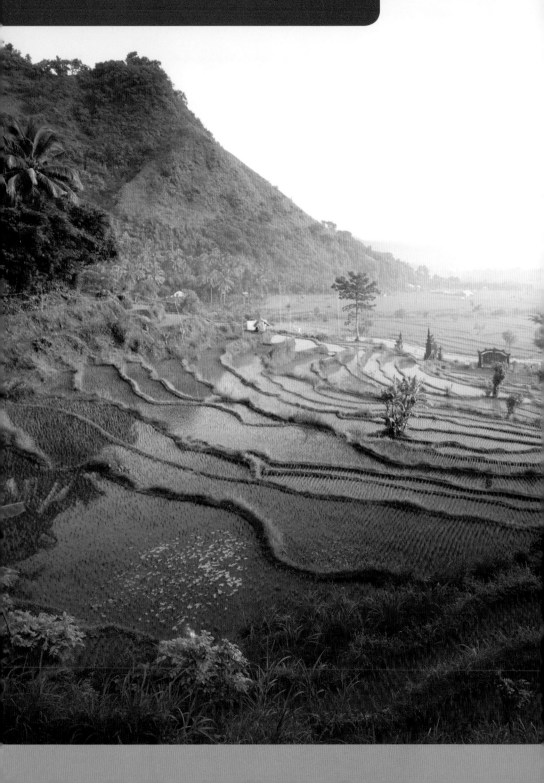

CHAPTER 5

A Global
Ripple Effect

About five years into my researching the world's longest-lived,
I realized that spry centenarians never *tried* to live to 100.
Longevity happened to them. It was not about discipline or
personal responsibility. It was about their environment.
—Dan Buettner

When I started Integrative Nutrition, I was just one person with a simple idea that if I could change what people ate, I could change the world. I started by moving to New York City because it's a global melting pot of people. At any time, day or night, you can walk around and experience any kind of food or people speaking almost any language. This energy is part of what makes it one of the greatest cities in the world. By living among so many different types of people and experiencing their culture, I felt more connected to the global community. I realized I didn't want to create just a school; I wanted to create a movement.

The phrase "Think globally, act locally" coined by the environmental movement encourages us to understand how our actions can impact the world. With a global mindset, we can create better health and greater happiness. The school's mission is quite similar: "to play a crucial role in improving health and happiness, and through that process, create a ripple effect that transforms the world." One of our core values is to "support each other in the global shift to better health." The world is really set up for this support and connection. At no time ever before have we had such easy and accessible means of communicating through social media platforms, online video calling or chatting, and affordable transportation.

I've already mentioned how the U.S. impacts trends around the world. I think we can also look at local cultures and see how they can influence our thinking about nutrition and health. I think it's fascinating to take a look at what the world is eating—and see what's working. People have been eating around the world for millions of years. Each day, we all wake up and have to decide what to eat. We've got a planet of 7 billion people who are full of wisdom and customs that we can all learn from. Now that you're familiar with many of the major dietary theories, you can continue to build on the wealth of information gathered from the global community.

And it's important to talk about not just the food, but the lifestyles and behaviors that contribute to our overall health in the world. I've seen so many cases where primary foods really override secondary foods. When people have a good life, they can often get away with eating whatever they want. Paris is a great example. People always wonder, how can the women there eat butter, bread and rich paté and still look so good? Well, they eat slowly and enjoy their meals. They talk to each other and give eye contact rather than constantly checking their phones. I think that eating and drinking in a more balanced and open way also helps them avoid cravings and binges. Many people today order only salads when they are out with friends but spend the night gorging on ice cream or chocolate.

The Secrets to Longevity

More scientific research backs up my idea of primary food—that living well is more than what's on your plate. I first read about the Blue Zones in a *National Geographic* article in 2005. The title of the article was, "The Secrets to a Long Life." I thought, who doesn't want to know those secrets? Just look at the market today. We are flooded with products that promise to make us look younger or defy our age. What if we could just live a long, happy life?

Author Dan Buettner wrote the article I read and subsequent book about these areas of the world that boast centenarians, or people who live to be 100 or more. And they don't just live longer but with a better quality of life, having very little disease or stress. As I mentioned in chapter 1, these areas include Sardinia, Italy; Okinawa, Japan; Nicoya Peninsula, Costa Rica; Loma Linda, California and the Greek island of Ikaria. What can we learn about these regions of the world that could help boost our longevity?

"In the United States, when it comes to improving health, people tend to focus on exercise and what we put into our mouths—organic foods, omega-3's, micronutrients," Buettner wrote in a 2012 *New York Times* article. "We spend nearly $30 billion a year on vitamins and supplements alone. Yet in Ikaria and the other places like it, diet only partly explained higher life expectancy. Exercise—at least the way we think of it, as willful, dutiful, physical activity—played a small role at best."[1]

One of the big factors that Buettner emphasizes is social structure. In the Blue Zones, they have different cultural attitudes about getting older—people stay engaged in the community through social activities and family life. Old people are celebrated and talked to rather than shunned or isolated. In Costa Rica they use the term "plan de vida," or life plan, which describes living with a lifelong sense of purpose. Buettner says purpose and love are essential ingredients to the Blue Zones lifestyle.

Some of the other qualities he's found in studying these areas that offer amazing health benefits include eating a plant-based diet, reducing stress in life, participating in spiritual communities, making time for family and finding your tribe. I know many students who enroll at Integrative Nutrition feel like they have found their tribe. I speak a lot about finding support in your life and surrounding yourself with people who share your values. Take a nod from the Blue Zones and start implementing some of these changes to your life.

The Jungle Effect

Along with these longevity hot spots, you can find many places around the world where the diets make you healthier. Family physician Daphne Miller, M.D., traveled to what she calls cold spots—canyons, deserts, islands, frozen lands, and jungles where people have few problems with chronic disease. She decided to learn more about how indigenous diets affect our health for her book, *The Jungle Effect: The Healthiest Diets from Around the World*. She found that getting back to the land could create better health for her patients in San Francisco, especially when they followed the diet of their ancestors. Our early ancestors relied on their intuition and experimentation to discover what plants tasted best, along with utilizing the freshest, local, natural ingredients.

Miller found clues to solve the diabetes dilemma faced by much of the modern world from the local diet in Copper Canyon, Mexico, home to 50,000 Tarahumara Indians living in remote canyons. Their diet consists of corn, beans, squash, eggs, chicken, chiles, berries, wild greens, cactus, oranges, tomatoes, avocadoes and the occasional wild game or fish. She was surprised that their diet was quite high in carbs, but they were unrefined and home-made. She learned that the glycemic index of corn is reduced when combined with beans and squash. Plus, many of the healing spices and plants in Mexico, including cactus, have been shown to help lower blood sugar. She realized that the high rates of diabetes in Latino populations living in the U.S. could be explained by losing these parts of the traditional diet along with eating too many highly processed, sugary foods.

In Iceland, people have low rates of seasonal affective disorder and depression, even though they have periods of winter with no sunlight and not a lot of vegetables growing on the island. People do eat wild fish and game, fresh milk and wild berries. In fact, Icelanders eat more fish per capita than anywhere in the world, according to Miller.[2] And even foods like lamb have high amounts of omega-3 fatty acids in them because the lamb eat tundra grass.

"They are able to get their antioxidants through surprising ways, like waxy potatoes, cabbage, and wild berries," Miller wrote. "I suppose they could import more greens, but they prefer their traditional foods. There is a feeling that this is what we do and we keep healthy." This example shows that the secrets to good health are really all around us when we choose to tune into our environment.

Miller also explored her own Ukrainian grandmother's recipe for borscht, which was made with canned sweetened beets, generous amounts of sour cream, and store-bought chicken broth. After a little digging, she found the recipe for borscht in her grandmother's hometown of Chodorov. Turns out the original recipe used fresh grated beets, light chicken stock, salt, pepper, and a spoonful of yogurt or clotted cream. You don't have to have a Ph.D. in nutrition to see how the modernization of these indigenous diets could create health problems around the world. Nutrition is not as complicated as the media can make it. Sometimes the best recipe is to keep it simple, nutritious and use whatever foods are freshest in your area.

PROFILE

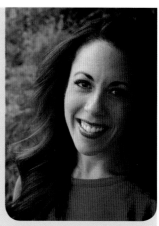

Melanie Woodrow,

Los Angeles, CA, USA

www.wholenatured.com

"I now stand wholeheartedly and confidently in my truth."

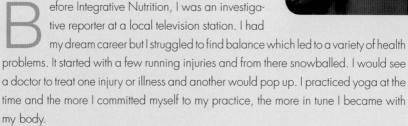

Before Integrative Nutrition, I was an investigative reporter at a local television station. I had my dream career but I struggled to find balance which led to a variety of health problems. It started with a few running injuries and from there snowballed. I would see a doctor to treat one injury or illness and another would pop up. I practiced yoga at the time and the more I committed myself to my practice, the more in tune I became with my body.

My body knew before my mind that there were things in my life I needed to change. As my awareness grew and I consciously made those changes, my body healed itself. Astounded by my body's ability to repair itself from the inside out, I decided to become a certified yoga instructor.

Integrative Nutrition was my way to bridge the gap between my investigative reporting career and yoga teaching. I remember saying to my childhood friend, who was also enrolled in the school, "Maybe I'll be on a health show one day or even have my own." By graduation, that maybe became my reality. The nationally syndicated daytime talk show, The Doctors, called me to discuss moving to Los Angeles to join them as an investigative health reporter. Now my investigations help viewers make informed decisions about their health, wellness and safety.

While Integrative Nutrition certainly helped me achieve new heights in my career it also shifted my life perspective. Listening to Debbie Ford's lecture was a pivotal moment for me. The idea that our shadows make us whole was something I had never considered before. This was a life changing moment for me. I now stand wholeheartedly and confidently in my truth. I think that was the balance I always sought.

It was always my dream to be a national correspondent. I never imagined it would be in quite this way or that my journey would bring me to Integrative Nutrition. In retrospect all of the dots line up. I guess that's the beauty of looking back, you get to see you were never really lost.

A Country Without McDonald's

While many fast-food chains are rapidly expanding throughout the globe, there's one country in South America where McDonald's did not survive. In Bolivia, people prefer their traditional foods to Big Macs. Citizens still love hamburgers, but they prefer to buy them from indigenous female street vendors called cholitas. The fast-food chain closed all locations in 2002 because it was simply not profitable. The failure piqued the interest of filmmakers, who made a documentary in 2011 called, "Why did McDonald's Bolivia Go Bankrupt?"[3]

"Fast-food represents the complete opposite of what Bolivians consider a meal should be," according to the blog El Polvorin.[4] "To be a good meal, food has to have be prepared with love, dedication, certain hygiene standards and proper cook time."

What I find most interesting about Bolivia is a culture where community values prevail. Bolivia's population values their food systems, food producers, and their ecosystems, so much so that food sovereignty laws continue to pass in the government to ensure that they preserve their food traditions and put less economic pressure on commodity crops. The country's first indigenous president, Evo Morales, even called U.S. fast-food chains "a great harm to humanity" at a United Nations General Assembly meeting in 2013. Talk about a slow food nation. I wonder what would happen in other countries if more of the population embraced longer, slower meals rather than quick, convenient foods.

The Healthiest Regional Cuisines

Many regions of the world are less reliant on processed, convenient foods and instead have amazing regional foods and customs that keep people healthy.

"Diets evolve over time, being influenced by many factors and complex interactions," according to the website of the World Health Organization.[5] "Income, prices, individual preferences and beliefs, cultural traditions, as well as geographical, environmental, social and economic factors all interact in a complex manner to shape dietary consumption patterns."

Africa

This large and diverse continent is home to root vegetables, leafy greens, beans and wild meats and fish. Okra and watermelon are native to Africa. The main grains found in Africa are couscous, sorghum, millet and rice. Researchers found that North Africans were possibly making yogurt around 7,000 years ago.[6] Pottery shards were discovered with traces of fat from a fermented dairy product, and scientists believe this method made it more digestible. Traditional Central and Western African meals are often based on hearty and aromatic vegetable soups and stews served over tubers or grains. Fufu is a dish made from starchy foods like cassava or yams usually served with grilled meat. Eastern Africa serves up more whole grains and vegetables, especially kale, cabbage and maize (cornmeal). Ethiopia and Somalia feature flat breads like injera (made out of teff or sorghum) and spicy beans like lentils, fava beans and chickpeas.

Australia/New Zealand

Traditionally, the diets in these island nations took their roots from the English diet with stewed meats, puddings and pies. Dinners typically consisted of lamb, beef, or chicken with potatoes or root vegetables. Seafood is certainly abundant in coastal areas. The indigenous Aborigine in Australia enjoyed meat from kangaroo, crocodiles and turtles, along with shellfish and native fruits like wild peach or riberry, similar to cranberry. The Maori in New Zealand took advantage of the many wild plants and roots like kumara (sweet potato) and taro. The world knows these areas for Marmite and Vegemite, food pastes made from yeast extract and used to spread on toast and sandwiches. With an intense flavor, these spreads are rich sources of B vitamins, niacin and folic acid.

Caribbean

Many local fruits and vegetables offer tons of nutrients and energy to the Caribbean lifestyle. Guava is a small oval-shaped fruit with a rough outer skin but with a sweet and sour taste inside that's high in fiber, potassium and vitamin C. Breadfruit can be boiled or mashed much like a potato and is an excellent source of fiber and potassium. Beans are another staple in the

Caribbean diet including lentils, chickpeas, kidney beans, black-eyed peas and split peas. Callaloo, the national dish of Trinidad and Tobago, consists of a stew made with green leafy vegetables, usually some kind of spinach variety.

India

India is famous for its aromatic cuisine. The country has some of the lowest rates of Alzheimer's disease in the world, thanks in part to some of its healthy spices. Curcumin, the yellow color in curry spice, continues to be studied for its health benefits that include cancer prevention and anti-inflammatory properties that help ward off the onset of Alzheimer's. Other spices like ginger, chilies and cardamom are also great for you. Indian dal is made with lentils and veggies, full of magnesium and can even help stabilize blood sugar. In a 2006 survey, about 40 percent of the population was found to be vegetarian, but demand for meat seems to be rising in recent years and with it, more of the health issues associated with it.[7]

The Nordic Region

Citizens of Sweden, Denmark and Norway boast some of the lowest obesity rates in Europe perhaps because their diet is full of cold-climate veggies like kale, cabbage and cauliflower. Their bread is made with rye grain, which is easier to digest than wheat and has more soluble fiber, helping to lower cholesterol and glycemic load. A small randomized study from 2010 tested the health of the Nordic diet using local foods like herring, rapeseed oil and berries on people with metabolic syndrome (a precursor to diabetes). Researchers found that those eating the healthy Nordic foods had significant improvements in their bad cholesterol/good cholesterol ratio and a marker for inflammation, which could result in a 20 to 40 percent decrease in developing type 2 diabetes.[8] While scientists felt confident the diet had health benefits, they also recognized it might be hard to replicate the diet outside of Nordic countries. It's just another testament to the power of local, whole foods.

The Middle East

Another region of the world known for its spices and healthy dishes is the Middle East, including countries like Turkey, Israel, Iran, Iraq, Lebanon,

Palestine, Jordan and more. Some of the most common ingredients here are olive oil, chickpeas, sesame seeds, dates and herbs like mint and parsley. This region is known for hummus and other healthy dips served with plenty of vegetables. Sumac, a dark red spice made from wild sumac berries, offers a tart flavor used as a rub on meats and kebabs, as well as marinades, dips and stews. Traditionally, the spice had medicinal purposes, too, helping promote good digestion, easing stomach pains and even reducing fevers. Sumac berries contain antioxidants and antimicrobial properties. The spice is also used in a spice blend called za'atar, which also includes wild oregano, thyme, toasted sesame seeds and salt. This health food dates back to the 12th century when the Spanish Jewish philosopher Maimonides is said to have used it with his patients to treat many ailments.[9]

Philippines

The Filipino diet includes rice with almost every meal, along with lots of fresh seafood and local vegetables like water spinach, eggplant and bitter melon. People tend to eat three meals a day along with a morning and afternoon snack. The food prep is usually quite simple—grilled, steamed or raw. Fish and veggies typically receive a marinade of vinegar or lime juice. More recently, American-style fast foods like hamburgers and pizza have become more popular, creating a similar rise in overweight and obese people as in the U.S.[10]

Japan

Japan is another place where obesity rates are low and people who live in the Blue Zone region of Okinawa live to be 100 or more. Food prep is usually light steams and quick stir-fries with fresh vegetables and fish. Of course, sushi is also easy to digest and can be high in heart-healthy fish oil. Some of the staple foods that contribute to that health are calcium-rich greens like bok choy, shiitake mushrooms, seaweeds and antioxidant rich green tea. Miso, tempeh, soy sauce and other fermented soy products are easy to digest and offer increased nutrition as rich sources of iron, magnesium and zinc.

South America

Another diverse continent, the 12 countries of South America make use of fresh vegetables, beans and fruit. A high protein seed that cooks up like a seed, quinoa is a superfood that grows abundantly here. Some areas like Brazil and Argentina are known for steaks and meat but also have healthier dishes like ceviche—a mixture of raw seafood, citrus juice and tomato. And the most basic South American meal of rice and beans with fresh cilantro and chile peppers is another healthy dish.

Southeast Asia

Fresh herbs, vegetables and fish prevail in this area. Using more water and broth for cooking is an easy healthy habit to take from Southeast Asian kitchens. Flavorings like cilantro, mint, ginger, tamarind, and chilies are all great for digestion and help fight inflammation in the body. In Vietnam, you find pho, an aromatic noodle soup full of antioxidant rich spices. Researchers at Thailand's Kasetsart University have studied the immune-boosting qualities of Tom Yum Goong, a soup made with shrimp, mushroom, coriander, lemongrass, ginger, and other herbs and spices. Incidences of digestive tract cancers are lower in Thailand than anywhere else in the world.[11]

Spain

Spain is synonymous with tapas—small plates of veggies, fish or meat. The rest of the world could certainly benefit from this ritual of eating smaller portions during a long, leisurely meal. Spanish food features fresh seafood, vegetables, and olive oil, a darling of the Mediterranean diet. Particularly healthy dishes like gazpacho are full of antioxidants and lycopene—known for its cancer-fighting properties. Paella is another great meal with seafood, rice, veggies and spices.

Wherever you are in the world, it's important to look at the whole picture and find balance with both primary and secondary foods. Healthy ingredients are great, but many people who eat relatively healthy still don't have the energy and zest for life as people who feel truly fulfilled in their lives. It's not just the food but also the lifestyle that contributes to the health of families, the environment and ultimately the planet.

Superfoods of the World

As I mentioned in chapter 1, many unhealthy habits get exported around the world. But a new trend has emerged around superfoods, or foods that are nutritionally dense and thought to possess super immune-boosting properties. It's a relief to see more nutrient-rich foods getting imported, exported and integrated throughout markets in the world. But like any trend, be curious about where your food comes from and don't forget your unique nutritional needs. We are all bio-individuals, even when it comes to superfoods. Some exotic berries or seeds might contain super nutrients, but the foods that grow right in your neighborhood usually contain the best nutrients for you.

The word "superfood" is not a scientific or regulated term. You might notice that many lists rate the top superfoods in the world with as many as 50 or 100 foods with everything from blueberries to seaweed. Don't forget the basics. Any food can become a superfood if it gives you energy and vitality. Eating a glamorous superfood every now and again cannot make up for nutritional or lifestyle mistakes happening day in and out. Right? You can't get by on a few hours of sleep and hope that a shake of superfoods will repair the damage. So don't get too swept away by these foods and remember to always listen to your body.

Technology todays has allowed for the exchange of information and ideas at a more rapid pace than ever before. People learn about superfoods and nutrition from articles on the Internet or a friend's recommendation on Facebook. We have seen some of the disadvantages of exporting certain foods, as the SAD diet has increased heart disease and obesity to the areas of the world that have embraced it.

But we also have the potential to improve the world's health by spreading more positive messages about food. If children in low-income families, for example, were taught about (or at least had access to learn about) superfoods, regional diets and concepts like the Blue Zones or the Jungle Effect, we could begin to make positive steps toward a healthier, happier world. Perhaps

Global Superfoods

ACAI – Region: Brazil
From the rainforests of Brazil, this small, bright purple berry is one of the most nutritious foods found on the planet. It's packed with antioxidants, amino acids and healthy fats. You can find it in powder or frozen form, which you can add to smoothies and juices for an extra punch of nutrients.

BEE POLLEN – Region: Worldwide
Found wherever bees roam, bee pollen is used throughout the world as a holistic remedy and superfood. It's the result of the accumulation of flower pollen, nectar and bee's salivary substances. It's rich in amino acids, B-complex vitamins and folic acid.[12]

CACAO – Region: Mexico and the Americas
Native to the Americas, the cacao bean was first cultivated in Mexico in 1500 B.C.[13] Now people use it to make raw chocolate or cacao powder because of its antioxidants and high amounts of magnesium, fiber and iron.[14]

CHIA SEEDS – Region: Mexico and the Americas
Aztecs and Mayans used chia seeds to gain strength and stamina starting around 3500 B.C. The health benefits of these small, dark seeds include antioxidants, fiber, calcium and more omega-3 fatty acids than salmon.[15]

GOJI BERRIES – Region: China
This berry is also known as the wolfberry and is a small, red berry known for its high level of carotenoids, which can help boost the immune system.[16] It has been used in traditional herbal medicine for about 2,000 years and in China they hold a strong belief that this fruit can significantly extend life.[17]

HEMP SEEDS – Region: Central Asia
The hemp plant originated in Central Asia as a food crop, but today it is grown all over the world except for the U.S. where it's banned.[18] The seeds come from a variety of Cannibis plant, but it contains very little THC—the part that is considered a drug in most countries. It's similar to the amount of opium in poppy seeds. Hemp seeds are very high in Omega-3 and Omega-6 essential fatty acids and an excellent source of protein.[19]

QUINOA – Region: South America
The Food and Agricultural Organization of the United Nations (FAO) declared 2013 as "The International Year of the Quinoa."[20] This seed is very high in protein, but cooks up like a grain, making it a great option for those looking to cut back on carbs. It's full of antioxidants and vitamins like manganese, magnesium and fiber.

MANUKA HONEY – Region: New Zealand
This honey, native to New Zealand, comes from bees that pollinate the Manuka bush. Honey has a healing reputation, but Manuka honey has been effective in scientific studies when used on top of wounds. It's also effective in fighting infection and promoting healing.[21]

MORINGA – Region: Africa/Asia
The leaves of this tree are thought to be a superfood because it's one of the world's most nutritious plant species with more than 92 types of nutrients and 46 types of antioxidants. It also contains protein and is a great source of iron, containing more iron than liver or roast beef.[22] It's usually available in powder or capsule form and can be brewed into a tea or added to a smoothie.

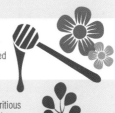

SPIRULINA – Region: Africa
This microalgae gets its name from its spiral shape, thriving in fresh and salt water throughout the world. It's a complete protein containing all essential amino acids and is one of the richest sources of B vitamins and iron.[23]

TEDx says it best with their mission of "ideas worth spreading." Understand that just one person—one person reading this book, just like you—can make an enormous difference for the health of yourself, your family and your community.

U.S. President John F. Kennedy said, "Ask not what your country can do for you, ask what you can do for your country." Well, it's time to expand this thought as we are so well connected. It's time to think about what you can do for your world.

Exercise

1. Think Globally, Act Locally

With a global mindset, we can create better health and greater happiness for all.

Consider how your actions impact the world and think about what you can do to get more of your food locally. Look into any farmers' markets, CSAs and food co-ops in your area. The more you know about how to find healthy food in your own area, the better impact you'll have on the environment and planet.

2. Become a Locavore.

What foods are local to your country or community? Create a recipe using as many local ingredients as possible. Recreate a favorite dish or try something new. Entrees, side dishes, smoothies and juices all count.

How do you feel after cooking with local versus store-bought, out-of-season ingredients? How do local ingredients affect the taste?

3. Experiment with Local Superfoods.

Superfoods add variety and color to your diet, in addition to providing an extra nutritional pop. What local superfoods do you have access to?

Experiment with what's available and add them into your daily diet.

Keep in mind, just because something is labeled a superfood, that doesn't mean you have to eat it every day. Rather than incorporating superfoods into your diet as a new food group, think of them as seasoning to compliment an existing healthy dish.

CHAPTER 6

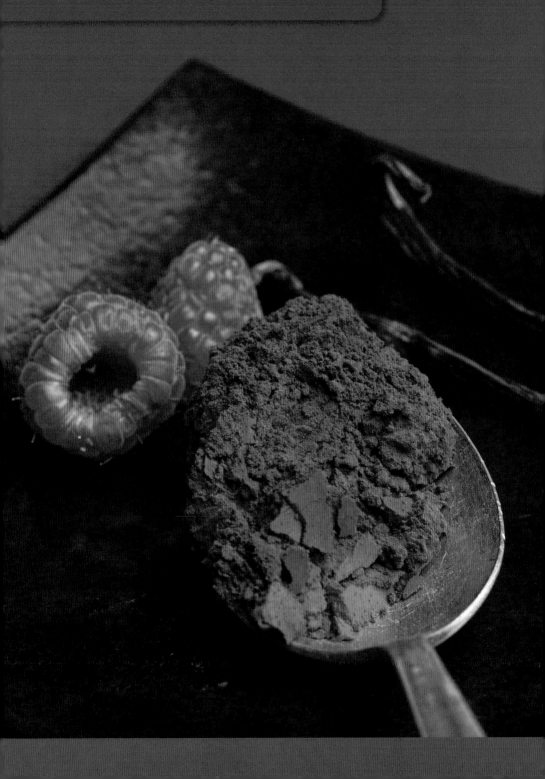

Deconstructing Cravings

> All I really need is love, but a little chocolate now and then doesn't hurt!
>
> —Lucy Van Pelt
> from *Peanuts* comic by Charles M. Schulz

Chocolate, bread, steak, eggs, french fries, candy bars, ice cream—
it really doesn't matter what you crave. The important thing is to
understand why you crave what you crave. Most people believe
cravings are a problem, but I have a different perspective. Once we realize
that the body is a reliable bio-computer that never makes mistakes, it's much
easier to conclude that cravings are critical pieces of information that help
you understand what your body needs.

I've been craving ice cream since I was a child, with a special sweet spot
for Ben and Jerry's Cherry Garcia, the perfect blend of dark chocolate, sweet
vanilla and tart fruit. I once noticed that on Sunday nights, after teaching
class all weekend, an alien force would take control of my body and drive my
car directly to the convenience store to buy a pint. As I watched myself eat all
this ice cream, I wondered, between delicious mouthfuls, "What am I doing
in my life that might trigger such an extreme craving?"

At the time, I was teaching many hours, eating a primarily macrobiotic
diet and drinking hot peppermint tea throughout the day to stay grounded
and focused. When I started investigating the craving, I noticed that my body
felt hot and tense when I had the tea, and shortly after, I began to daydream
about chocolate-covered cherries smothered in rich, cold vanilla ice cream.
The hot tea was causing my craving for cooling foods. I started drinking more
water, stopped asking for water without ice at restaurants, and increased my
intake of vegetables, which have a cooling and relaxing effect on the body. I
also realized that after gorging on ice cream, I felt extremely satiated. Knowing
that fat is what makes us feel full and that my macrobiotic diet did not con-

tain much fat, I incorporated more olive oil into my cooking to provide an alternative source of fatty satisfaction. Long hours of teaching can be stressful, and the fact that I was having these cravings on Sundays indicated that I was using the ice cream as a reward or de-stresser after teaching all weekend.

Lo and behold, within a few weeks of making these changes, my cravings passed and my Sunday night ice cream binges ended. Of course, I still look forward to a few bites every once in a while, but the days of empty pints in the backseat of my car are long gone. By observing my own behavior and trusting that my body needed something from the ice cream, I was able to modify my diet and lifestyle to get what I needed in a more health-supportive way.

Sugar Addictions

Many years ago, a successful female dentist came to me for help with her sugar cravings. She confessed that all day long she told clients to avoid sugar, but every afternoon she would sneak into her back office and secretly binge on sweets, particularly candy bars: Butterfingers, Snickers, Milky Ways, Twix bars. She was a sincere, intelligent woman who knew that consuming large amounts of sugar destroys teeth, but was helpless when it came to her own cravings. She was puzzled and felt helpless, not for a lack of understanding or discipline, but because willpower is not enough when it comes to food dependencies, especially those involving sugar.

"I'm addicted and I feel like an absolute hypocrite," she told me.

"You're not a hypocrite," I said. "Humans naturally crave sweet flavors, but there is something you can do about it. Let's get some milder sweet foods into your diet on a more regular basis to avoid these afternoon binges."

I explained the distinction between simple and complex carbohydrates, advising her to reduce processed foods—except pasta, which she loved—and increase grains and vegetables. I knew, however, this alone would not be enough to beat her intense sugar cravings. So I introduced her to two new products, rice cakes and rice syrup. Rice syrup is a sweet syrup made from rice that contains many complex, as well as simple, sugars. It has a milder impact on the body than standard sugar, candy bars, donuts and other processed, sweet foods. Rice syrup is delicious on rice cakes, which are made of puffed brown rice, and also rich in complex carbohydrates. I told her to buy a big supply of rice cakes and rice syrup and put them in her back office for when she was craving something sweet. In two months, her sugar cravings had diminished remarkably. Months later, she was urging her own clients with sugar addictions to switch to rice products as a substitute for chemicalized sweets.

These days, a lot of natural options are out there to help you transition from refined, processed sugars, and more research is addressing how much we all need to make the leap. At the forefront of the research is Dr. Robert Lustig, a pediatric endocrinologist from California, who believes sugar is downright toxic and addictive. He's authored dozens of scientific articles, but in May 2009 Dr. Lustig made headlines with a lecture he gave called "Sugar: The Bitter Truth," which was later posted on YouTube and has been seen by more than 3 million people. In it, he argues that sugar is the primary cause of our worldwide health crisis due to its potential for abuse, its toxic nature and its growing prevalence in the Western diet. He brings to light that sugar is hidden in almost all processed foods today from bread to peanut butter to canned sauces and dressings, especially in the form of high fructose corn syrup.

Dr. Lustig says evolution has taught us that sweet things are safe to eat. But fructose, the naturally occurring sugar in fruit, comes with fiber and other important nutrients, which is a far cry from the sweet stuff we are consuming today. A study published in 2013 linked increased sugar consumption with increased rates of diabetes in 175 countries worldwide.[1] Researchers found that increased sugar in a population's food supply was linked to higher rates of diabetes. As sugar has become a bigger part of the daily diet around the world, so have chronic diseases.

Simple and Complex Carbohydrates

Nearly everyone craves sugar. When experiencing such cravings, most people go right for the most accessible sweet treat: candy, chocolate bars, cake or cookies. But what these people don't realize is that many healthy alternatives can help alleviate sweet cravings.

A sugar craving is simply the body asking for energy. When sugar is digested, it becomes glucose. Glucose is fuel for all of the body's cells.

When you eat sugar, it enters the bloodstream and is converted into glucose at different rates, depending on the type of sugar you consume. All carbohydrates contain sugar, but depending on their chemical structures—simple or complex—they are processed differently. Most simple carbohydrates are highly processed, contain refined sugars and have few vitamins and minerals. Processed foods contain short chains of sugar, which enter the bloodstream almost momentarily after they are ingested. This causes a rapid rise in the glucose levels in the body—a sugar rush. The rush is shortly followed by a crash. The body sees the high level of sugar as an emergency state and works hard to burn it up as quickly as possible. Then blood sugar drops precipitously. Other natural foods, like fruit, contain naturally occurring simple sugars. Fruit is high in fiber, which helps slow digestion, limiting the amount of sugar that flows into the cells.

Carbohydrates that appear in nature, in whole foods like vegetables and whole grains, are complex. Complex carbohydrates are composed of long chains of sugars. These long chains are bound within the food's fiber. The body processes the sugars by breaking the chains and releasing fiber into the bloodstream. This process is relatively slow; therefore, the sugars are absorbed into the bloodstream at a steady rate for many hours, providing long-lasting energy.

If you eat a whole grain—a complex carbohydrate—for breakfast, you will likely have energy throughout the morning and then experience a mild dip around noon, just in time for lunch. If you eat an Oreo cookie, a candy bar or white bread—all simple carbs—the bloodstream will be suddenly flooded with sugars, providing a quick burst of energy. But shortly after, your blood sugar will drop and you will be hungry again. Your body wants to maintain balanced blood sugar, so it is telling you to eat something to bring your blood sugar back up. Most people go for more sugar, and this experience of sugar ups and downs continues throughout the day. Blood sugar often drops around 3 p.m., a few hours after lunch—the time when most people seek sugar or caffeine to get them through the rest of the afternoon.

In today's modern nutrition world, high-protein diets are fashionable and "carbohydrate" has become a dirty word, associated in many people's minds with the obesity crisis. This is absurd. Carbohydrates provide much of the energy needed for normal body functions—such as heartbeat, breathing and digestion—and for exercise. Carbohydrates are in everything from candy bars to grains and even vegetables. The problem is that people are not eating the types of carbohydrates nature intended. They're eating carbohydrate-rich foods that have been deformed and denatured. Simple sugars can lead to weight gain because our cells do not require large amounts of glucose at one time, and the extra sugar is stored as fat. The anti-carb movement should really be an anti-simple-carb movement.

Overconsumption of simple carbohydrates has led to an abundance of hypoglycemia in America. Hypoglycemia is the body's inability to handle large amounts of sugar. It's common among people with diabetes but can also be caused by an overload of sugar, alcohol, caffeine, tobacco and stress. Hypoglycemia is triggered when the pancreas secretes too much insulin in response to a rapid rise in blood sugar, which in turn causes blood sugar levels to plummet, starving the body's cells of needed fuel. A person with hypoglycemia may feel weak, drowsy, confused, dizzy and hungry, especially around 3 p.m. when blood sugar is naturally at its lowest. When your blood sugar is low, you are vulnerable to cravings because your body urgently needs something to spike its glucose. If a hypoglycemic episode hits you between meals, a healthy choice would be to nibble on a carrot or celery stick, not grab a bagel with cream cheese or wolf down a chocolate chip cookie.

Sugar cravings are as natural as our desire for air. Throughout two million years of evolution, humans have been programmed to desire sweet-tasting foods. Long before food processing, the only source of sweet tastes was plant foods such as squash, tubers, roots, grains and fruit. In order to get the sweet taste their bodies desired, people had to eat plants. It is no coincidence these sweet foods are also great sources of nutrients, energy and fiber—everything we need to maintain our health. So, the best way to curb or alleviate intense sugar cravings is to provide the body with the sweetness that it needs by regularly eating naturally sweet foods.

Hungry for Nutrition

A student of mine once talked to me about her "problem child," Kevin, who was addicted to processed foods like sugary cereals, peanut butter and jelly on white bread, pizza, fast food and all kinds of sodas and salty snacks. The more Kevin ate, the hungrier he got. This ravenous 11-year-old was clearly eating too much, and was overweight as a result.

"Maybe he's not hungry for calories," I said to her, "Maybe he's hungry for nutrition."

"What do you mean?" she asked. "I'm feeding him all day long. I would think he's getting too much nutrition."

I explained that the food he was eating was all processed, and rich in simple sugars but deficient in nutrients. Sugar is fuel for cells, but they need vitamins and minerals to do their jobs properly. He was fueling his body, making his cells work, but not giving them the raw materials they needed. Kevin was craving more and more food because his cells were starving for vitamins and minerals. He was suffering from malnutrition.

"He's on a very inefficient diet and needs to eat a lot of food just to get enough nutrients to operate his body," I told her.

"But what can I do?" his mother asked, looking a bit stunned.

"He's got to reverse the formula," I said. "Eat foods that are rich in nutrients and low in calories, the exact opposite of what he's doing now."

I then laid out a program for her son, which did not take out any of his foods, but rather added nutrient-rich foods, especially vegetables and whole grains to his diet, suggesting leaner choices of meat and plenty of exercise. I spoke to her about making home-cooked food that might appeal to her 11-year-old. He could still have his favorite peanut butter, but on a celery stick instead of white bread with sugary jelly. He could still eat pizza, but homemade pizza with vegetable toppings. She had to take it slowly. Kevin wasn't going to immediately start wolfing down collards and brown rice. Getting a child who is hooked on sugar and processed foods to eat natural foods can seem impossible. His taste buds were accustomed to artificial flavors. Natural foods would probably taste bland.

I sometimes tell students to pour chocolate sauce on greens at first, if it will get their kids to actually eat them. Do whatever it takes to get kids accustomed to natural foods. It takes most people, both children and adults, three times of trying a food before they really begin to enjoy it. I suggested that Kevin's mom make greens and have him eat just a few pieces the first time,

PROFILE

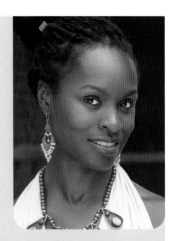

Latham Thomas, New York, NY, USA

www.mamaglow.com

"We all have that power within us to create what we desire."

Before Integrative Nutrition I was a new mother with a dream of healing others but I had no real map for how to harness and achieve my vision. I knew that I wanted to work in the wellness arena but didn't know exactly how to go about it. I had seen the Integrative Nutrition catalog in a health food store over a period of years, then one day I visited the website and felt a strong urge to learn more. Something about the school resonated with me and I knew that if I was going to make a difference I had to invest in myself and go!

Today I am a full-time prenatal wellness expert, speaker, and author. My practice, Tender Shoots Wellness, is a boutique holistic lifestyle practice for women during the childbearing years. Based in New York City, we offer culinary services, nutritional coaching, yoga, and birth doula services. I work with clientele that inspire me every day and love that I am making a huge difference in the lives of so many. My personal mission is to help women feel empowered, experience optimal wellness—by feeling and looking their very best, and prioritizing self care as a daily practice. I hope to constantly evolve and heal through my work with women in transformation.

My book, *Mama Glow*, is a modern holistic guide to pregnancy and was published in the Fall of 2012. I also am starting work on my follow up book and DVDs. I have been featured twice on the *Dr. Oz Show*, NBC, ABC News, and *Fox News LIVE*. As well as in publications that I love, including *Martha Stewart's Whole Living*, *Vogue* and *The New York Times*.

My life is grand! I've designed a lifestyle and career that I love. We all have that power within us to create what we desire. I'm able to spend time with my son, take vacation when I want, and work with my ideal clientele. My work has been endorsed by my mentors who are giants in the wellness community: Dr. Christiane Northrup, Dr. Mehmet Oz, and my sister Kris Carr.

I am so grateful for the work that Joshua and Integrative Nutrition does to grow wellness professionals into wellness warriors. My experience at Integrative Nutrition ignited a spark in me and now I'm trailblazing!

the second time and the third time. After that, he was helping himself to the greens. Six months later, Kevin had lost 30 pounds.

Like a lot of people, Kevin was stuffing himself with sugary foods and becoming sick and overweight. He kept eating because his body was craving nutrients, not simply food mass.

The body is smart. It tells you when you are not feeding it properly. If you feed it fats, oils and sugar, it is going to send you messages that it needs more food. It needs protein; it needs vitamins; it needs minerals. But if you are not accustomed to eating vegetables, whole grains, and other nutrient-dense foods, you're not going to decipher this message as a specific craving for something healthy. So Kevin, for example, was just getting the hunger signal and grabbing the foods he'd been brought up on: meat, pizza, bread, sugar, Big Macs, or whatever.

Kevin was lucky that his mother sought help. A heartbreaking number of children in this country are struggling with their weight and obesity. They are addicted to sugar and processed food. Most people don't realize that they keep eating because their bodies are hungry for nutrition.

Contracting and Expanding Foods

Your body naturally wants to be balanced. The food you eat is a major contributing factor to the overall balance of the body. Certain foods, such as vegetables and whole grains, have mild effects on the body. Other foods, such as meat, milk, sugar and salt, have more extreme effects on the body, throwing off its natural balance. This struggle eventually leads to a craving for whatever the body needs to regain balance. I call these foods extreme foods and I divide them into two categories: contracting and expanding.

Contracting Foods

The most common and powerful contracting food is salt, which many of us consume regularly in large quantities. Salt is used commonly as a preservative, especially in artificial junk food. Other extreme contracting foods are animal foods, including beef, pork, ham, hard cheese, eggs, chicken, fish and shellfish. The main benefit of animal foods is that they are rich in protein

The 8 primary causes of cravings

1. **Dehydration** The body doesn't send the message that you are thirsty until you are on the verge of dehydration. Dehydration occurs as mild hunger, so the first thing to do when you get a strange craving is to drink a full glass of water.

2. **Lifestyle** Being dissatisfied with a relationship, having an inappropriate exercise routine (too much, too little or the wrong type), being bored, stressed, uninspired by a job or lacking a spiritual practice can all contribute to emotional eating. Eating can be used as a substitute for entertainment or to fill the void.

3. **Yin/Yang Imbalance** Certain foods have more yin qualities (expansive) while other foods have more yang qualities (contractive). Eating foods that are either extremely yin or extremely yang causes cravings in order to reestablish balance. For example, eating a diet too rich in sugar (yin) may cause a craving for meat (yang).

4. **Inside Coming Out** Oftentimes, cravings come from foods that we have recently eaten, foods eaten by our ancestors or foods from our childhood. A clever way to satisfy these cravings is to eat a healthier versions of one's ancestral or childhood foods.

5. **Seasonal** Often the body craves foods that balance out the elements of the season. In the spring, people crave detoxifying foods like leafy greens or citrus foods. In the summer, people crave cooling foods like fruit, raw foods and ice cream, and in the fall people crave grounding foods like squash, onions and nuts. In winter many crave hot and heat-producing foods like meat, oil and fat. Other cravings, such as turkey, eggnog or sweets, can also be associated with the holiday season.

6. **Lack of Nutrients** If the body is getting an inadequate amount of nutrients, it will produce odd cravings. For example, inadequate mineral levels produce salt cravings, and overall inadequate nutrition produces cravings for non-nutritional forms of energy like caffeine.

7. **Hormones** When women experience menstruation, pregnancy or menopause, fluctuating testosterone and estrogen levels may cause unusual cravings.

8. **De-evolution** When things are going extremely well, sometimes a self-sabotage syndrome happens, where we suddenly crave foods that throw us off balance. We then have more cravings to balance ourselves. This often happens from low blood sugar and may result in strong mood swings.

and give us feelings of strength, aggressiveness and increased physical and mental power. However, when we eat too much of these foods, we create an imbalance and quickly feel bloated, heavy, sluggish and mentally slow. The more contracting foods we eat, the tighter our bodies become. As a result of eating contracting foods, the body naturally craves expanding foods as a way of maintaining balance.

Expanding Foods

The predominant extreme expanding food is refined white sugar. Expanding foods provide feelings of lightness, elevations in mood and relief from blockages and stagnation. However, refined white sugar also causes rapid elevations in serotonin, followed by rapid declines. When serotonin levels fall, we typically experience feelings of depression, low energy, anxiety and loss of concentration. We crave extreme contracting foods to balance the equation and again find ourselves in the throes of the ping-pong diet, using one type of extreme food to alleviate the effects of the other.

Our bodies can enjoy a certain quantity of extreme foods without creating too much imbalance. But when we exceed our personal limit—and it varies with each individual—there are consequences. If you eat extreme foods daily, your body will become exhausted and depleted as it frantically tries to rebalance itself. To get out of this cycle, you need to deconstruct what you are craving, and seek out less extreme, healthier alternatives to satisfy you.

Hunger and Binging

Sometimes cravings come in the form of extreme hunger. You don't know what you're hungry for; you just know that you're starving. Most people avoid hunger at all costs, and many develop habits of overeating and/or constant eating just to avoid ever feeling hungry. When we habitually overeat, a high proportion of our available energy is always directed toward digestion. If we eat when we are not hungry, we compromise our digestion of the food. You may want to consider the idea, almost heretical in this day and age, that it's okay to be hungry now and then. I'm not talking about a drastic form of starvation dieting—just an experiment to see how it feels. It's not going to kill you, and it may make life more interesting.

On the other hand, many people today try to go hungry all day, ignoring the body's cravings for food. This habit creates a backlash, which I call the "binge eaters diet." In an attempt to lose weight, these people skip breakfast, go off to work, maybe grab a mid-morning cup of coffee to keep going, and then settle on a salad for lunch. Somehow they make it through the afternoon, but by the time they get home in the evening they discover that they are ravenous. The hectic activity of the workday may have distracted them from urgent messages emanating from their stomachs, but as they slow down they realize, "I am so hungry!" Then they overeat heavy foods at dinner, until they feel stuffed and uncomfortable. The next morning they start the cycle over again, not eating breakfast because they feel full from last night's binge, which is still undigested.

I do not believe in trying to override natural instincts. Of course, it helps to have discipline around food, but trying to control the body by using the mind is very challenging in the long term. For one thing, the head often makes mistakes. Remember when you went shopping for a fabulous new outfit and spent a lot of money but never wore the clothes? Remember when you met a good-looking guy and thought, "Wow! This is the right person for me!" and he turned out to be a complete jerk? Another mistake your head can easily make is to decide, "This is the right diet for me. I can handle this one." Our bodies don't really care what our heads think. Our bodies are built to survive and thrive. Your head can say, "I am not eating this food because it is fattening," and your body may cooperate for a while. At some point, though, it will start murmuring quiet messages like, "Hmm, we definitely need some more fat in here, to keep the brain thinking and make me feel satiated." The next thing you know, you're holding an empty pint of ice cream.

Learning to listen to your body is essential. The longer you ignore your body's messages, the more extreme the backlash. Just as a crying child will use increasingly extreme measures to get attention, the body will heighten your cravings and create disease if you don't listen to it.

Crowding Out

One solution to cravings that I've found to be quite effective over the years is to add more to your diet rather than taking away from it. For years, I did not eat bread at home. I just ate whole grains. But when I was in restaurants and they put bread on the table, I would wolf it down very quickly. I realized that bread was a part of my upbringing. It was what my parents grew up on and what I grew up on. Rather than have the white bread version at restaurants, I started to incorporate healthy breads at home. Now when I'm out eating, I can take the bread or leave it. It's no longer as if I have a parched throat in the desert and bread is my water. Bread is now just another food.

Many dietitians and nutritionists give their clients a list of foods to avoid and foods to eat, which explains why so many people are turned off by nutrition. People think they'll have to give up their regular diet and start eating things they know are "good" for them but that they don't enjoy. Taking away people's favorite foods is like taking heroin away from a heroin addict. The food is giving them something they need. I have found that one of the most effective methods to overcome habitual consumption of unhealthy foods is to simply crowd out these foods. It's hard to eat five fruits and vegetables a day and binge on ice cream at the end of the day. The body can only take so much food. If you fill your body with healthy, nutrient-dense foods, it is only natural that cravings for unhealthy foods will lessen substantially.

By eating and drinking foods that are good for you earlier in the day, you will naturally leave less room and desire for unhealthy foods. This method is most evident when you increase your intake of water. Fill a water bottle or pitcher with clean, filtered water, or buy a liter of pure spring water, and sip it steadily throughout your morning. As the day continues, you'll have less room for coffee, black tea and soft drinks. Really, it's that simple. You will immediately begin to cut down on other liquids if you keep yourself well hydrated. You may need a second bottle for the afternoon. People's need for water varies, so you should listen to your body to determine how much you need to drink in a day. Not only will water crowd out more unhealthy drinks, it may also improve your health in other ways.

Just as drinking water crowds out unhealthy beverages, eating healthy foods can crowd out junk foods. Vegetables are high in vitamins and minerals, and you can eat a lot of them without gaining weight. When you increase your intake of nutritious foods, such as dark leafy greens and whole grains, your body will have less room for processed, sugary, nutrient-deficient foods. And the beautiful part is that once you start adding these foods into your diet, your body will naturally begin to crave them. The trick is to organize your life so that you have access to these healthful foods at all times, especially when you feel like snacking at work or when you are traveling. Then you can make it to your evening meal without impulsively eating junk food because that's the only thing available. It takes a little practice to make this happen, but it's definitely possible.

Cravings Are Not the Problem

The lesson here is to look for the foods, deficits and behaviors in your life that are the underlying causes of your cravings. Many people view cravings as weaknesses, when in reality they are important messages meant to help you maintain balance. It all comes down to trusting your body, instead of thinking of your cravings as an enemy, to be ignored or defeated.

How much do you trust your body? When I ask people this question, most tell me, "Not very much."

"Why not?" I ask.

"Because it's always craving foods that get me into trouble," they say, shaking their heads sadly, disappointed at their own perceived weaknesses.

"What do you mean?" I ask.

"Well, whenever I'm on a diet my body wants foods that I'm not supposed to eat, foods that make me fat or sick."

"Why do you think your body craves such foods?" I ask.

"I don't know," people say, genuinely puzzled. "I guess I've got some built-in flaws. I can never do the right thing when it comes to food."

We have been taught to believe that our inability to stick with a diet is our fault, a flaw of our body and our will. This is absolutely incorrect. Diet book authors claim that if we want to lose weight and regain health we must conform to their rules and control our cravings for foods they deem unhealthy. To do this we must develop deep discipline over our natural instincts. We accept these ideas even though every other diet we have been on was unsuccessful. We start the newest program with the best of intentions, determined to make good this time. Again and again we repeat this cycle, blaming ourselves when the part of us that directs our food choices asserts itself, showing once again that it cannot be disciplined, controlled, suppressed or denied.

Increasingly, we find ourselves craving "illegal" foods until one day we fall off the diet, giving in to our cravings for bread, chocolate, meat, sugar, whatever foods have been forbidden. Afterward we feel guilty and worthless, and blame ourselves for failing to stick to the diet, which seemed so simple, so promising just a few weeks ago. It's never the program's fault; it's always our fault. Or so we think. It never dawns on us that there's nothing wrong with us, that maybe the diet itself is flawed—that it actually sets us up to fail, and then unfairly lays the responsibility on our shoulders when we do.

Why is the human instinct that determines food choices so powerful and unruly? Why can't it be easily controlled and disciplined? And what motivates these choices and cravings? Clearly, this is not a cerebral process. So what is it?

In my experience, the part of us that cannot be controlled is actually our inner guide to health and happiness. This innate wisdom is always trying to make us feel better by urging us to eat foods that will dissipate, at least temporarily, our physical tension, give us more energy and lift our moods. In essence, this part of us is always monitoring our physical, emotional and psychological conditions and struggling to create balance, harmony and happiness. Cravings are the body's solution to underlying imbalances, and food becomes a kind of medicine to regulate our current inner state.

Let me give a few examples. When we don't sleep well and wake up feeling lethargic, we often crave coffee to boost our energy and clear our minds. If we experience loneliness or mild depression, we often reach for chocolate or some other sweet food to boost our mood. After a stressful day, many of us want to eat something sweet or drink an alcoholic beverage to release tension. Afterward, we often feel weak and empty, and want something nutritious and strengthening. We crave eggs, steak, chicken or fish, which can leave us feeling bloated and heavy. It's a vicious cycle as we ping-pong from sweet, processed foods to excessive amounts of animal foods, from one extreme food group to another. Our minds, bodies and spirits are drained of energy with no apparent way out.

Trust Your Crazy Cravings

Whenever your body is craving something, pause for a moment and wonder, "What's really going on here?" Whenever you find yourself impulsively reaching for something you know is not good for you, take a moment to slow down, breathe and reevaluate the situation. Consider what your body is really asking for. Start with the flavor.

Are You Craving Something Sweet?

Sweet foods vary widely in nutritional content, from chocolate, cookies and pastries, to sweet vegetables, fruit and fruit juice. As much as possible, try to satisfy your desire for sweet flavor with a milder, less extreme food that doesn't contain refined white sugar. Like my dentist client, you might try eating a rice cake with rice syrup on it. You'll be surprised how satisfying this treat can be and how quickly it can eliminate your need for extreme sugary foods. If something stronger is desired, try various cookies or pastries made from whole-grain flour and sweetened with fruit juice or barley malt, a sweet syrup made from barley.

Certain vegetables have a deep, sweet flavor when cooked, like corn, carrots, onions, beets, winter squash (butternut, buttercup, delicata, hubbard or kabocha), sweet potatoes and yams. Eating a lot of sweet vegetables will satisfy your natural cravings for sweet foods, and reduce your cravings for sugary, processed junk food.

Natural sweeteners can also help with sugar cravings. My favorite, and the favorite of most of my students, is raw wild honey, which is made from the pollen of plants and trees. Unprocessed honey is one of nature's richest sources of antioxidants with a plethora of health benefits. Due to the presence of live enzymes, raw honey is easily digestible for most humans. The sweetness comes from natural fructose that is absorbed slowly by the body, so there's less of a sugar rush. It's great to have around the house to use in tea or salad dressings, or when baking.

Another sweetener that has gained recognition and sparked controversy is agave nectar. Agave nectar is made from the juice of the agave cactus, the same plant that gives us tequila, and is a traditional sweetener for Native Mexicans. The controversy stems from the fact that agave nectar is typically made using a chemical process that converts the starch into a refined, fructose-rich syrup that can be compared to high fructose corn syrup. While it contains small amounts of calcium, potassium and magnesium and ranks lower on the glycemic index than many other sweeteners, it is still best to limit consumption. As with all sweeteners, I recommend to use them sparingly.

When choosing a sweetener, it is always best to understand how it got from the source to you, because often times the marketing of products can be misleading. Other popular alternatives to sugar are brown rice syrup, barley malt and stevia, an herb native to South America. All of these can be found in your local health food store. Try them and find the ones that work best for you. For a complete list of sugar alternatives, see chapter 10.

Quality also makes a big difference. If you decide to have an extreme sweet food, choose the best quality you can buy and chances are good that you'll be satisfied with much less. Eat the food consciously, chewing it slowly and thoroughly enjoying it. Take chocolate as an example. Many of us crave chocolate and end up inhaling packages of M&M's while on the run or during a crunch time at work. It's a much different experience to quietly indulge in a small piece of organic dark chocolate, thoroughly chewing each morsel. If you're a chocoholic, check out the chocolate section of your health food store and you will find many brands of organic chocolate, with many wonderful flavors, such as ginger, currant, lime and my personal favorite, lavender.

Are You Craving Salty Foods?

Cravings for salty foods often indicate mineral deficiency. All salt originates in the sea, and natural sea salt contains 60 different trace minerals, which are the basis for the formation of vitamins, enzymes and proteins. Most of us use common table salt, which has been refined and stripped of many of these minerals. People's diets are generally lacking in minerals because much of our food has been highly processed and chemically grown, hence the popularity of salty foods. Before you go out and have a bag of pretzels or chips, try eating a wide variety of vegetables, especially leafy green veggies, which are very high in minerals. These foods often satisfy the craving for salty foods, which is really a desire for more nutrition. You may also want to purchase a high-quality sea salt to use in your cooking and incorporate sea vegetables, which have a naturally salty flavor and are high in minerals.

Are You Craving Bitter Foods?

Remember the old saying, "It's the bitter pill that cures you"? Well, this is a good rule to live by, especially because most modern diets don't contain many healthy bitter foods. Bitter foods enhance digestion, so a craving for bitter flavor may actually be a craving for nutritious foods to cut through fat and stagnation in the body's organs and digestive tract. Most people satisfy bitter cravings by drinking coffee and dark beers. If you find yourself craving bitter tastes, try eating dark leafy greens, such as dandelion, mustard greens, arugula, kale and collards. These greens will unblock stagnant organs and promote healthy assimilation and elimination.

Are You Craving Pungent Flavors?

Chinese cooking often incorporates pungently flavored foods that act as digestive aids. In traditional Chinese medicine, ginger is an herb for the large intestine and lungs. It enhances the function of, and promotes healing in, both organs. So, if you have a craving for heavy, saucy Chinese food it may be your body asking for the healing properties of pungent flavors. When this happens, try grating fresh ginger on your vegetables or in your soup. Other foods that will quench this craving are cayenne, scallions, onions, leeks, garlic and pepper.

Are You Craving Spicy Foods?

Are you looking for an array of flavors, both subtle and strong, or are you looking for hot spices? So much processed food is lacking in flavor because it's been on the shelf for such a long time and is stale, bland and tasteless. This kind of food lacks vitality, energy and aliveness and includes added fat and cholesterol. When people eat this kind of diet for years, the body can become overweight and stagnant. Blood becomes thick, or viscous, and circulation slows. As circulation weakens, organs and extremities become cool. At this point, the body may start craving spices.

When people crave spicy foods they often turn to pizza or hot Mexican spices. These extreme foods warm the body but also create a lot of stressful, chaotic energy. Instead of eating a pizza, with its dry, hard crust and heavy cheese, or refried beans and hot jalapeño peppers, try a bowl of noodles, such as soba, mixed with green vegetables and a nice marinara sauce with oregano, basil, red pepper flakes, onions, garlic and celery.

You can use a variety of spices and condiments to add kick to your food. Two popular choices are ground cayenne and hot pepper sesame oil, both of which you can find at any health food store. You can also chop jalapeño peppers and add them to a salad or stir-fry for that extra bit of spice.

What Texture or Consistency Are You Craving?

When craving something creamy, consider if you've had a lot of bread, crackers or other baked flour products recently. When eaten in excess, these foods create feelings of dryness and stagnation, and can also make us feel stuck, hard and irritable. When we reach that state of imbalance, we very often crave creamy, relaxing foods, such as ice cream, milk products or oily foods. Try eating porridge made from whole grains, such as amaranth or brown rice. You can also make cream of broccoli soup, or cream of watercress soup, and use oatmeal rather than cream to get the consistency you desire.

If you are craving chips or pretzels, it may be the crunch that you actually desire. I think when the body wants crunch it's probably because you're not chewing enough. The act of chewing actually enhances digestion. Instead of grabbing the chemicalized, artificial snack products, try satisfying your crunchy cravings with raw carrots and celery, or organic versions of potato chips and hard pretzels without added sugar. And don't forget to chew all your foods to assure proper digestion of your food.

Are You Craving Something Moist or a Liquid?

When craving liquids, ask yourself if you've been eating an excessive amount of salty foods or dry, baked flour products. Do you feel dry or tight? Are you thirsty? Many physical problems, including headaches, urology problems and kidney stones, are the result of chronic dehydration. People typically just don't drink enough water. Instead of quenching thirst with sugary and caffeinated beverages, try drinking water at least three times a day. Put a bottle or a cup of pure spring water on your desk and sip it throughout the day. As you drink, notice how your body responds. If you suddenly awaken to how thirsty you are, then you know you've been ignoring your thirst. If you don't want the water, you will feel your body resist it, signifying that you are well hydrated.

Are You Craving Something Crispy and Dry?

If you are craving something crisp and dry, you may be drinking too many liquids. If this is the case, try to keep away from chips because they are rich in fats, especially saturated and trans fats. Avoid crackers that are highly processed and will elevate both glucose and insulin levels. To fulfill your craving for crisp and dry foods, choose rice cakes, high-quality crackers without oil or sugar-free sesame sticks. You can also bake your own potato chips or sweet potato chips, which are much healthier than the store-bought versions.

Are You Craving a Light or Heavy Food?

If you crave heavy foods, ask yourself if you've been eating a lot of salads or fruit. Are you cold, especially your hands and feet? Salads, fruit and other raw foods make the body feel light. They also cool the body and may give rise to cravings for heavier, warming foods, such as fish, beef or hard cheese. Fish is rich in protein, low in fat and high in omega-3 fatty acids, which boost immunity and prevent heart disease.

Sometimes when you're not hungry enough for a meal but need something light to eat, you'll go for a snack. The snack food shelves at supermarkets and even health food stores are full of tantalizing items chock full of sugar. When you're craving a light snack or meal, why not eat some raw or steamed vegetables instead of a sugary snack? If you are hungry and nibbling on a raw carrot doesn't satisfy, try a handful of trail mix, an avocado sandwich or a fruit smoothie.

Are You Craving a Nutritious Food?

When I check in with my body to see what I am actually craving, I often realize that what I really want is something nutritious, something of substance, especially when I am working hard and utilizing the nutrition my body is getting from my diet. This craving also happens when I travel and my routine of eating home-cooked food becomes unavailable. At these times, I long for plain vegetables and simple foods.

Non-Food Cravings

Sometimes we also crave food for emotional reasons. Maybe we are looking for excitement in our lives or looking for comfort after a stressful situation. This nourishment is a kind of emotional feeding. It's not really about the food, but about the emotion it creates.

Are You Craving Entertainment?

We often use food to distract us from boredom. It's important to decipher true cravings from eating as a form of entertainment. If you are bored, try to deal with the issue directly rather than distracting yourself by snacking and munching to fill time. Boredom is a challenge to be more creative with your life. The prime example of this craving is at work. Many people snack or eat just to take a break from staring at the computer. The next time this happens, try taking a walk around the block with a coworker. Or close your office door and stretch for five minutes.

Are You Craving a Hug?

One of the biggest problems with diets today is that people attribute their cravings to appetite and hunger, when these cries are usually from another part of their being that is starving. These cravings have nothing to do with physical nutrition. They are for love, affection and fulfillment. Food can fill you, but not fulfill you. Touch is an important part of the human experience. Don't be afraid to ask for a hug when you need it. Try it with your friends, your kids, your sisters or brothers or whomever you are close with in your life. You might be surprised at how many hugs you've been missing.

Are You Craving Movement?

Stress, hard work and lots of thinking create tension in the body, which can lead to chronic aches, tightness and constipation. Many people try to alleviate these symptoms with alcohol and sugar, which only serve to dampen their unease and anesthetize the body. Exercise is an ideal way of releasing a buildup of physical tension. Developing a regular exercise program to suit your particular body type and lifestyle will have numerous rewards. Start small. Go out for a walk or check out a gentle yoga or karate class. Listen to your body about what kind of movement it desires.

Your Body Loves You, Unconditionally

Physical health is the foundation of our lives. Once we free ourselves from extreme foods, the healing mechanisms of the body can be harnessed to overcome our deeper physical and emotional issues. That's when healing miracles happen. When people learn how to deconstruct their cravings, they can reclaim the sense of balance and bodily harmony that they were haphazardly seeking through indulgence or willpower.

Our bodies are like crying babies. The child is crying but it can't talk, so the mother has to figure out what has disturbed her child. Did it hurt itself, not get enough sleep or wet its diaper? Is it teething or does it have allergies? The mother goes through a process of elimination until she finds the real problem. It's a similar situation with your body. Your body can't talk, but it can send you messages through discomfort or food cravings that need to be decoded. If we acknowledge and accept our cravings, they will point us toward the foods and lifestyles we need. For example, if you have a headache, try to figure out what caused it before taking an aspirin. Did you work too much in front of the computer yesterday? Did you not drink enough water? Did you drink too much wine at a party? Did you sleep with the window closed and deprive yourself of oxygen?

We can, and must, develop dialogue with our bodies. They're talking to us all the time and their messages are too important for us to ignore. And please remember, your body loves you. It does everything it can to keep you alive and functioning. You can feed it garbage, and it will digest it for you and turn it into energy to fuel your life. You can deprive it of sleep, but still it will get you up and running the next morning. You can drink too much alcohol, and it will process it through your system. It loves you unconditionally and does its best to allow you to live the life you came here to live. The real issue in this relationship is not whether your body loves you, but whether you love your body. In any relationship, if one partner is loving, faithful and supportive, it's easy for the other to take that person for granted. That's what most of us do with our bodies, and it's time to change. Working to understand your cravings is one of the best places to begin to build a mutually loving relationship with your own body.

Exercises

1. Craving Inventory

For one week, keep a journal of every food you crave each day. Rate the craving on a scale of 1 to 10, with 10 being the strongest level of desire. Write down your thoughts next to each entry on how that craving is a response to an imbalance somewhere in your diet or life.

Craving rating:

Time of craving:

Type of craving:

Thoughts:

2. Dearest Body of Mine

Write a letter to your body, announcing your intention to listen more carefully to its messages and to act in a more loving way toward it. The following list of suggestions may be helpful to include, but be sure to make your letter personal to your own body. Set a specific period of time aside when you can sit quietly by yourself, undisturbed and in pleasant surroundings, and then begin to write. You don't need to complete the letter in one session. It is sometimes helpful to come back to your letter after a day or two, review the contents and make additions or subtractions. Write from your heart, as well as from your mind.

Dearest body of mine,

After careful thought and consideration, I hereby promise to:
Accept you and be grateful for you just the way you are
Love and appreciate you for what you do
Offer you healthy foods and drinks
Overcome the addictions that hurt you
Realize that laughter, play and rest help you feel good
Exercise regularly and appropriately for my body type
Adorn you with nice, comfortable clothes and shoes
Understand that my unexpressed emotions and thoughts affect you
Listen to the messages you are sending me when you are tired or sick
Accept that I have the power to heal you
Realize that you deserve to be healthy
Honor you as the temple of my soul

I love you so much,

_____

Please Sign here

CHAPTER 7

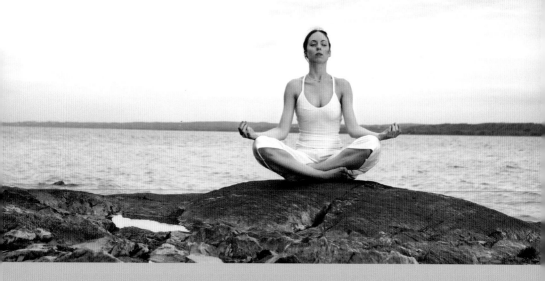

Primary
Food

This chapter explores the differences between ordinary food and what I call primary food. Recall from chapter 1 that primary food is more than what is on your plate. Healthy relationships, regular physical activity, a fulfilling career and a spiritual practice can fill your soul and satisfy your hunger for life. When primary food is balanced and satiating, your life feeds you, making what you eat secondary. But what is primary food?

Please think back to a time when you were passionately in love. Everything was exciting. Colors were vibrant. Intimacy was magical. Your lover's touch and feelings of exhilaration sustained you. You were floating on air, gazing into each other's eyes. You forgot about food and were high on life.

Recall a time when you were deeply involved in an exciting project. You deeply believed in what you were doing and felt confident and stimulated. Time fell away. Hours passed. You developed single-pointed focus. Mealtime and sleep time were irrelevant.

Remember when, as a child, you were playing outside, having fun? Suddenly, your mother announced dinner was ready, but you were not hungry at all. The passion of play took all your attention.

Sometimes we are fed not by food but by the energy in our lives. These moments and feelings demonstrate that everything is food. We take in thousands of experiences of life that can fulfill us physically, mentally, emotionally and spiritually. We hunger for play, fun, touch, romance, intimacy, love, achievement, success, art, music, self-expression, leadership, excitement, adventure and spirituality. All of these elements are essential forms of nourishment.

The extent to which we are able to incorporate them determines how enjoyable and worthwhile our lives feel.

Modern nutrition—carbs or proteins, fresh produce or fast food—is really just one source of nourishment, which I call secondary food. If we are not starving, other dimensions of the human experience are generally much more important to us than what we put in our mouths. Secondary foods don't come close to giving us the joy, meaning and fulfillment primary food provides.

When we use secondary food as a way to alleviate or suppress our hunger for primary food, the body and mind suffer. Weight gain is just one of the consequences. Diet-related disorders such as heart disease, cancer, obesity, high blood pressure and diabetes are national epidemics, and one of the main reasons is because we are stuffing ourselves with secondary foods when we are really starving for primary food.

Chronic depression is also widespread in our society. Globally, an estimated 350 million people suffer from depression, according to the World Health Organization.[1] More than one in 10 people ages 12 and older, in the U.S. alone, take antidepressants.[2] Many also experience frustration, anger, disappointment, sadness and isolation. These conditions and emotions are all cries for primary food, but instead of giving ourselves what we really need, we often turn to secondary food for comfort and solace. The problem is that this substitution does not work. If you are not getting the primary food you need, eating all the food in the world won't satisfy your hunger.

The concept of primary food became clear to me while working in a small natural food store. All day, every day, I watched customers moving through the aisles, shopping, asking questions, giving great care and attention to the quality of the foods they would be consuming. Then, after work, I would often go out into my neighborhood to chill out. Sometimes I would go to the movie theater next door, where many of the popcorn-munching, soda gulping moviegoers were laughing and enjoying themselves with their friends or a romantic partner. I began to notice that the people I saw in the evening often looked healthier, happier and more alive than the people shopping in my store. This got me thinking. It wasn't just about the food.

Once a client came to her coaching session crying about her marriage. While working with her, I saw that eating more fruits and vegetables was not going to make the issue disappear. And then later I found other clients who made great improvements in their health by smoothing out their relationship issues. Creating more positive relationships made them happier and healthier than any dietary changes could have made them. The idea of holistic health is to look at the integrated system rather than one or more separate parts, which includes the physical, mental, spiritual and emotional parts of life. I encourage you to look beyond the food on your plate and consider these other forms of nourishment that truly feed you.

Relationships

During the course of a lifetime, we have relationships with parents, grandparents, children, husbands, wives, boyfriends, girlfriends, extended family, friends, teachers, coworkers—the list is endless. The quality of these relationships explains a lot about the quality of a person's life and his or her health. Just as no one diet is right for everyone, no one way of relating works for everyone. What's important is to cultivate relationships that are healthy and support your individual needs, wants and desires.

Friendships

I believe a key ingredient in personal fulfillment is community. Today, people in the modern world lead overly isolated lives spending large amounts of time with media—watching television, playing with apps on iPads and surfing the Internet. The extended family is gone. You can eat all the broccoli and brown rice in the world, but if you feel isolated and lonely, you are not going to be living life at full capacity. Having high-quality friendships adds depth and meaning to life. Friends who truly listen and care and are open to new ideas can be difficult to come by, but you can take steps to create a positive, supportive community.

I invite you to look at your relationships the same way people look at their wardrobes. You've probably kept many clothes hanging in your closet that you haven't worn for years. Maybe you are hoping they'll come back into style, or maybe they don't quite fit, but you keep them in the back for sentimental reasons.

It's the same with friends. If you think of everyone you know, chances are you will find at least a few people from your past who don't really belong in your present. In fact, if you're honest with yourself, you'll admit you find their company draining, but you keep them in your wardrobe of friends even if they have little to offer in return. Perhaps they are smokers, drinkers or drug users, and you've moved on from that scene. They could be past lovers who keep hanging around, or people whose lives are always in crisis, requiring large amounts of time or energy from you, never to return the favor. Remember, you're their friend, not their therapist.

I suggest you determine which of these people you can let go of. If breaking off all contact seems too drastic, you can downgrade your relationships with them. You may want to keep them in the back of your dresser rather than the central part of your closet. You can see them less often, give them less of your energy or stay in touch by email. If this seems scary, don't worry. You will be maintaining your quality friendships while at the same time clearing space for new people to come into your life.

I once had a client who was struggling with low self-esteem and confidence, due to her upbringing in a dysfunctional family setting. Most of her friends did not treat her very well. Then one day, through our coaching, she woke up and saw the whole picture. She had unconsciously recreated her parents in her circle of friends. She was always the one calling to set up times to meet; she was the one who was listening to most of the problems. The friends were the ones canceling at the last minute or asking for favors, and it just wasn't working for her.

So step-by-step, for months, she let go of people. She took them off her cell phone, stopped sending them email and created a vacuum in her life. At first it felt lonely. Eventually, it felt new and exhilarating to have free time to think and feel. Slowly but surely, she found herself meeting new people and making friends with inspirational people she admired.

Please think of two or three people you would enjoy spending more time with—people who are more of a contemporary mirror for you and have qualities with which you resonate. Maybe you're thinking of someone outside your social strata, but you are excited by the idea of spending more time with them. Contact them. One of the easiest ways to do this is to invite them out for tea or lunch. The worst that could happen is that they say no, but if you set an intention, the universe will deliver. Once you are clear about who they are, be proactive and take initiative to see them more often.

Like all relationships, friendships take work. They can also be hugely rewarding. Remember, friendship is primary food. It should nourish you.

Love and Intimacy

We all have a need to give and receive love. Love is food for the soul. Love nourishes body, mind and spirit. To bring more love and intimacy into your life, I suggest improving connections with everyone. Being well connected with others—husbands, wives, boyfriends, girlfriends, parents, children, friends, family and coworkers—is an essential part of life. We all feel a sense of comfort, safety and connection when we are free to express our hopes and dreams, fear and anger, joy and struggles with others.

When examining relationships, try to understand your personal preference in regard to how much intimacy you want in your life. Some people love being alone; they feel energized by the experience and require plenty of time to catch up with themselves. These people are relatively introverted and develop ways to be on their own with great ease. They usually prefer to relate with one or two people and are finicky about their choices in friends. At the other end of the spectrum are those who love being around people. They are more extroverted, become energized by social interaction and often create an extended family and a network of friends. They have hundreds of people on speed dial and their email list is very extensive. They look forward to seeing everyone at parties, holidays and group events.

Most people fall somewhere in the middle. It may be helpful to think about your own social needs and preferences on a scale of 1 to 10. Where do you fall on this scale? Please avoid making judgments about what is socially acceptable or superficially desirable, and take time to reflect about who you really are and what style of relating works best for you. No rules, just what is genuinely true for you at this point in your life. Vive la différence!

When I suggest improving the quality of your relationships, I am not suggesting everyone should be more social or get married. I am saying, find a type of love and intimacy that is appropriate and nourishing for you. It's a bit like establishing the amount of protein, vegetables or exercise that is appropriate for your body. Each person needs to find the right balance of togetherness and aloneness, and know that these needs will change with time, just as dietary needs change and just as everything in life changes.

For single people who are dating, experiencing love and intimacy can be tricky because you don't have a set agreement with one person or an established routine. Each person is new and you have to navigate these new relationships. In these new situations, be clear with yourself about what you are looking for. Confusion often arises when one person is looking for a life partner and the other person is looking to meet a lot of different new people. Wouldn't it be so much easier if you were honest about this up front? It greatly reduces confusion later.

For singles: Take some time to get as clear as possible with yourself about what kind of experience you want to have with dating. Are you looking to meet a lot of different people? Are you looking for deeper intimacy, but only for a short period of time? Are you looking for a life partner? As you are dating, what you want will probably change, so keep checking in with yourself about your priorities. This is much more effective than just throwing yourself out there to see what happens or going along with whatever your friends are doing or whatever your date wants. When you are clear about your priorities, you can communicate them clearly to the people you date. In the end, you will find yourself spending time with the people or person who want the same kind of relationship or relationships that you do. Also, spend some time assessing your personal boundaries. What are some healthy expressions of love that you want to experience? What kinds of behaviors and attitudes are you not comfortable with? The better you understand your own boundaries and desires, the more you'll be able to make healthier choices for you.

People with boyfriends or girlfriends often feel they have a "go-to" person to experience love and intimacy. In my opinion, open communica- tion is extra important at this stage of relationship. Everyone has different ideas of what it means to be in a relationship—how much time you spend together, how serious you are, when to meet the parents, etc. Often our ideas come from our families or from the media, but your ideas about relationships may differ drastically from those ideas. So be open and share your needs and ideas with your partner. Some couples like to set time frames. For example, they might say to each other, "This seems like it's working—let's do this for three months and then check-in again." Sometimes it's going great, sometimes it's not working out so they make some changes and keep going, and sometimes they separate. In all those cases, both partners know what the other one wants and needs in order to enjoy and be nourished by the relationship. Whether you are with your boyfriend or girlfriend for three months or three years or forever, talking things through in a gentle, honest and caring manner will make the whole experience more loving and less stressful.

People who are married often have a bond that goes beyond personal needs. They often have children together, a community of friends in common and share ownership of cars, houses or businesses. I've noticed many married people eventually get stuck in a rut. They may care strongly for one another but have no time to spend together. Or they may have "lost that loving feeling" and focus solely on the external trappings of their relationship. In the U.S. only about 50% of marriages last. Marriage relationships need to be nurtured by both partners. I strongly encourage married people to find time to spend alone together, and to find more time to have fun. Sit down every so often and evaluate how things are going and if any changes need to be made. Small resentments that build up over time can erode the foundation of any relationship.

Flexibility and growth in marriage is also important. It's kind of crazy to expect the person you married to stay the same for 5, 10 or 20 years of marriage or to expect this person to fulfill all of your needs. Many married couples live together, vacation together, go out to eat together, spend all their free time together. No matter how much you enjoy one person's company, over time you can grow tired of one person if you are constantly together. Work to find balance between activities you enjoy together and activities you can enjoy with other friends or on your own.

It is natural and healthy for everyone to change and grow. If one partner is not open to growing and learning new things, or if only one partner is putting energy into the relationship, it might be healthiest for the marriage to end. But often, you can find a way to work it out. Many, many resources are available for learning how to communicate well and deepen intimacy. If you are concerned about your relationship, find a coach who specializes in helping people in long-term relationships and find one you like. Look for a coach who is happily married. If you don't make progress with one, you may want to try another one before giving up on the process. Take the initiative to create the marriage you really want.

For people at any stage of a relationship, you can increase the level of love and intimacy in your life simply by setting new intentions. Explore what you really want from your relationships. You can journal, meditate or talk to a friend about it. Make a list of what you are looking for from your current relationship or from a new relationship. Look at your list every day and know that you are a unique being who is worthy of love and intimacy. When we are clear about our intentions, the universe very often delivers.

Touch, Hugs and Cuddles

Children who aren't held and touched enough won't grow to their full potential. Babies thrive on human touch, and holding them helps them become healthy, happy and well-adjusted. This holds true for adults as well. Most of us feel nourished by human touch, warmth and intimacy. Yet most adults are touch-starved. We can get along without it, but in time we will feel the lack and crave connection.

It feels good to be touched, to be massaged, to feel physically connected to other people. However, our society tends to confuse touching with sexuality so that many people today actually fear touch. In certain cultures, it's common for women to walk arm-in-arm and for men to hold hands, but in Westernized countries this behavior is much less acceptable. Two men holding hands are assumed to be gay, and if women are too affectionate, people raise their eyebrows.

Sexual concerns aside, touching makes many people feel uncomfortable because it is an open expression of love, care and appreciation. If someone is not accustomed to expressing their feelings or to giving and receiving love, a layer of embarrassment and awkwardness around physical contact may exist. You've probably noticed this barrier even between family members or close friends.

You can break through this social barrier by finding comfortable, non-threatening ways to connect. Human touch helps us realize we're all in this crazy, modern world together. Think of it in the same way as a supplement. Be sure to get your recommended daily allowance of positive human interaction and touch. It's not as difficult as you may think. You can find people who are aware that modern life is increasingly isolating, and who want to connect and say hello in a warm way. Talk with one or two people you currently feel close to, such as a partner, parent, child or friend, about exchanging neck and shoulder massages. Even a five-minute neck rub can have a positive impact on your day. A little touch goes a long way.

Sensuality and Sexuality

Another level of physical contact, beyond massage, hugs and cuddling, is sensual touch and sexual interaction. These experiences can be very nourishing, and it is important that people understand what they're looking for in these delicate areas. Sex is a major part of life, but issues around sensuality, sexuality, love and relating are rarely discussed in an open, intelligent manner.

None of us would be here without sex. Sex created me. Sex created you. So, it's completely natural and normal that most of us are fascinated by sex. It doesn't mean there is anything wrong with us. If we weren't meant to enjoy sex, we would just touch index fingers or lay eggs to make babies. Or, at the very least, we would not be so full of hormones, that from adolescence on, we feel continually drawn toward sexual contact. Indeed, within the deepest and most primal part of our brain, we are programmed to seek pleasure.

For many centuries sex has been considered primarily a means of reproduction. The idea of sex as a nourishing, pleasurable and recreational experience, unrelated to childbirth, is relatively new, especially for women. Since the Woman's Movement, women have enjoyed economic independence and access to birth control, and having a baby is a choice. Sex is not just for making babies. Sex can be fun. Sex doesn't even require a partner. People have always pleasured themselves but usually in secret and cloaked in guilt. Recently, this has expanded to include full permission for both women and men to spend time alone, finding ways to create sensual and sexual pleasure in their own bodies.

The freedom we now experience, living in a relatively liberal, democratic society in the 21st century, has given men and women more opportunities to feed their bodies and souls with positive sexual experiences—whether alone, with a friend or with a committed partner. At the same time, our communication skills about sex haven't quite caught up to our freedoms.

People are often confused about what they're looking for in terms of sex and relationships. This confusion increases the likelihood of misunderstanding, exploitation and frustration. Someone comes into our lives and gives us attention, maybe a warm hug. One thing leads to another, and we feel like we're at the beginning of a relationship. We get excited, making plans for the future and telling all our friends. Next thing we know it's over, and we're sobbing into a half-eaten pint of ice cream.

Sexuality and sensuality are exciting parts of the human experience and can be deeply nourishing if you are clear about what you want. Whether you are casually dating or in a serious relationship, take some time to investigate what you want and need. If there is something you need that you are missing, try to ask for it. If you often find yourself in unhealthy situations, I encourage you to determine what boundaries you need to set for yourself and others and to stick to them. Once you start speaking about your needs in a clear, kind and mature manner, you will see that it is like discussing any other topic. Don't be afraid to express yourself. Others will appreciate your good communication skills and respond to your needs.

It may seem strange to be talking about sex in a book on nutrition, but we can eat an awful lot of green leafy vegetables and not get anywhere near the healing effects that come from having great sex.

I once had a female student in her early 20s who had just recovered from cervical cancer and was suffering from amenorrhea, or loss of her period. She hadn't had her period in more than a year and couldn't figure out why. Doctors wanted her to take birth control, but she wanted to heal naturally. When she shared this with me, I asked her about other parts of her life. She was eating really well, exercising, had an active spiritual practice and a loving, supportive family. She was, however, not having sex. In talking with her further, she admitted she was a highly sexual person but also a monogamous person, not interested in casual sex. She was also raised Catholic and not very comfortable talking about sex. Since there was no man in her life for the past year or so, she was not expressing her sexuality. I advised her to express her sensuality by dressing in a way that made her feel hot, by dancing or flirting. I reminded her she didn't have to have sex to express sexuality. After a few months, she really blossomed into a woman, owning her sexual power, and her periods came back.

Communicating in Relationships

When it comes to relationships, especially intimate relationships, effective speaking and listening are key in staying connected and nourishing one another. But you've probably noticed that it's very rare to have a conversation with someone who actually listens to what you're saying, without interruption or judgment.

Most people live in their heads, thinking about what they have to do tomorrow, what happened yesterday or an hour ago—pretty much anything except the present moment. Have you ever been to a party where someone asked you a question and then didn't listen to a word of your response? These interactions happen all the time. It is equally unusual that we listen to another person without interrupting them, judging or planning what we're going to say next.

We are all starving to be heard. Healing occurs when people listen to us, and when we listen to them. By harnessing the power of listening, you can greatly improve all your relationships. When in conversation with others, try to concentrate and listen to what they are saying. While they are speaking, put all thoughts about yourself out of your head and be present for them. The other person will feel heard and appreciated. This habit will greatly improve the quality of your communication.

Many, many loving and caring couples struggle in their relationships because of communication problems. Sometimes one partner does all the talking, and the other partner does all the listening. Perhaps they only talk about their problems and not about what they love about the other person. Maybe they never talk about their problems but save them up until one day it all comes out in a hurtful manner and the relationship ends. A helpful exercise for any couple is to speak regularly about the positive and negative elements of their relationship and to practice listening to one another.

I recommend scheduling a specific time when both people have enough time and space to discuss delicate issues in a calm and sincere way. You should plan to talk in a space that feels private and safe. You can help establish a healing, positive environment by lighting a candle, playing your favorite music or sharing a meal together.

Begin by looking at the positive. Take turns. Each partner should speak, uninterrupted, for as long as he or she wants about everything that is going well in the relationship. Some things to mention might be how the other person makes you feel, qualities of your partner that you appreciate, gratitude for specific ways in which your partner has supported you lately, and admiration of the other person's appearance. Brag about all the aspects of your relationship that are going well, and allow yourself to fully verbalize and appreciate the other person. One partner should listen carefully and take in all that the other person is saying without interrupting. Then switch so that each person has a chance to speak and to listen.

Take as much time as you want to cover everything that is going well. The bond you share is something worth acknowledging and celebrating. When you have both spoken, take a short break. Sit silently for a few moments, absorbing what each person has said.

Next, take note of one or two aspects of your relationship that you would like to improve. Maybe it's something simple, like household responsibilities, or maybe it's something deeper and sensitive, like wanting more quality time for intimacy and togetherness, or the opposite, maybe a little bit of space would be refreshing. Repeat the same structure as above, allowing one partner to speak openly about his or her feelings and perspective while the other partner listens carefully, and then switch. You can remedy problems more easily once each of you clearly understands what the other wants.

During this exercise, practice communicating without blame to offer solutions and to explain how you would like your relationship to grow. Remember, the aim is to strengthen the flow of nourishing energy that passes between two people. You are each other's primary food, and you are fine-tuning the recipe for long-term satisfaction.

Sometimes a partner may want what the other cannot give. When this happens, don't fall into the trap of resignation. Instead, consider the possibility of asking for outside help. We are not islands. We all have the same basic issues and we don't have to deal with them in isolation. Counseling and support groups are available for every aspect of personal relationships. Once you view your relationship as a form of nourishment, it becomes natural to seek out ways to improve and sustain it so both you and your partner can feel satisfied.

Physical Activity

People need to exercise. Our bodies thrive on movement and quickly degenerate without it. An emerging field of inactivity research suggests that sitting is actually lethal. Most people sit all day at a job, and researchers estimate that people who sit too much are easily shaving a few years off their lives.[3] For those people who work at a desk all day, be sure to get up every hour or so and stretch, walk around your office or even consider a standing desk. When it comes to working out, the challenge is to find the types of exercise you enjoy most, and then build them into your life. Physical activity can take simple and modest forms, like getting off the subway or bus one stop earlier and walking to your destination. It can be taking the stairs, instead of the elevator, to your office or apartment. It can be taking your dog for a walk or your children to the park. A 30-minute brisk walk every day may be all you need to keep yourself in shape. It's good to find something you can do every day without altering your schedule too much. Making physical activity a simple, daily habit greatly increases your chances of staying active.

Something interesting I've noticed is people's inclination to choose exercise that aggravates their current condition. In gyms, the bulky, aggressive people tend to lift weights, which makes them even bulkier and more aggressive. Yoga classes are often full of delicate, vegetarian-type people who would probably be grounded and strengthened by doing some weightlifting, just as a yoga class would lighten weightlifters. I am a big proponent of creating balance, and exercise is a great way to do that. Different forms of exercise will give you different types of energy, and by listening to your body you can find the movement that will work best for you.

After living at Kripalu Center for Yoga & Health, doing yoga every day, I realized I was all stretched out. I was practicing a very relaxing style of yoga, and I needed to get more grounded. So I stopped practicing yoga and switched to weightlifting and running. It provided great balance and stability in my life. In this way, movement is a lot like food. Once you understand how different types of movement nourish your body, you can put together a menu of activities to keep yourself in balance. For example, if you have been feeling frail and unfocused, you could choose vigorous exercise to make you feel stable and powerful, such as kickboxing or running. On the other hand, if you feel tight and tense, you can choose gentler exercise to increase lightness and flexibility, such as swimming or yoga.

Consider what time of day is best for you to get physical activity. Just as some people think more clearly in the morning and others think more clearly at night, some people prefer to exercise first thing in the morning, while others prefer to exercise later in the day. There's no right or wrong; it's simply a matter of personal preference.

Different people require different types of exercise to stay healthy, and your exercise needs will change with time. Stay open to all the options. You can go rock climbing, paragliding, surfing, in-line skating or canoeing, or you can take up Pilates, karate or ballroom dancing. You can find team sports like baseball or volleyball, which have the added benefit of human interaction. Maybe exercising outside in nature is more pleasurable for you. If you are a quiet person who likes a lot of alone time, consider buying a small trampoline or a set of hand weights so you can move in the comfort of your home. Your options are endless. Be experimental and find a routine you can nourish yourself with on a regular basis.

Career

In today's society, most of us spend eight to 10 hours a day at work and very little time with our loved ones. While we are choosy about who we relate with intimately, we spend years doing work we can't stand and that may be completely opposed to our personal values. Think about it for a moment. We have 24 hours each day. We sleep for eight hours, work for at least eight hours and have six to eight hours left for other activities. More than half of our waking hours are spent working—and even more if we include commuting. Work is a huge part of our daily routine, yet how many of us really enjoy it? How many of us complain constantly about what we do but feel powerless to change it? This feeling of helplessness is not a nourishing lifestyle.

A great example of this connection between job satisfaction and health is weight gain. I've known many people who were struggling with their weight, wanting to lose those last 10 pounds. They had tried many diets, and some were even very healthy eaters. But the weight would simply not come off. What they had in common was being unhappy at their jobs. And when they finally found work they liked, the extra weight came right off.

We don't realize the extent to which our lives would improve if we were doing work we loved. We have little to no understanding of our ability to walk away from a particular job or career and begin a new one. In the flexible, fast-moving job market of today's business-oriented society, we can easily have three, four or five careers in a lifetime. Most of our parents and grandparents didn't have such choices. They knew one craft, one skill, and that was all they did. They were dedicated to the company, and the company was dedicated to them. But the modern business environment is different. Each of us has the power to try working for different companies, reinvent our careers and seek out jobs that we find personally and financially satisfying.

We all know someone who has made a satisfying job change—a banker who quit Wall Street to open a bakery; a plumber who retrained as an IT consultant; an editor who started her own publishing company; a salesman who became a stay-at-home dad. Although the modern work world is challenging, it is also a world of opportunity. We have the luxury of creating work that nourishes us and gets us excited about each day. I encourage you to think about your current job—some of your likes and dislikes of what you do each day. Finding work you love is essential to living a healthy, balanced life.

Entrepreneurial pursuits are on the rise. Worldwide, more people than ever are starting their own businesses. Almost 400 million people in 54 countries are considered entrepreneurs, according to the Global Entrepreneurship Monitor Global Report.[4] I'm not surprised, as it's easier than ever to start a business. Launching an online business has very little start-up costs, and connecting with new customers through social media and blogging is a great way to begin. One interesting trend in the U.S. is the rise of senior entrepreneurship. About 25 million Americans ages 44 to 70 are interested in starting their own business or non-profit venture, according to research by Encore.org.[5]

Finding the Work You Love

"Finding the work you love, loving the work you find" is a well-known exercise in the field of job reeducation.

For the first part, "Finding the work you love," take a sheet of paper and list all the things you love to do, including your hobbies, activities you enjoy in your leisure hours, and subjects you read about with great curiosity. This list may include food, massage, exercise, coaching, fashion—almost anything. Take your time; make sure the list is exhaustive. Somewhere in this list lies the key to your new career.

Now review your list. If you could spend eight hours a day thinking about or working with some of these subject areas, which ones would you pick? Circle your top five. Use these as indicators of the kind of work you might find enjoyable. For each item list as many job titles you can think of that relate to a subject area. You might need to do some research. Look up jobs in that field on the Internet. Call someone you know who works in that area. Find out all you can about it.

Once you've listed possible jobs, circle three that are the most appealing to you. You may be strongly drawn to jobs in several areas. In that case, brainstorm how you can blend these together into one career that you would love.

You now have in your hands a key to a new, exciting career. When you have identified and selected your strongest interests, start taking steps to make your new job a reality. It may take some time and effort, but the benefits to your health and quality of life will be enormous. Keep in mind that what you need from a job may change with time. You can always use your creativity and intelligence to create a new situation.

Loving the Work You Find

The other half of this exercise is "loving the work you find." Sometimes it is simply not optimal to go out and create a new career. Or perhaps you like your career, just not your current work environment. This exercise can help you improve your current job as a source of pleasure and nourishment.

PROFILE

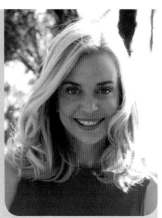

Holli Thompson, Washington, DC, USA

www.HolliThompson.com

"My goal was and still is, to help people heal themselves."

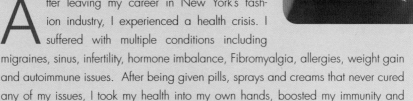

After leaving my career in New York's fashion industry, I experienced a health crisis. I suffered with multiple conditions including migraines, sinus, infertility, hormone imbalance, Fibromyalgia, allergies, weight gain and autoimmune issues. After being given pills, sprays and creams that never cured any of my issues, I took my health into my own hands, boosted my immunity and cleaned up my diet with whole foods and lots of home cooking.

My goal was and still is, to help people heal themselves, just as I was able to do for myself. I named my company Nutritional Style, and my dream became a reality. Of course I was nervous the first time I posted a blog, unsure about sending my first newsletter, and when I was asked to appear on camera for TV, I was terrified. Thankfully, the Institute for Integrative Nutrition gave me the confidence to work through my fears and to reach higher than I thought possible.

I now blog weekly for a number of well-known sites, offer virtual individual and group programs and I have partnered with the American Heart Association, Less Cancer and the Georgetown Hospital Lombardi Cancer Center.

Having my own company allows me to pursue what I want to do and design programs that are in line with what I've been called to do. I'm able to take time out to take on new projects, but most importantly, being an entrepreneur allows me to design my own lifestyle. I'm a wife, a mother and a daughter, and primary foods are an important part of my nutritional style. I make sure that I balance time with family and friends, and I always remember why I became a Health Coach to begin with.

I never imagined that I could have a second big career after leaving my position as a Vice President for Chanel; I couldn't have imagined that I would be appearing on network TV, or that I would someday write my own nutrition book to share my journey. IIN gave me the certification necessary, and the confidence to pursue those dreams.

Take a piece of paper and make a list of everything you like about your work. On the back of the piece of paper make a list of everything you don't like. Think about the content of your work, the structure of your day, your colleagues, your salary, your work environment, opportunities for advancement, any successes or disappointments you have experienced, and how deeply you feel about the importance of the work. What is working and what is not working?

Now imagine you have a job offer from another company. This other job may pay you more, be in a better location or offer more exciting projects. Imagine going to your supervisor's office to give notice. Imagine that when you come out of your supervisor's office you have decided to stay with your current company. Why? What did your supervisor offer you? A raise? A nicer office? A more flexible schedule? A new project? Circle these items on your list.

By making adjustments in these few key areas, you could make your job more exciting and rewarding for yourself. Your job could become a positive influence in your life instead of a drain. By using good communication skills you can enlist the support of your coworkers and supervisor to try to make these improvements. Ask for a raise or for flex time, redecorate your office or request to join a new project. It is up to you to ask for what you need. You may be surprised by how easily you get it.

For example, I think many of my students enroll at my school because they want to work in holistic health instead of their current jobs. They start seeing clients, enjoy the process, graduate, develop momentum to break through to a new career and go to their bosses to give notice. I can't tell you how frequently they walk out with a pay raise. Usually when this happens, they realize they actually enjoy the stability of their full-time job, and choose to do coaching after work or on the weekends as a part-time supplementary career. Sometimes all you need is a 20% pay increase to have renewed appreciation for your job. If you desire a higher salary, and if you are a responsible, intelligent and hard-working employee, there's a good chance you'll get it if you ask.

One of my students was working for a large brokerage firm for many years, and her working hours were just under the requirement for full-time employment because this allowed the company to avoid paying for her benefits and insurance. She was fed up with the way they were treating her, and after months of thinking it through, she decided to quit. She walked into the office and announced she was leaving in two weeks. They immediately gave her the extra hours, switched her to full-time staff and bumped up her pay, saying they'd been thinking of giving her new responsibilities and more money anyway. She decided to stay on.

"I wished I'd done it two years earlier," she confided in me.

Whatever it is you need to make your job a more positive place to be, I encourage you to go after it. Feeling happy and productive in the place you spend most of your time will dramatically increase your sense of well-being.

The Meaning of Work

Too often we equate work with a paycheck. We may think of our jobs only as a means to earn money. Having money to take care of yourself and your family is obviously very important, but it's a limited view of work. For example, some people go to work to make the world a better place. They may be involved in a project that improves the lives of a few people, hundreds of people or the whole planet. For others, work is a form of creativity and self-expression; whether in a corporate office or an artist studio, work is a place to hatch new ideas and to put their personal stamp on the world. Few things are more rewarding in life than meaningful and exciting work. You feel confident and stimulated. Time stops, and the outside world fades away. You are totally absorbed and energized by it. Doesn't it make sense to work on something you are passionate about?

Maybe you are interested in finding work that you can dedicate yourself to, but you haven't come across something that seems worthy of your time. I encourage you to try out new hobbies or interests. Join a club, volunteer with an organization or start a study group with a few close friends. As you explore your interests, you will discover whether or not you really enjoy this new area and, if you do, you will make contact with people who could help you start a new career.

Another way to identify meaningful work is to notice what you already spend your time on. Many of my students have been doing health coaching for years without knowing it. They have been coaching their friends, family members or coworkers about their diets and lifestyles—they just haven't been paid for it. This is a good clue that they will be happy making health coaching their career. Our school helps them take their natural talents and make a career out of it. Once they build confidence and learn the basic skills, they find they are much happier working hard for their own businesses rather than working for someone else.

There is no one right answer about what work means or how to find happiness in your career. Maybe you love working hard in a corporate environment. Maybe you need a less conventional, more flexible relationship with work. Everyone is different. Be honest about what works for you. Remember that we all need to nourish ourselves by finding work we love and being paid fairly for it.

Spirituality

Spiritual nutrition can feed us on a very deep level and dramatically diminish cravings for the superficial rewards of life. We all search for meaning in our lives, and feeling at one with the world can help satisfy that longing. I encourage clients and students to develop and deepen their spiritual practice, whatever that might be. Some people follow their traditional religion of birth. Others explore Eastern religion or New Age spirituality or evolve an integrative approach.

I was raised in an orthodox Jewish family, which valued ritual, tradition and the sacredness of daily life. We celebrated the holidays and fasted and traveled to Israel. I was taught to value of "tikun olam," of trying to make the world a better place and felt connected to this value. It felt good to be one of the "chosen" people. However, it all kind of fell apart when I went to a Catholic college, and I found out they thought they were the chosen people. So, I decided to let it all go and find a path for myself that made sense to me, which took many, many years to evolve.

For me, spirituality means seeing myself as a microscopic part of the cosmos. I believe that whatever force makes the day turn into night and night turn into day, and winter become spring and fall become winter; whatever keeps all the stars and planets going around perfectly in their orbits, creates new buds in spring and moves old leaves to drop away in autumn, can surely look after this one little life of mine. So I take steps to keep myself in harmony with the order of the universe. I eat naturally grown foods, spend time outside, rise when it is light, sleep when it is dark and adjust my activity level according to the season of the year. By doing this I tend to increasingly be in the right place at the right time, doing the right thing, just like all the other major elements in the universe.

Harmonizing with nature is my spiritual practice. For you it may be something different—daily meditation, attending religious services, reading inspirational texts or walking in the woods. Whatever it is, I encourage you to commit to and deepen your practice. Developing spiritual openness and sensitivity can add depth and meaning to your life in a way that nourishes you on a profound level.

Synchronicity

Carl Jung popularized the term "synchronicity," indicating the subtle interaction between individual will and universal law (or God's will or the movement of the cosmos, depending on your perspective). A spiritual practice can help a person become more attuned to synchronicity—to read the signs, to see the way the wind is blowing, to feel the direction in which life wants to go, and then use his or her creativity and intelligence to help it happen in the best possible manner. Once we develop a knack for noticing and welcoming synchronicity, life becomes more interesting and rewarding. We start to meet the right people at the right time to lead us to the next station in life.

It's easy to embrace synchronicity when things are going well, but there are times when events seem to conspire against us. Some days the computer system decides to crash at the very moment I am about to complete an important document, and then I get stuck in a huge traffic jam when I'm in a hurry to get somewhere. Three or four things all seem to conspire against me, preventing me from doing whatever I think I need to do. At such frustrating moments all kinds of interpretations can pop into my mind, including the self-defeating attitude that life is against me.

Life is never against me, or anyone else. In these situations, the most effective strategy is to pause for a few minutes and reflect on the balance between the apparent antagonism of life that is disrupting our plans, and how much or how urgently we want to achieve our goals. Maybe, upon reflection, it's to our advantage that the goals are delayed a little. Maybe we're trying to push events faster than they can go out of fear that things won't turn out the way we want. Take a break. Step back. Reflect. Might there be a reason that life is intervening at this moment?

At the same time, paying attention to synchronicity doesn't mean we should give up on our efforts and goals. It doesn't mean that every time something goes wrong we are on the wrong path. We shouldn't let the negative or challenging influences in life justify procrastination or allow us to abandon our goals in favor of temporary pleasures and distractions.

A spiritually healthy life is lived in delicate balance between these two extremes: will and letting-go, goal-orientation and spontaneous impulse, personal desire and the cosmic plan. We need to learn how to walk a middle path, to be sensitive to the natural flow of events while not throwing away our own determined idea of where we want to go.

Some helpful tools are available, if you desire to become more attuned to synchronicity. These tools include the Chinese masterpiece, *The I Ching*, or *Book of Changes*, astrology, numerology and tarot cards. They can all help you learn to read the signs and signals of life, but don't take these tools too seriously; otherwise you may wind up relying on them to make simple, ordinary decisions.

If you want to explore the same phenomenon without such tools, try creating a record of all the moments in your life when you felt synchronicity was happening to you: the people you met at pivotal moments by coincidence, the chances you took on a gut feeling, the decisions that somehow happened by themselves, the dreams you had that eventually happened during waking moments. When you have finished, see if you can apply this understanding to your daily life now, paying more attention to little synchronous happenings, like when the phone rings and it's the right person at the right time. You'll soon get the hang of it.

Awareness

Almost all forms of spiritual practice come down to one thing: the more we bring our individual lives into alignment with the whole of existence, the more we feel nourished and at peace. Awareness practices can help connect that alignment. They are designed to quiet the busy mind, relax the body, and bring a sense of attunement with existence. Prayer, meditation and ritual meals are all common awareness practices found in many religions and spiritual traditions.

Here is a simple awareness exercise that anyone can do. Sit in a relaxed, comfortable position, breathe through your nose and notice how the air is slightly cooler going in and slightly warmer going out. Place one hand over your heart and one hand over your belly. Feel your heart beating and thank your heart for being there for you all day every day, pumping your blood and keeping you alive. Feel your belly, noticing the rise on the inhale and the fall on the exhale. Thank your belly for digesting all the food you eat. Sit silently, with your eyes closed, and allow yourself to be with yourself. When you feel ready, take a deep inhale and exhale, open your eyes, rise and move back into your day.

I encourage you to incorporate simple practices like this one into your life on a regular basis. As you deepen your connection to the greater processes of life you may find yourself coping with stress and emotions more easily, relating more lovingly with others and finding more joy in life.

Exercises

1. The Circle of Life

This exercise will help you to discover which primary foods you are missing the most. The Circle of Life has 12 sections. Look at each section and place a dot on the line marking how satisfied you are with each area of your life. A dot placed at the center of the circle, or close to the middle, indicates dissatisfaction, while a dot placed on the periphery indicates ultimate happiness.

When you have placed a dot on each of the lines, connect the dots to see your circle of life.

You will have a clear visual of any imbalances in primary food, and a starting point for determining where you may wish to spend more time and energy to create balance and joy in your life.

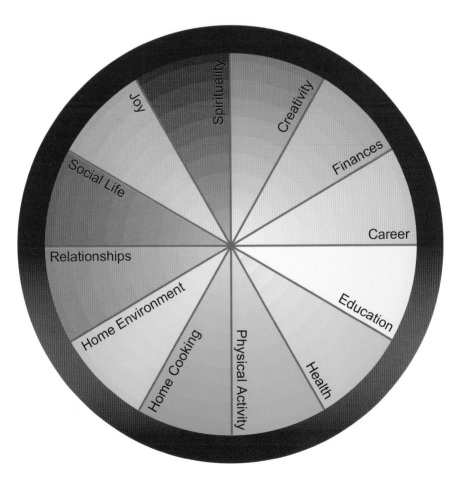

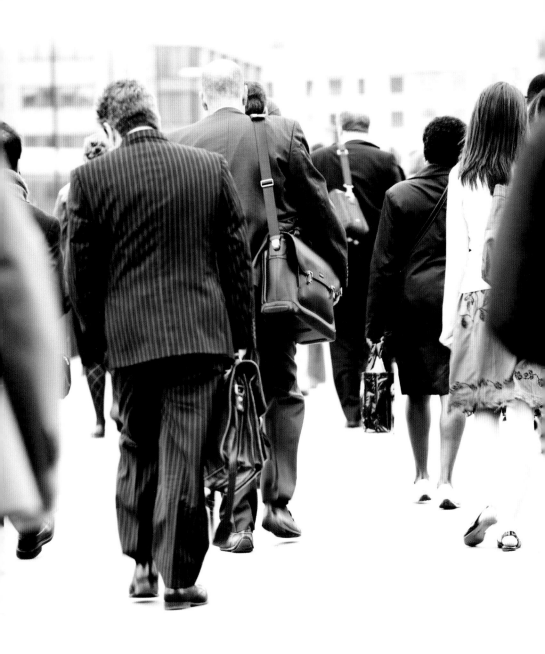

CHAPTER 8

Escape
the Matrix

Most people now begin realizing that they live in the matrix. What most people don't realize is that the matrix lives in them. Whenever we permit sodas, candy bars, junk food and cigarettes to enter our body, we're letting the energies and vibes of corporations, factories, offices, CEOs and executives into our very being. These are the active ingredients of the matrix.

—ZEMACH ZOHAR, www.alokhealth.com

We may live a large portion of life never questioning what we've been taught. We go along with this sort of matrix mentality, unaware of what other realities are possible for our lives. Escaping the matrix and reclaiming our own individuality and lifestyle is the task at hand. It is extremely challenging and rewarding. And, when you start to wake up and look around, you will find many other intelligent people on the same path.

What is the matrix? As Morpheus said, "The matrix is everywhere." We are completely surrounded and enveloped by it. It's the accepted beliefs and false concepts about the world that drain our life force. It's a kind of mental, emotional and spiritual programming. It's more than the corporate agenda; it's from the government, the church, big business. It's the persistence that we all should get married, have children, join a church and buy stuff. You can feel it at work, at church or at the grocery store.

It creates our collective beliefs about food, fashion and most aspects of life. It's the constant drum that calls us to produce, process, sell and buy. It's the voice in our heads that tells us not to rock the boat, not to take risks. It's the treadmill many of us feel we are running on, which we can never move forward on. The matrix is what's familiar and even comfortable to most people, yet the beliefs and practices it demands steal our happiness, our authenticity and our future. The matrix dictates to us its rules about our food, our health, our relationships, our spirituality and how we should live.

Think about what the matrix looks like. It's slender women who are young forever, virile men who are wealthy and powerful. It's an endless parade of things to buy, to play with, to wear and to consume. The matrix pushes fast food, mass-produced junk, caffeine, sugar, white flour, meat, alcohol and medications to temporarily anesthetize us from feeling our feelings. The matrix has us running on stress, in survival mode, and always tells us we're not enough and we need more. The matrix says we never look good enough. It insists that we are really alone in this world. It tells us not to trust others. And it hypnotizes us in forgetting our true essence and greatness.

We may show our independence by making cynical, sophisticated remarks about aspects of the culture that surrounds us, about TV commercials or certain products, but in the end it is nearly impossible not to succumb to the overwhelming forces that bombard us every day with these messages. Millions of dollars are spent every day to persuade us to do things and to buy things that we would never otherwise buy.

We allow clothing companies to brand us, abandoning our individuality and covering ourselves with logo-emblazoned sneakers, pants, shirts, purses and jackets. Then we parade ourselves in front of each other, trying to gauge who has been branded best. We equate these brands with lifestyles. They represent youthfulness, luxury or fun. These brands even fill needs, like the need to belong or to feel respected.

I have no desire to replace the free market economy or the democratic system with some revolutionary utopian ideal. But it's ironic that in the years when Soviet and Chinese communism were viewed as a threat to the free world, intellectuals pointed out how brainwashing techniques and other forms of social programming were used to control the behavior of millions of people. Yet we rarely pause to think about what's happening now. The matrix is also a form of corporate "social-ism." It is an extremely powerful set of attitudes, beliefs and thoughts that are relentlessly imposed on the public, every day, through many media channels. And the business-oriented motives that drive it are escalating and causing damage to the mental and physical health of millions of people and the planet.

Corporations have developed their own self-interested economic laws and dynamics because their survival depends on it. A fundamental economic law is that the corporation must always do what is best for the corporation, which is to maximize profits, outperform competitors, expand, grow and keep shareholders happy with high-performance stocks and regular dividend payouts. The health and welfare of the consumer is irrelevant.

Top Ten Advertising Categories of 2012[1]

RANK	COMPANY	YEAR 2012 ($ MILLIONS)	YEAR 2011 ($ MILLIONS)	% CHANGE
1	Retail	$16,345	$15,866	3%
2	Automotive	$14,840	$13,848	7%
	Manufacturers	$8,859	$8,582	2%
	Dealers	$5,981	$5,266	14%
3	Local Services	$8,978	$8,736	3%
4	Telecom	$8,660	$8,348	4%
5	Financial Services	$7,889	$8,074	-2%
6	Personal Care Products	$6,836	$6,535	5%
7	Food & Candy	$6,567	$6,433	2%
8	Direct Response	$6,342	$6,224	2%
9	Restaurants	$6,185	$5,912	4%
10	Insurance	$4,860	$4,949	-2%
	TOTAL[2]	$87.502	$84,916	3%

SOURCE: Kantar Media
1. Figures do not include FSI, House Ads or PSA activity
2. The sum of the individual companies can differ from the total shown due to rounding

Escaping the cultural matrix of needing to look, dress and eat a certain way means mustering the courage to step away from outside influences, to look inside and ask yourself, "Who am I, and what do I really want from my life?" As an example, look at the U.S. One of the most fundamental concepts embedded in the American psyche is freedom. Americans like to think we are the freest people in the world, and, in a way, we are.

But I see two types of freedom: freedom from and freedom for. Where "freedom from" is concerned, we are doing well. Through our democratic institutions, particularly the U.S. Constitution and the Bill of Rights, we have achieved a great deal of freedom from religious persecution, from monarchy, from undemocratic political systems like communism, fascism and military dictatorships. But what is "freedom for"? Freedom for what? To work our butts off all day and then sit in front of a TV, computer or PlayStation until it's time for bed? To stuff our mouths with processed food until our pants burst or our bodies deteriorate? To chase after the latest products that will make us feel complete? Isn't there something more to life? Our "freedom for" habits have spilled over to the rest of the Western world and I urge everyone to consider what freedom means to you.

Hungry? Why Wait?

One of the most insidious features of the matrix is that it tells us that life is about instant gratification. And if life is about getting what we want as fast as possible, then so is eating. In fact, our nutrition woes today can be summed up in a one-liner from a Snickers commercial: "Hungry? Why wait?" Introduced to the market in 1930, Snickers has global sales of more than $2 billion and is the world's best-selling candy bar due to savvy marketing techniques based on giving people what they think they want—fast, convenient, colorfully packaged food. [1]

As the slogan implies, there's no need to wait until the next meal, no need to cook food or wait for other family members to get home to sit down together for a meal. Just grab the nearest tasty thing and pop it in your mouth. Modern marketing and distribution have ensured that when we feel hungry, many products are lining the shelves of the local stores or stacked in the office vending machine. Almost all these foods are loaded with calories, fat, refined sugar, processed salt, dairy products and artificial chemicals—making them foods that are not really fit for human consumption. Just look at the ingredients listed on the Snickers wrapper. They are as follows: milk chocolate (sugar, cocoa butter, chocolate, lactose, skim milk, soy lecithin, artificial flavor), peanuts, corn syrup, sugar, skim milk, butter, milk fat, partially hydrogenated soybean oil, salt, egg whites and artificial flavor. I have nothing against Snickers bars. I even ate one a few years ago, but I'm using Snickers as an example of the way people are being seduced into buying foods that, when eaten regularly over time, increase weight and decrease health.

The less healthy a food is, the more money companies spend on its marketing. Advertising is a multibillion-dollar industry charged with stimulating the buying impulses of the biggest consumer society on the face of the earth. We are constantly bombarded with ads encouraging us to eat and drink more.

From the billboard on the side of the bus to the back cover of a stranger's magazine on the subway, from commercials slotted between songs on the radio to the pop-up ads on our social media and Internet searches, we are inundated by commercial messages every day.

For children, it's even worse. Every Saturday morning, children are bombarded with junk food ads for high-sugar and high-fat foods like Pop-Tarts, cereal bars and many types of processed cookies, cakes and snacks. Is this really what we want to teach young people today? Good nutrition is crucial in the formative years, but our kids are eating junk, especially in the school system, and it shows. In the U.S., childhood obesity rates have tripled in the last 30 years.[2] Scientists predict our children are the first generation in American history to live shorter lives than their parents.

The number of 30-second TV commercials seen in a year by an average child is 16,000, and the number-one ranking advertiser for child-oriented advertising on television is the junk food, fast food industry.[3] Most parents would be shocked to see ads for cigarettes or alcohol during the Saturday morning lineup. They should be equally upset by junk-food advertising, especially as childhood obesity rates continue to skyrocket.

It's no surprise that obese children are also more susceptible to food ads seen on TV, which makes them more likely to eat, according to a 2012 study published in the *Journal of Pediatrics*. The study's authors also found that companies spend more than $10 billion each year on food and beverage ads for children and that 98 percent of those products are high in fat, sugar and salt.[4]

Small strides have been made with children's television networks like Walt Disney Co., Nickelodeon and the Cartoon Network, who have begun reworking ads to meet federal guidelines for nutrition and restricting their characters from promoting unhealthy products.[5] Schools are also making slow improvements. In 2010 Congress passed the Healthy, Hungry-Free Kids Act, which in addition to improving the health of all school meals, it all also requires competitive foods—the ones sold outside the school meal program, which include fast food items, sodas and junk food in vending machines, etc. But in April 2013 public health lawyer Michele Simon wrote that the "USDA's narrow focus on nutrients such as grams of fat and sugar will still result in highly-processed junk food with only slightly improved nutritional profiles." I would say we still have a long way to go to help kids escape the junk food matrix.

I'd like to make it clear that I am not against fast, convenient food. I think it's a great idea. But I long for the day when the colorful packages on our supermarket shelves and the papery wrappers from fast food restaurants contain good, wholesome, nutritious foods that keep us healthy. It is possible. All we need is enough people to demand it. Then instantly, overnight, the companies whose existence depends on knowing what we want and supplying it will switch to healthy products in order to guarantee their own survival. It's really up to us.

I've said it before and it's important to remember that what we're dealing with today is something totally new. Nothing like this massive-consumer society of ours has ever happened in the history of humanity, and it's very possible nothing like it will ever happen again. This message may seem simplistic. Maybe you think you're aware enough to see beyond the glitz and hype? But the ads keep coming, they keep entering your brain, and their influence is powerful and escalating. Can you be vigilant enough in your own life to filter out the useless messages the matrix communicates?

Think of how its influence affects your own moods and feelings. Compare the way you feel after spending a few hours in the park versus watching a few hours of TV. Or think of a time when you were chasing things outside yourself to fulfill you. Consider your relationship to food after spending the morning at a local farmers' market talking to the people who grew the food versus sticking a few quarters into a vending machine to satisfy an afternoon craving.

The Pressure to Be Thin

The idea of being thin enters girls' minds very early in life. Increasingly, young girls say they want to be thinner. About half of girls in the United States between the ages of 11 and 13 see themselves as overweight.[6] Most of these girls own a Barbie doll, and Barbie has a body shape that is impossible to attain. If Barbie were a real woman, she would be about 6 feet tall with a bust measurement of 39 inches, a waist of 18 inches and hips of 33 inches. Her

PROFILE

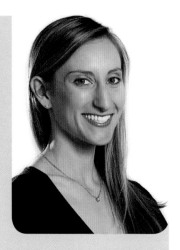

Sheri Oppenheimer, Atlanta, GA, USA
www.100womenproject.com

"I learned how to manage my stress and anxiety once and for all."

My lifelong struggle with anxiety began when I was in second grade taking timed math tests. I would freeze under pressure and fail every single test, despite my proficiency in math. Although I went on to achieve straight A's throughout high school and Dean's List in college, my anxiety hovered over me. Growing up, my mom always struggled with her weight. She always says she is the incredible expanding woman, having lost 1,600 pounds—40 pounds, 40 times! She tried every diet under the sun. I had learned to rely on exercise and a vegetarian diet as a way to manage my anxiety, and began helping my mom overcome her struggle by supporting and educating her.

After college, I worked at several Fortune 100 companies, balancing 60-hour weeks, long commutes and fast-paced environments. I wasn't passionate about my career and my health was suffering. I was burned out and ready for a change.

I turned to my mom for help with the anxiety I was experiencing, who at this point had lost close to 90 pounds thanks to our long walks and healthy dinners together. She had just enrolled at Integrative Nutrition and shared her knowledge with me in an effort to help. After looking through the class materials, I knew I had found my calling! I enrolled the next day. Throughout my time at IIN, I learned how to manage my stress and anxiety once and for all. In 8 short months, I built a thriving health coaching practice, earned back my tuition, left my corporate job, ended a relationship, moved to a new city, and opened an office in an organic day spa in Atlanta, GA.

Over a mother/daughter weekend to New York City, my mom and I decided that if we could help each other overcome our health challenges, we could empower millions of other women around the world to do the same. We started with 100 women and The 100 Women Project was born. The Project took off immediately and there is no stopping us! To date, we have women involved in every state in the U.S. and more than 20 countries, and we're growing every day. I feel incredibly grateful to have this opportunity to help women around the world reach their health and happiness goals, once and for all.

weight would be about 110 pounds.[7] If women were really built like Barbie, they would not be able to walk, have a menstrual cycle, give birth or breathe. If young girls see this doll as an image of what it is like to be a woman, what kind of message does that send to them about how they should look?

Despite the many strides women have made in recent history, we still live in an overly masculine modern society. The world needs strong, powerful, nurturing women to balance this energy. But many women are limited and silenced by their insecurities because of the messages they have received throughout their lifetimes about what it means to be female.

Read any women's fashion magazine and you will see that the content and advertising are incessantly inflaming, and cashing in on, obsessions with measuring up to media-driven images. The pages are covered with emaciated women, who our society agrees are beautiful. These models are idealized, and the advertisements make us want what they've got so that normal-size women will go and buy those Louis Vuitton handbags or Ralph Lauren sunglasses to feel attractive.

What is shown in magazines, however, is not reality. The magazines don't publish disclaimers announcing that the models work for hours with the world's best hair and makeup artists, that the clothes are tailored to fit their exact shape or that professionals retouch the photos. Blemishes are removed, cellulite airbrushed, and any extra fat from the belly, thighs, and arms is erased.

Women see these ads and begin to believe they are supposed to roll out of bed being as beautiful as these models on the pages of the magazine. Men also see these ads and impose their unrealistic ideals onto women.

Supermodels represent the cutting edge of all that is supposed to be beautiful and desirable in a woman. But they come from another planet. Typical models are thinner and taller than 99.9% of women. The average model is 5'11" and weighs 117 pounds. In the U.S., the average woman is 5'4" and weighs 164 pounds. To keep their jobs, models must maintain as little body fat as possible. The human body, especially the female body, is simply not designed to operate without body fat. It's an inhuman concept. Small wonder that, on any given day, more than half the women in this country are on a diet, trying to mold themselves into an artificially created cultural concept of what it means to be beautiful.

Even now, in the 21st century, women are squeezed between two powerful cultural forces. One is the pressure to consume readily available, unnecessarily fattening foods, and the other is the pressure to conform to a female stereotype that demands slimness as a prerequisite for beauty. In both cases, advertising is the key to unlocking their minds and purses. Marketing is the catalyst, the trigger that stimulates and provokes them to buy both the unhealthy food and the unhealthy ideal of beauty.

Advertising encourages women to substitute food for love, while glamorizing images of borderline anorexic women. The media is reluctant to examine the impact of advertising on the public's health because it depends on advertising for commercial viability and cannot afford to bite the hand that feeds it. As discussed in chapter 1, governments are compromised by the power of corporate interests. Left to ourselves, we can just drift along with the collective cultural mindset and try to make the best of it, or we can choose to stand up for what we know is the truth, regardless of what the media pushes us to believe.

Superwoman Syndrome

Liberated from the confinement of traditional female roles, with increasing opportunities to explore areas once exclusively for men, modern women frequently end up leading chronically stressful lives as they struggle to balance all their options. They want to be successful in business, have a great marriage, beautiful children, a dynamite figure with a flat belly, involve themselves in the arts and maybe even run for office someday. Phew! Just thinking about it makes me stressed out. I know many women who suffer from the Superwoman Syndrome, trying to maintain this stressful lifestyle, and then wondering why it's not making them happy.

I am a great believer in encouraging people to slow down. I understand why women want to explore all the possibilities open to them, having been denied them for so long, and I admire those who manage to do so. But sooner or later anyone who maintains such a high-powered lifestyle, man or woman, is bound to see that an intelligent selection of priorities is required. Courage is also needed to stand up and say, "Okay, everyone. You can pass me on the fast track to success. I've tasted it, understood it, and I am no longer interested in keeping up because I know now that the price is too high. I want to stay true to myself, and I want to enjoy myself. These are my priorities."

Superman Syndrome

Men also face sexual oppression in our society. Men today have enormous pressure to be strong, to provide for their families and to be there for their wives or lovers. In recent years, marketing geared toward men has dramatically expanded to include images of men with fit bodies, including six-pack abs, who are also highly successful in their careers.

When I teach about sexual oppression at the school, I am always reminded of the pressure men feel to be successful in their professions. Just as women are seen as "sex objects" in our society, men are seen as "success objects." Somehow, men in our culture get the message that if they don't "bring home the bacon," and in large quantities, they are failures. The drive to be a success object often causes men to override their bodies. They don't listen to the wisdom of their cells, to the gentle voice inside that would have them go slower and be more self-loving. After all, by our culture's standards, this isn't very manly.

In helping men overcome the pressure to be "perfect" by our society's standards—to have a fit body and a well-paying job, and to be open, but not too sensitive—I encourage men to seek support. I urge them to create communities where they feel comfortable, free from the pressure to conform to other people's ideals of who or what they should be and where they can express their emotions openly, without judgment. Lastly, I support them in letting go of any guilt or responsibility for things that may have happened in the past.

Men in our culture are ready to learn that they don't need to sacrifice their bodies for success. Males are often expected to lay it all on the line, to sacrifice their health to toxic jobs and to the military, to push themselves with pride and take injuries or wounds "like a man." Yes, men can be strong, but they can also be vulnerable. Many men want to nourish themselves and be caring around their own health. They need encouragement and permission, not only from the women around them but also from their fellow men.

The Individual

Even though I look at the big picture, at the structure of the matrix surrounding us, my focus is always on the individual sitting in front of me, and on listening carefully with an open mind to what she or he is saying. This perspective is from Zen Buddhism. It's called "Beginner's Mind" and refers to the art of approaching something with an innocent attitude, in a fresh, receptive and inquiring manner. This is a wonderful way to starve the matrix and let your beauty and truth shine through.

I look at the person in front of me—whether a student, client or friend— as a *tabula rasa,* a clean slate, and I ask them, "How are you? What is your health concern?" A lot of evidence exists in the counseling and coaching worlds that a person will get themselves well just by speaking about their problems and receiving love without the listener making any recommendations. This approach takes time and runs counter to mainstream healthcare, in which the focus is to get the job done quickly by diagnosing symptoms, identifying diseases and prescribing medications.

Looking back, I notice that many of my clients have recovered quickly without the need for medications or other interventions. I attribute this to my careful listening skills, my sincere appreciation for them and my deeper knowledge that they need not suffer. In fact, many of my clients and students could probably have worked out their problems on their own, without my help, if they were willing to put as much attention and intelligence into their own healthcare as they do into their professional lives. But this rarely happens. Society, culture and media all shift people away from caring for their own health, drawing the focus away from what's "inside here," to what's "out there." Fashion, the lives of celebrities and gossip take precedence over our own physical health and well-being.

I like to remind my students to love and respect themselves and to take time to listen to the needs of their bodies, minds and souls. I encourage people to notice the issues that are troubling them, and then invest time and energy into fixing them. Our method makes people focus on themselves and address the issues that are bothering them. Once this happens, the solution is usually quite obvious, and the person with the answers is usually the individual, not the professional. But having that person there, a trained listener who is devoted to helping them get better, is how people discover their answers.

Fitting Out

One of the more powerful ways we can free ourselves from the matrix is to learn to "fit out" rather than trying to always "fit in." We are all susceptible to the age-old social pressure to conform, be accepted and keep up with the Joneses. Who cares about the Joneses? This need to fit in keeps us locked into the matrix, which pushes for a poor diet and fast foods. Its illusions push us to work harder, relying on addictive stimulants, like coffee, sugar and cigarettes. As a slave to our own ambitions, we feel compelled to push forward with all our life force. Getting off this treadmill requires a willingness to stand on our own and disregard others' opinions.

I am personally sensitive to this tendency because, being raised in an Orthodox Jewish family, I grew up with a need to fit in, not attract unnecessary attention, and pretend I was just like everyone else. That's why it's easy for me to spot the same tendency in others. I have noticed when people shift to significantly different lifestyles, they sometimes try to hide it or play it down for similar reasons. So as you're starting to make healthier food choices or quit drinking or whatever new things to nurture yourself, I encourage you to come out of the closet, be open about it and let people know what you're about.

Many Integrative Nutrition students do not fit into average society. In one way or another, they live on the periphery and don't want to attract too much attention, so they mimic the customs and habits of their families and neighbors, despite feeling like the black sheep of their families. They tell me, "I'm nothing like my brother or my sisters, my parents, or my next-door neighbors. I see myself as being quite different from the society around me." But they'll blend in with the crowd, chatting about the latest election, sporting event or social happening, and wear the same clothing, just to be acknowledged as part of the collective. Others may have an interest in healthier eating habits but feel that they don't want to interrupt their usual routines, whether it's lunch at a fast-food restaurant with coworkers or food served at family events. Our eating habits—at home, at the office or in the restaurant—are sure to reflect our willingness to compromise for the sake of social harmony. I suggest starting small. Experiment with bringing a healthier dish to a family function or let your coworkers know about a new healthy place that just opened.

Another area in which people, including myself, often compromise for the sake of appearances is in relationships. After three years of marriage, I felt mine wasn't working, but I stayed married for another three years because my parents were so happy that I had married a Jewish woman. I couldn't imagine disappointing them. This same pressure manifests in a thousand different ways in other parts of our lives. I often refer to sections of the newspaper to illustrate this topic. We have a section for wedding announcements with smiling, happy couples. But we don't have a divorce section with pictures of smiling women or men who have decided to take their own path. Are you caught in your own picture, trying to uphold something that's not working? Maybe it's a relationship, a job or a way of eating.

I'd like you to pause for a moment and reflect on how much of your intelligence and creativity is being channeled into "fitting in." My own experience is that if you put the same amount of effort into "fitting out"—giving yourself permission to be spontaneous, natural and authentic in the way you live and behave—you'll immediately become much happier and more content.

Escaping the matrix is a key step in creating true health and happiness. Start by noticing the places in your life where you feel inauthentic. Are there certain people who you have difficulty expressing your true self around? In what circumstances do you try to fit into other people's expectations? Without self-judgment, begin to notice when and where this occurs, and start building the confidence to express your true self at all times, to embrace what makes you different from the norm. By loving yourself completely, you will reach a new height of health that no food could ever give you. And by expressing your authentic self, your life force will soar, your heart will open, and the world will never look the same.

Exercises

1. Turn Off the Media

I encourage you to experiment with turning off the media for a day, a week or a month. Hide the TV, skip the magazines or newspapers and avoid the Internet. Notice how your thoughts about the world and about yourself change without constant media messages. Notice that you have more time for the people you love or to face the fact that you are overly isolated.

2. Tracking Media Messages

Write down all the media you are exposed to on an average day and all the messages you receive. Be sure to include radio commercials, television commercials, billboards, Internet ads, subway ads and so on.

What are the major messages you are receiving?

3. Wish List

This is a tool for you to let go of societal ideals of what your life should look like and connect with your deepest desires for your future. Write down the elements that are most meaningful to your future, such as relationships, children, career, health and spirituality. Write what you want to accomplish or obtain, the places you want to go, the people you'd like to meet or become closer with, or anything that your heart, mind and soul truly desire.

Start listing your desires. Begin with the simple and obvious, and you will notice that more ideas come to you once you start writing. Allow yourself to go crazy—write down all that you desire. Use any language you're comfortable with, such as "I want . . ." or "I desire . . ." or "I intend . . ." Allow yourself to have fun with it.

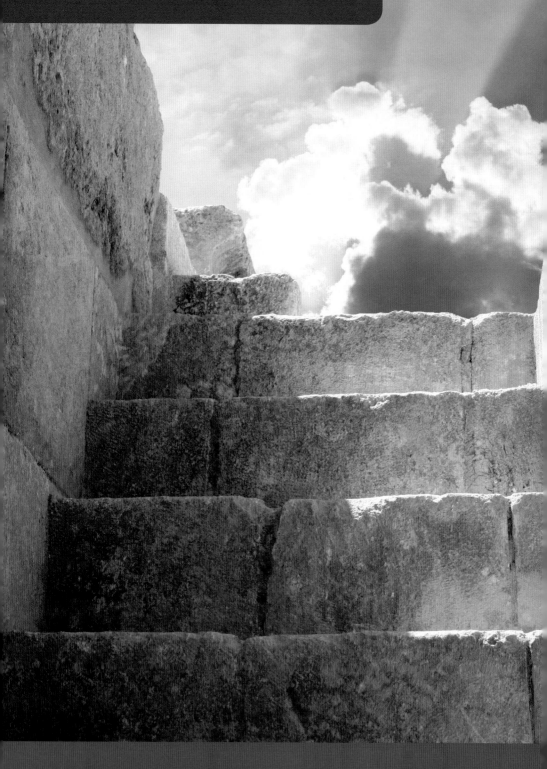

CHAPTER 9

The Integrative Nutrition Plan:

12 Steps to Health

To get through the hardest journey we need take only one step at a time, but we must keep on stepping.
—CHINESE PROVERB

We've examined the politics surrounding the food industry and the difficulty of breaking out of contemporary cultural attitudes that influence our eating habits. We've looked at the innate wisdom of the body, learning to trust it and to understand the importance of the signals it sends to us in the form of cravings. We've examined dietary theories and looked at the pivotal issue of primary food. Now it's time to integrate this knowledge in the form of a plan. No one way of eating will work for everyone, but this is a program of general principles and suggestions, not rigid rules. This approach has flexibility according to each individual's needs, recognizing that no two people are alike and no two people have the same food preferences.

I do not expect you to change your way of eating all at once. On the contrary, I have found that drastic, sudden shifts are difficult to maintain because they force people to repress their food cravings and imbedded eating habits. The more habits are repressed, the more powerful they become, leading to internal stress that builds until people fall off the wagon and the diet fails. A gradual introduction of basic changes allows people to create a larger shift without as much effort or strife.

Even by choosing to follow just one step from this chapter, significant changes will happen for you. Think about it like climbing a ladder. You have to take one rung at a time or you might fall off. I'm offering many suggestions, but it is up to you to find the ones that fit. Most diet books recommend that you completely alter your current way of eating and follow their strict rules. I say choose the things that you most want to do and leave the hardest ones for later. As you start doing the easier ones, your body's energy will kick in and you will pick up momentum. You will then find yourself doing the hardest things with greater ease because you're not starting from zero. If you like the idea of a hot towel scrub, do that. If it's appealing to you to eat more sweet vegetables, do that. Whichever suggestion you want to follow is the right one for you. One thing I can tell you is they all work.

The Integrative Nutrition Plan has 12 steps, but there is no special significance to this number. You do not need to follow the steps in order. Pick one and then go on to another when you are ready. Go at a pace that's suitable for you. You could tackle one new step a day, a week, or a month. This isn't a short-term diet; this is a long-term lifestyle. Trust your instincts, and know that each change you make has a tremendous impact on your present and your future.

Integrative Nutrition Plan: 12 Steps

1. Drink more water
2. Practice cooking
3. Experiment with whole grains
4. Increase sweet vegetables
5. Increase leafy green vegetables
6. Experiment with protein
7. Eat less meat, dairy, sugar and chemicalized, artificial junk foods; consume less coffee, alcohol and tobacco
8. Develop easy and reliable habits to nurture your body
9. Have healthy relationships that support you
10. Find physical activity you enjoy and do it regularly
11. Find work you love or a way to love the work you have
12. Develop a spiritual practice

1. Drink More Water

The body is 75% water, so it makes sense that this essential fluid must be continually replenished. We can go for a month without food, but we can live only two or three days without water. Water is crucial to our survival.

Many people are confused by how much water they should be drinking; they are always told to drink more. What is more? What is the correct quantity of water for your body? Some experts recommend eight glasses a day, but this begs the question, how big is one glass? Eight ounces? More? Less? The answer must come from your own experience. Much will depend on size. A smaller person will need proportionately less water than a bigger person. It also depends on your level of physical activity, the climate in which you live and your diet.

Drinking more water increases yin, making the body light and airy and expanding energy through the whole system. If you are too yang—too tight or contracted, suffering from stress, headaches and bodily tension—you may want to try increasing your water intake to balance these symptoms. In addition, cravings for sweet (yin) foods may actually be signals of dehydration. Drinking water may reduce or eliminate the cravings.

The late Dr. Fereydoon Batmanghelidj, an Iranian-born physician, gained international attention with his claim that regularly drinking water can treat a vast array of illnesses. "You are not sick, you are thirsty," he asserted in his best-selling 1992 book, *Your Body's Many Cries for Water*, which attributes most pain and sickness to chronic dehydration. Through years of reading and research, Dr. Batmanghelidj concluded that ordinary water prevents and cures depression, asthma, arthritis, back pain, migraines, high blood pressure, multiple sclerosis and many other illnesses. He also opposed the use of costly drugs for treating illnesses, saying that you "don't treat thirst with medication."

Dr. Batmanghelidj was jailed as a political prisoner in Iran following the Islamic Revolution in 1979. Because he was a medical doctor, other prisoners came to him with medical problems. Having no access to medicine or drugs, in desperation he told an ulcer patient with severe abdominal pains to try drinking two glasses of water. To his surprise, the patient's pain receded within minutes. During three years in prison, he treated more than 3,000 fellow prisoners who suffered from peptic ulcers, viewing the prison environment as an "ideal stress laboratory." After his release in 1982, he came to the United States and continued to explore of the role of water metabolism in the human body until he passed in 2004.

A large majority of the American population is dehydrated, which contributes significantly to a poor state of health. Regularly flushing out the kidneys and bladder with water ensures that dead cells and other waste products can be expelled before they reach toxic levels. Maintaining hydration can prevent premature aging, eliminate pain and headaches, lessen hypertension and promote weight loss. Some people say they can't drink water because they don't like the taste. I advise them to add some fruit juice, a squeeze of lemon, a slice of cucumber or anything that creates an appealing flavor.

People always ask me what kind of water I recommend. This issue has become increasingly complex. In the past few decades, bottled water has become one of the most popular beverages in the world. In 2011, global bottled water consumption was almost 61 billion gallons.[1] That's a lot of plastic! It's fascinating to me that people, including holistically minded ones, drink water flown in from Fiji, Holland and other parts of the world. Many times the cost of the water is for the brand, and the water is not much different from what comes out of your tap. Federal standards for tap water are actually higher than those for bottled water.[2] Plastic water bottles are also a huge strain on the environment. The amount of fuel, not to mention plastic, used in these bottles is tremendous. I'm not saying everyone should drink only tap water, but drinking solely bottled water is simply not sustainable for our planet. When you're out and about, sometimes drinking bottled water is the only option. I recommend you try different kinds—don't just settle for the cheapest one or the prettiest bottle. Good water is like good wine; it requires careful selection and sensitivity to how your body responds. You can also look for options in glass bottles and even eco-friendly boxes.

Most tap water does contain chlorine, fluoride, and sometimes lead. So if you are going to drink tap water, I recommend getting some kind of filter system. A wide variety of filters are on the market and they vary in price as well as quality. Most people are familiar with the pitcher filters or faucet filters, such as Brita, which are relatively inexpensive. You can also try a carbon water filter or a reverse osmosis filter, both of which are more expensive but are known for eliminating a higher amount of toxins. You can research the different kinds of filters online to find one suited for your needs and your budget. If after researching water filters you decide to invest in one, be sure to change the filter regularly.

Timing is also important in water intake. After waking up in the morning, it's good to drink one or two glasses of water immediately to hydrate the body. Many people realize late in the day they didn't get enough water, so they drink a lot right before bed. Good sleep is integral to health, and you don't want to disrupt it by waking up to go to the bathroom. Complete regeneration occurs only when we sleep deeply. If you notice that you are waking up at night to go to the bathroom, I suggest drinking most of your water in the morning and early afternoon.

Many health experts say water is the only liquid that can hydrate the body, and that juice and tea don't count. As far as I'm concerned, caffeinated drinks, like coffee, soda and black tea, don't count because they are dehydrating. Herbal tea, soup and juice all help hydrate the body, although not as much as pure water.

Others recommend drinking hot water with lemon first thing in the morning, claiming it's good for cleansing the liver. If you try this, notice how your body reacts. If you're already a stressed and tight kind of person, lemon may pucker you up and make you tighter. Experiment and see what really works for your body. The same thing applies to ice water and hot water. A lot of people refuse ice in their water, thinking it's unhealthy because the water used is poor quality or the coldness disrupts digestion. These people may think nothing of drinking pints of hot tea, creating an overheated condition. The body, through its natural wisdom of seeking balance, will need to compensate by eating something cooling, such as ice cream. Ice water can often help restore the imbalance caused by drinking excessive hot liquids without sugar's side effects.

Remember to look at your whole day's intake when deciding how much water you need. Certain foods are more water-dense than others. Cooked grains are two parts water, one part grain. Vegetables also have high water content. Steaming or boiling vegetables, as opposed to frying or baking them, further increases their water content. If you eat a dry breakfast cereal or bread, a muffin or cookies, you will take in little or no water from these foods. In fact, they may create a water deficiency, while cooked grains, vegetables and soups may create a surplus.

Considering the proven impact of water on human health, it amazes me that people remain so unaware and uneducated about this subject. They spend most of their lives dehydrated, needlessly suffering from low energy, cravings and symptoms, not realizing they could feel much better by merely drinking more water.

2. Practice Cooking

It's a well-known paradox that only a skilled cook knows how to prepare a meal in just a few minutes. You would think expertise would bring complexity, but making a meal can actually be divided into two simple stages: preparation time and cooking time. Preparation time for rice is short—about a minute. Take it out of the bag, measure it, rinse it and put it in the pot. The cooking time is longer, but this doesn't mean you need to hang around the kitchen, impatiently testing the rice every few minutes to see if it's ready. Just flip on a timer and go about doing whatever else you need to do.

Vegetables, which are seriously lacking in most people's daily diet, are especially easy to prepare. Making a salad involves rinsing and chopping. Cooking vegetables takes a couple of minutes of prep time to rinse and chop and then a few minutes of cooking time to steam, sauté, boil or roast. Juicing is an instantaneous way to prepare vegetables; all you need is a juicer and a few minutes to clean it once you are done. Other easy ways to eat vegetables are buying bags of baby carrots or celery sticks, or simply washing vegetables and eating them in their natural, crunchy state. Dip them in hummus, yogurt or nut butters. The key is to have them available and ready for snacking.

Learning the art of simple meal planning will help you get all the nutrients you need as well as release you from dependency on restaurant food, fast food and other processed foods. We eat differently when we are feeding ourselves than when we are out and about. Restaurant food is usually very salty and highly flavored, as it's designed to be a taste sensation. It often comes in very big portions, more than enough for the average person. By buying and preparing our own food, we eat in accordance with our body's actual needs and we are less likely to overeat or consume excess salt and flavoring.

Cooking delicious, satisfying meals in a brief period of time is a skill worth learning. It's not difficult, but it takes practice. At first, you may burn the rice or overcook the kale but that's okay. You may go through an initial period of trial and error. Give yourself permission to make mistakes. It's like starting a new office job. The first few weeks seem complicated because you have to figure out how the phone system works, how the photocopy machine works, where the bathroom is and who's who in the office. In the beginning it seems like a huge task, but a month later you are doing it without even thinking about it. You know it all by heart. Cooking is just like that.

For many people, the task of cooking seems daunting. They are puzzled, and ask questions like, "How do plain, ordinary vegetables turn into such a delicious meal in a few minutes?" A chef is like an alchemist, turning simple ingredients into gold, transforming a caterpillar into a butterfly. But few cookbooks talk about the initial, most-challenging period. They don't mention that cooking a meal takes much longer when you are an inexperienced chef than when you have had some practice. It is a great gift to be able to cook with ease and confidence. It just takes some patience and practice. In a short time, you will be effortlessly washing, chopping, cooking and nourishing yourself and others.

Creatively selecting combinations of foods is similar to a painter choosing colors from a palette. Cooking is the only art form that actually enters the bloodstream. You can look at a painting and find it inspirational or listen to a piece of music to create a mood, but homemade food has a much deeper effect because it goes into your body. A very intimate relationship exists between a meal and the person who consumes it.

3. Experiment with Whole Grains

Many fashionable diet theories advise people to avoid carbohydrates, naming them as a culprit in our obesity crisis. This advice is a huge and faulty generalization. By looking at the delicate, thin bodies of Japanese people, who consume high-carbohydrate diets composed of large amounts of rice and starchy vegetables, it's impossible to conclude that all carbs lead to weight gain. Still, the subject of whether or not to eat grains does stir up emotions for many. Some people live on brown rice and oatmeal, others do better with less grains, and some swear by getting off grains altogether. No foods are inherently "good" or "bad," so I encourage you to experiment with whole grains and see which ones work best for you, if at all.

Whole grains have been a central element of the human diet when we stopped hunting and gathering and settled into agrarian communities. Until very recently, people living in these communities on all continents had lean, strong bodies. In the Americas, corn was the staple grain, while rice predominated in India and Asia. In Africa, people had sorghum and millet. People in the Middle East enjoyed pita bread and cous- cous. In Europe, it was corn, millet, wheat, rice, pasta and dark breads. Even beer, produced by grain fermentation, was considered healthy. In Scotland, it was oats. In Russia, they had buckwheat or kasha. For generations, very few people eating grain-based diets were overweight.

People are gaining weight today because they eat too much chemicalized, artificial junk food, and consume too much caffeine, sugar, nicotine and alcohol. It's not the carbohydrates. Oddly enough, people today will eat all kinds of junk food, while skipping natural, whole grains, which might significantly benefit their health. Whole grains are some of the best sources of nutritional support, containing high levels of dietary fiber and B vitamins. Because the body absorbs them slowly, grains provide long-lasting energy.

Whole grains can especially help people who struggle with maintaining a steady level of blood sugar. Whole grains release sugar into the bloodstream slowly, in contrast to the sudden rush and energy crash caused by refined sugar foods and sodas.

Sally Fallon Morell points out that people traditionally soaked or fermented their grains, often for a few days before cooking. Soaking grains, or fermenting them by soaking in hot water with vinegar, neutralizes the phytic acid and makes the grains easier to digest. All grains contain phytic acid in the outer layer of the bran. Phytic acid combines with certain minerals in the body, such as calcium, magnesium, copper and iron, and can block absorption in the intestines, which may lead to digestive disorders, mineral deficiencies and bone loss. Eight hours of soaking in warm water will neutralize the

Creating Great Grains

- Measure the grain. Rinse. Remove any unwanted material.
- Optional: Soak for 1 to 8 hours, to eliminate phytic acid and make the grain more digestible. Drain the grain and discard the soaking water.
- Add grain to recommended amount of water and bring to a boil.
- A pinch of sea salt may be added to all grains except amaranth, kamut and spelt (it interferes with cooking time for these).
- Reduce heat, cover and simmer for the recommended time.
- Check your grains halfway through and near the end of cooking to determine if they are done or if more liquid is needed. If too much liquid has been added, remove the lid and boil off excess. You can change the texture of grains like quinoa, millet and buckwheat with different cooking methods. Bringing the liquid to a boil before adding the grain will keep grains separate, like rice. Boiling the grains and liquid together will create a softer, porridge-like consistency.
- Tip: To reheat cooked grains, simply add a bit more liquid and reheat on low on the stove.

phytic acid and greatly improve the nutritional benefits of grains. Even an hour of soaking will help. If you have difficulty digesting grains, you may want to try soaking them overnight.

The most common grain in our culture is wheat. Many people are allergic to wheat but don't know it. Wheat products are heavily subsidized and promoted by the government in the dietary guidelines, and the food industry incorporates it into almost all breakfast cereals, cookies, cakes and crackers. Gluten, a protein found in wheat, barley, rye and oats, is difficult for many people to digest. If you are sensitive or allergic to gluten, you can experience bloating, constipation or gas after eating wheat and other glutenous grains. Other related problems are allergies, celiac disease, brain fog, chronic indigestion and candida. Sometimes the symptoms occur immediately after eating, but they can also take time to manifest. If you think you have sensitivity or allergies, I recommend removing all wheat and gluten products from your diet for four to six weeks and seeing how you feel. During that time, stick with gluten-free grains, such as amaranth, brown rice, buckwheat, millet, quinoa, sorghum and teff.

4. Increase Sweet Vegetables

Almost everyone craves sweets. Instead of depending on processed sugar, you can add more naturally sweet flavor to your daily diet and dramatically reduce sweet cravings. Certain vegetables have a deep, sweet flavor when cooked— like corn, carrots, onions, beets, winter squash (butternut, buttercup, delicata, hubbard and kabocha), sweet potatoes and yams. Some lesser-known vegetables that are semi-sweet are turnips, parsnips and rutabagas. And there is another group of vegetables that don't taste sweet but have an effect on the body similar to that of sweet vegetables. These include red radishes, daikon

Sweet Sensation

A simple way to cook sweet vegetables is to follow a recipe I call "Sweet Sensation." It has few ingredients and preparation time is minimal.

- Use one to five of the sweet vegetables mentioned above.
- Chop the hardest ones, like carrots and beets, into smaller pieces.
- Softer vegetables, like onions and cabbage, can be cut into larger chunks.
- Use a medium-size pot and add enough water to barely cover the vegetables. You may want to check the water level while cooking and add more water if needed. Remember, vegetables on the bottom will cook more quickly than the ones on the top. Cook until the vegetables reach your desired softness. The softer the vegetables get, the sweeter they become.
- Try adding any of the following ingredients: spices, salt, seaweed. You can add tofu or a can of beans for extra protein.
- When cooked to your satisfaction, empty the ingredients into a large bowl, flavor as desired and eat. The leftover cooking water makes a delicious, sweet sauce and is a healing tonic to drink by itself.

radish, green cabbage, red cabbage and burdock. They soothe the internal organs of the body and energize the mind. And because many of these vegetables are root vegetables, they are energetically grounding, helping to balance out the spacey feeling people often experience after eating other sweets.

Other delicious ways to incorporate sweet vegetables into your daily diet include eating raw carrots, baking sweet potato fries, roasting squash, making soup with corn and onions or boiling beets to put on top of your salad.

5. Increase Leafy Green Vegetables

If vegetables are the scarcest food in the American diet, leafy green vegetables are lacking most of all. Learning to cook and eat greens is essential for creating lasting health. Greens help build our internal rainforest and strengthen our circulatory and respiratory systems. The color green is associated with spring, a time of renewal, refreshment and vital energy. In Asian medicine, green is related to the liver, emotional stability and creativity. Nutritionally, greens are high in calcium, magnesium, iron, potassium, phosphorous, zinc, and vitamins A, C, E and K. They are crammed with fiber, folic acid, chlorophyll and many other micronutrients and phytochemicals.

Some of the benefits gained from eating dark leafy greens are:

- blood purification
- cancer prevention
- improved circulation
- immune strengthening
- subtle, light and flexible energy
- lifted spirit, elimination of depression
- promotion of healthy intestinal flora
- improved liver, gallbladder and kidney function
- clearing of congestion, especially in lungs, and reduction of mucus

When most people hear "leafy green vegetables," they probably think of iceberg lettuce, but the ordinary, pale lettuce in restaurant salads doesn't have the power-packed goodness of other greens.

Cooking Greens

Try a variety of preparation methods like steaming, boiling, sautéing in oil, water sautéing, waterless cooking or chopped in salads. Boiling makes greens plump and relaxed. I recommend boiling for under a minute so that the nutrients in the greens do not get lost in the water. You can also drink the cooking water as a health-giving broth or a tea, if you're using organic greens. Steaming makes greens more fibrous and tight, which is great for people who are trying to lose weight. Raw salad is also a wonderful food. It's refreshing, cooling and soft, and supplies your body with live enzymes.

You can choose from a variety of greens. Broccoli is very popular among adults and children—each stem is like a tree trunk, giving you strong, grounded energy. But remember to be adventurous and try greens you've never seen before. Rotate between bok choy, napa cabbage, kale, collards, watercress, mustard greens, broccoli rabe, dandelion and other leafy greens. Green cabbage can be included as a green, either as sauerkraut, which provides the body with live enzymes, or as an ingredient in the Sweet Sensation recipe. Arugula, endive, chicory, lettuce, mesclun and wild greens are generally eaten raw. Spinach, Swiss chard and beet greens are best eaten in moderation because they are high in oxalic acid, which depletes calcium from your bones and teeth. Cook these vegetables with something rich like tofu, seeds, nuts, beans, butter, animal products or oil to balance out the impact of the oxalic acid.

Get into the habit of adding these green vegetables to your diet as often as possible. Nourishing yourself with greens will naturally crowd out foods that make you sick. Try it for a month and see how you feel.

6. Experiment with Protein

Protein is the basic building block of the human structure, helping our bodies form muscles, skin and hair. Because of our bio-individuality, protein requirements vary dramatically from person to person. I recommend experimenting with reducing or increasing your protein intake and trying different sources, animal and vegetable, and noticing the impact on your body. The majority of Americans today eat way too much protein. Some people, especially O blood types and men, need more protein-rich foods more often. Low protein can lead to low energy and a variety of cravings.

On the other hand, many people feel lighter and clearer, and notice a decrease in physical symptoms when they reduce animal protein in their diet. Animal foods are rich in fat and cholesterol. Disorders such as heart disease, cancer, obesity and high blood pressure can all be linked to an excess of animal foods. People often find that reducing animal protein consumption helps clear up constipation, low energy, body odor and sugar cravings.

Vegetarian and vegan people often attempt to get their protein needs met through beans and bean products. Although beans contain protein, that protein is not easily assimilated. Beans are one of the most difficult foods to digest, and vegetarians must learn to properly prepare their beans to get maximum nutritional benefit and reduce gas and indigestion. Usually, this means choosing smaller beans and cooking them longer than you think is necessary.

In Mexico and Central America, where beans are a fundamental part of the daily diet, the most frequent bean dish is refried beans. The beans are cooked once and then refried in oil or butter to ensure easier digestion. A similar situation exists in Japanese cuisine with soybeans. Rarely, if ever, do the Japanese eat soybeans unless the beans have first been fermented or aged. They convert the beans into foods like miso, soy sauce and natto. They also eat tofu in small amounts.

Out of all the beans, soy is the most difficult to digest. After wheat, soy is one of the most common allergens, though people don't realize this because soy is highly touted as a health food. Remember, just because something is sold in a natural food store does not mean that it's healthy. Americans beware: about 90 percent of soybeans grown in the U.S. are genetically modified.[3] Even if you think you're not eating soy, more than 60 percent of packaged and processed foods contain soy ingredients.[4] Many vegetarians and vegans rely on tofu, soy milk (which is really tofu that has not been coagulated) and other soy products as their main sources of protein. They pour soy milk on their cereal, have soy smoothies and cook tofu as part of their dinner every night.

Tofu is a good source of protein, but I recommend it be eaten in moderate quantities. Eating edamame, the young, whole soybean is preferable because it is relatively easy to assimilate compared to processed food products, such as soy dogs, soy milk or soy ice cream.

Soy has also been linked to thyroid disease due to its naturally occurring isoflavones, which can suppress thyroid function and can be particularly detrimental to infants who consume soy-based formulas.[5] Soy products can cause allergic reactions and digestive upset because most of them are highly processed.

Some research shows that a certain chemical found in soy, called genistein, can potentially damage fertility, especially in men. Traditionally, in Zen monasteries, men would eat tofu to help reduce their sex drive so they could sustain a celibate lifestyle. So men, if you want to be celibate, tofu is a great food for you. However, if that is not your mission, you may want to avoid eating too much tofu. Soy isoflavones can also increase estrogen activity, and some research shows that consuming soy products during menopause can ease some of the negative symptoms that some women experience during menopause. But other research links increased estrogen activity to higher risks of developing breast cancer. In general, much research is still needed on the effects of soy. My basic advice is to eat soy in moderation and listen to your body.

For those who refuse to eat animal meat, but are okay with eating animal products, eggs may be a good source of protein. High-quality yogurt may also be a good option for those who are not lactose intolerant. I strongly encourage buying organic eggs and dairy that are free from hormones and antibiotics.

Many Americans prefer beef as their main source of protein. Try other animal meats, such as duck, pheasant, buffalo, lamb, chicken and fish, and rotate these in your diet to avoid the stagnancy and health concerns associated with excess beef consumption, including heart disease, high blood pressure, constipation, high cholesterol and mad cow disease. Quality of meat is really important, and organic is always the best option. Generally, animals on organic farms are treated much more humanely than on factory farms. As I mentioned before, we take in an animal's energy when we eat it. Wouldn't you rather take in the energy of an animal that was treated humanely throughout its lifetime?

When deciding how much animal food to eat with a meal, I urge you to follow the guidance of Dr. Barry Sears. He recommends eating a piece of meat "no bigger and no thicker than the palm of your hand." This is about 4 ounces per portion and a much healthier choice than having a huge slab of meat as a main course.

We intuitively know that animal food increases our sense of personal power, self-esteem, and confidence. Many people eat excessive amounts of meat for these benefits but pay the price of poor health and life-threatening illnesses. Those who eat a plant-based diet are likely to be more balanced and healthy, but can become too set in their ways. Life stops becoming fun because they don't have the energy to go out, hit the town and enjoy themselves. They are more like plants. They just want to sit still. Look at what most CEOs, politicians and athletes eat—not too many vegetarians in those circles!

Again, there is no right and wrong here. Food is not religion. No special heaven is reserved for vegetarians. So please find the fuel that is most suitable for your current needs. Finding the optimum protein intake is a key to a balanced, healthy life.

7. Eat Less Meat, Dairy, Sugar and Chemicalized, Artificial Junk Foods; Consume Less Coffee, Alcohol and Tobacco

I would rather add than take away from any individual's diet. However, most people who reduce meat, dairy, sugar, chemicalized, artificial junk food, coffee, alcohol and tobacco in their daily diet feel more energized. If they are already sick, cutting back on these foods helps them to recover their health and vitality. The effects of consuming too much dairy, sugar and coffee are covered in the next chapter. The impacts of smoking and drinking on the body are well known and could fill an entire book.

8. Develop Easy and Reliable Habits to Nurture Your Body

The tongue cleaner, hot water bottle and hot towel scrub are three of my favorite daily tools to establish a loving relationship with your body. This relationship is a key component of overall health and often overlooked by the medical community.

The tongue cleaner, an inexpensive yet transformative tool, is a simple, thin, U-shaped piece of stainless steel with a blunted edge to remove gunk from the surface of the tongue. Dentists recommend the tongue cleaner more and more because it helps fight cavities by removing bacteria from the mouth. It also prevents bad breath, especially for people who eat a lot of dairy and build up mucus in the mouth, nose and throat. The tongue cleaner comes from the tradition of Ayurveda, which says people who use them are better at public speaking, expressing themselves more thought- fully and speaking more sincerely and authoritatively. Some people ask if the same effect can be gained by brushing the tongue with a stiff toothbrush. Brushing the tongue moves the coating around and is helpful, but a tongue cleaner is more effective, as it clears out the deep deposits and generally keeps the area more clean, stimulated and alive.

The tongue cleaner also helps with cravings by cleaning the tongue of leftover food residue that could lead to cravings for those foods eaten previously. A clean tongue has fewer "food memories" on its surface. A tongue cleaner reverses the process of desensitizing your taste buds, which happens to everyone to some extent. It allows you to taste more subtle flavors in food so that you can eat vegetables, fruits and whole grains with greater enjoyment. When old residue remains on the tongue, we aren't able to taste the natural flavors in whole foods. When you have a clean tongue, you will be better able to taste your food and won't need to eat as much since you will have gained greater satisfaction from your meal.

A big advantage of using a tongue cleaner is that it enhances kissing by making the tongue sweeter, fresher and more sensitive. If you are in a relationship, I invite you to check this out with your partner. Make an agreement

PROFILE

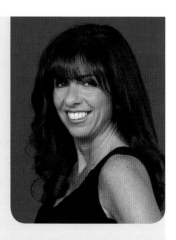

Randi Dukoff, Muttontown, NY, USA

www.coreandmorehealthandfitness.com

"My life just keeps getting better."

In 2003, I changed careers and chose to be a personal trainer, and became fascinated with Holistic Nutrition. I had lost 30 pounds by beginning to exercise with free weights and by eliminating processed foods and gluten from my diet 85% of the time. I began to drink more water, cook better, eat cleaner food and sleep more. I learned that: 'Yes' has no value until you learn to say 'no.' Training clients opened my eyes to the fact that food has a bigger impact on health and weight loss then exercise. I became licensed as a Holistic Nutritionist and Life Coach. I had so much information and education, but I was still struggling to get clients.

One of my closest friends became interested in nutrition because of what I had taught her. She found Integrative Nutrition and within 10 months she had so many clients who were finding success. I wasn't sure I would learn more than what I knew already, but I felt this was the right choice for me. I learned so much from IIN! I learned goal setting, how to follow through, how to empathize and listen to people and how to make all of the information manageable and teach it in a way my clients would feel successful. I also learned how to set up my business and where to go for support.

My career has taken off since attending Integrative Nutrition. I learned how to get clients and succeed in the New York City corporate market and I love it. I was able to give a 15-minute fitness break at the 2010 IIN Conference for over 2000 people. I was nervous at the number of people, but Joshua and John Douillard taught me to embrace and overcome my fear to grow. I loved the experience and want to do it again! Now I love presenting to large groups of people.

My inspiration comes from knowing you can overcome any diagnosis with the right mindset, therapies, healers, food and attitude. Change your thoughts and you can change your life. I did it and each day is a gift, a present we are given to enjoy.

My life just keeps getting better. My job doesn't feel like work because I love it that much. I live the way I teach and I think that comes through. I look forward to more growth, new ventures and more new experiences.

to scrape twice a day for one week and feel the difference. The tongue cleaner takes just seconds to use, and can easily be worked into your morning and nighttime rituals. You can purchase tongue cleaners at most health food stores or online.

It's an ancient and natural feeling for both men and women to seek some kind of warm coziness at night. Even if there isn't someone in the bed with you, then a hot water bottle can help create this feeling. It's also an easy and inexpensive way to heat up your bed before sleeping. For years, I've recommended people try using a warm compress on their bellies. The lower belly is the home of your Hara, the central balance point of your body and, according to Asian philosophy, is the center and source of your life energy. The Hara is the gate, the doorway to the universal energy surrounding us. Heat from a water bottle brings more energy and more blood circulation to the digestive organs in this area, which are really the engine of your body. It aids in digesting food and in unblocking energy that may be stuck after a heavy meal.

At bedtime, place an old-fashioned hot water bottle on your belly for about 15 to 20 minutes. Most hot water bottles today are plastic, so you'll want to put the bottle in a pillowcase or get a cover before placing it against your skin. On a psychological and emotional level, warmth on the belly may promote absorption and digestion of whatever feelings or mental input are left over from the day's events.

I get a lot of feedback from single people about how they dread getting into a cold, empty bed at the end of a busy day. After being introduced to the hot water bottle solution, some of them even start using two or three of them to create a soothing, comforting feeling that helps them relax and sleep better. It's a simple and effective way to feel nourished.

Women can also use a hot water bottle, similar to a heating pad, to help relieve the pain and tension associated with menstrual cramps. It conforms to your body and you can use it at night and not worry about falling asleep with it. British scientists have proven that applying heat to your abdominal region actually deactivates pain at a molecular level, similar to the effect of taking over-the-counter painkillers. The heat from the bottle blocks pain messages to the brain.

The hot towel scrub is an incredible tool for relaxation, circulation and detoxification. The skin is the body's largest organ of elimination. More dead cells, toxins and waste products from the body get eliminated through the skin than through urinating and defecating. Stimulating the pores of your skin with a rubbing action allows them to eliminate better. The only thing separating you from your external environment is your skin. The hot towel scrub rejuvenates this living organ, creating a better two-way flow of sensory information between you and your environment. It's a great source of primary food because it creates a loving connection between you and your body. Also, the heat and friction helps to melt away subcutaneous fat and break down cellulite.

Here's how it works: take a wash cloth, dip it into hot water or hold it under running hot water, wring it out, and then rub your entire body for five to 10 minutes. There is no right direction in which to rub. Try head to toe, toe to head, toward the heart, away from the heart, whatever feels easy and natural for you. It's invigorating if you do it in the morning, relaxing if you do it in the evening after work or at night before you go to bed. It has a neutralizing and balancing effect on the mind.

Some people say it's similar to using a loofah or skin brush, but the added effect of using heat to open pores and break down fat is very important, so don't settle for brushing. Also, take the trouble not to do this in the shower. Instead, stand by a sink. It makes a difference because showering is such a routine, mechanical act. By the sink, you are looking in the mirror and seeing your body, and you are more present to the sensations the hot towel scrub is creating in you.

When I show a washcloth to my students and say, "This will change your life," they are naturally skeptical. But after, I get a lot of positive feedback, like, "I can't believe how well this works!" and "I feel my skin opening up, vibrating," and "I've fallen in love with my body." If you use it for a few minutes every day, or even once a week, your body will thank you.

These simple tools really speak to improving the quality of each day. The tongue scraper, hot water bottle and hot towel scrub are three of the fastest, easiest and least expensive means of creating a loving relationship with your body and, in turn, a new level of health.

9. Have Healthy Relationships That Support You

It's rare that I meet someone who feels entirely supported by his or her family, friends, coworkers, boss and significant other. Sometimes the answer to getting the support you need is as simple as asking for help from these people or from a professional. Other times, the answer may lie in creating new relationships and letting go of the old ones that no longer serve you. Start by developing the relationship you have with yourself. When you find ways to nurture and love yourself, you will be better able to communicate your needs to others.

Figuring out what kind of love relationship works best for you is crucial. For some, a happy marriage early in life is their main goal. They are clear that they want to have children and build a firm structure for their whole life and for future generations. Others look for alternatives to marriage or wait until later in life to marry or settle down with one person. Many people feel pressure from their families or society to get married and have children, while this is simply not the right path for some. It is important that you take time to determine what you want, and then work practically and positively toward it. Having a dream is one thing; making it happen is another. And again, don't hesitate to ask for help with this if you need it. We all need support on this very important issue, so find people in your life that can offer it to you.

10. Find Physical Activity You Enjoy and Do It Regularly

A lot of people go to great lengths to make sure they are eating healthy food, but they don't bother to exercise regularly. Movement aids digestion, assimilation, circulation and respiration and is a crucial part of any healthy person's regimen. Many people don't like exercising. It's challenging for them to find an exercise they enjoy. Think about what you loved to do as a kid. Did you dance, bike or hike? This is a good place to start when looking for a new exercise routine. Look for a gym or yoga studio near your home or on the way to the office where you can work out. It's important to find a location that's convenient, and where the atmosphere is pleasant, comfortable and welcoming. This will enhance your chances of going regularly.

Exercising can be an opportunity to reconnect with nature, perhaps by going to a large park if you are a city dweller. Getting out to a rural environment—somewhere you can breathe clean, fresh air, hear the birds and see the sky—on a regular basis can be very healing. We can live without food for months, and without water for days. However, we cannot live without air for more than a few minutes, so it makes sense that air quality is essential to life quality.

11. Find Work You Love or a Way to Love the Work You Have

Career can be one of the most dysfunctional areas of adult life. Many people resign themselves to doing tedious work in jobs, offices and corporations that are not in alignment with who they are. They do this not for a day, a week or a month, but for years and even decades. Sometimes they are working in fields that are diametrically opposed to their own personal values. As a long-term lifestyle, this is bound to affect their health. If you are one of these people, I encourage you to be more courageous and proactive in remedying the situation. Do you believe we are spiritual beings in a material world? If so, I think you'll agree that what we do all day, every day is central to why we are here.

Many people feel trapped in jobs because they have a retirement fund, 401(k) plan or accrued benefits. They know they should leave, but they have a mortgage or bills to pay, and they just need to work a few more years before they can quit or retire. If this describes you, the challenge is to find a way to love the work you have. You can try making your office environment more attractive, identifying people at work who can be allies and avoiding people who are irritating. Get an office with a nice view if you can, use a comfortable chair that supports your back and take stretch breaks every hour.

You can also try to identify what isn't working in your job on a personal level and find ways to address these issues. Maybe your deadlines are too quick and you have problems with procrastination or maybe you have a hard time communicating with large groups because you are shy. Maybe you feel you are overqualified for your position and feel bored at work. Instead of putting all the blame on your work environment, see what you can learn from your current situation and how you can make changes. Research local seminars on organization, public speaking or continued learning in your field. You may be surprised to find that when you make changes in yourself, your job may feel more fulfilling.

12. Develop a Spiritual Practice

Spirituality is what gives depth and meaning to life, creating the feeling of divine order and harmony that exists above and beyond human limitations. For some, this means embracing their religion of birth, following the traditions of their ancestors and seeking depth through prayer and with God. Others feel discontented with the past and explore new avenues, such as Eastern religions, meditation or the religion of their partner. For people who are agnostic or atheist, being spiritual may mean going for a walk in the late evening and feeling the vastness of the night sky, or walking by the ocean and enjoying the sense of infinite, endless space. It has been my experience that when people feel connected with the big picture, they get healthier faster.

Exercises

1. Your First Step

Choose one of the 12 steps to try for a week. What will your first step be?

What are three things you can do to support yourself in making this happen over the next week? Great! Now go and do them.

Check back in with yourself after one week. How did it go? What worked and what didn't? Are you ready to add another step? If so, pick the next one that resonates with you. If not, focus on maintaining the first step until you are ready to add the next. Continue this process until you are doing all 12 steps. Go at your own pace. You will see and feel the difference in your body, mind and spirit.

2. Daily Journaling

For more support on incorporating these steps into your daily life, check out *The Integrative Nutrition Journal: Your Guide to a Happy, Healthy Life.* This book contains daily, weekly and monthly exercises to keep you on track with your personal goals around health.

CHAPTER 10

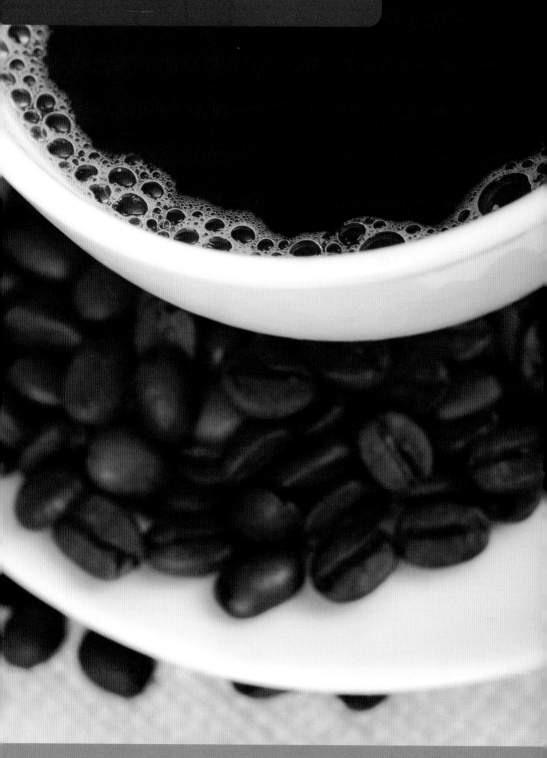

Foods to Avoid or Minimize

No foods are forbidden except when your body tells you so.
　　—LIMA OHSAWA

By now you've grasped the fundamentals of maintaining a healthy diet. In spite of the enormous amount of confusing and contradictory information that regularly floods the world of nutrition, the basics are simple. Most people would be much better off consuming less meat, milk, sugar, chemicalized, artificial junk food, alcohol, caffeine and tobacco and increasing their consumption of water, whole grains and vegetables, especially dark leafy greens.

I want to emphasize, however, that no food is innately bad. If you really want to have fried chicken, a burger, a chocolate chip cookie or ice cream, it's okay within the overall context of a healthy diet. I am not in favor of fanaticism or extreme food practices. As I said before, it's not what you eat some of the time; it's what you eat most of the time that makes a difference.

This chapter looks at some extreme foods to give you a clearer understanding of their effects on the body. We'll start with the most challenging of all: sugar.

Sugar

It's no surprise that the United States is the largest consumer of sweeteners and one of the largest global sugar importers. Starting in 1689 when the first sugar refinery was built in New York City, colonists soon began to sweeten their breakfast porridge with refined sugar, and within 10 years individual consumption had reached 4 pounds a year. The average American now consumes more than 130 pounds of sugar and sweeteners per year.[1] In contrast, Americans consume an average of about 5.6 pounds of broccoli.[2] The USDA recommends no more than 9 teaspoons per day, yet most Americans eat about 22 teaspoons per day—that's more than twice the liberal recommended daily value.[3]

Humans love sweet things. Even before we started refining sugar, we sought out foods with sweet tastes. Sugar is a simple carbohydrate that occurs naturally in foods such as grains, beans, vegetables and fruit. When unprocessed, sugar contains a variety of vitamins, minerals, enzymes and proteins. When brown rice or other whole grains are cooked, chewed and digested, the natural carbohydrates break down uniformly into separate glucose molecules. These molecules enter the bloodstream, where they are burned smoothly and evenly, allowing your body to absorb all the good stuff.

Refined table sugar, also called sucrose, is very different. Extracted from either sugarcane or beets, it lacks vitamins, minerals and fiber, and thus requires extra effort from the body to digest. The body must deplete its own store of minerals and enzymes to absorb sucrose properly. Therefore, instead of providing the body with nutrition, it creates deficiency. It enters swiftly into the bloodstream and wreaks havoc on the blood sugar level, first pushing it sky-high—causing excitability, nervous tension and hyperactivity—and then dropping it extremely low—causing fatigue, depression, weariness and exhaustion. Health-conscious people are aware that their blood sugar levels fluctuate wildly on a sugar-induced high, but they often don't realize the emotional roller-coaster ride that accompanies this high. We feel happy and energetic for a while and then suddenly, inexplainably, we find ourselves arguing with a friend or lover.

Sugar qualifies as an addictive substance for two reasons:

1. Eating even a small amount creates a desire for more.
2. Suddenly quitting causes withdrawal symptoms such as headaches, mood swings, cravings and fatigue.

Today sugar is found in many of the usual suspects, like cakes, cookies and candy. But you will also find it in canned vegetables, baby food, cereals, peanut butter, bread and tomato sauce. It is often disguised in fancy language, labeled as corn syrup, dextrose, maltose, glucose or fructose. Even some so-called healthy foods contain sugar. A crunchy peanut butter Clif Bar has 21 grams of sugar, or 5 teaspoons.[4] Compare that to a chocolate-glazed cake donut from Dunkin' Donuts, which has 14 grams of sugar, or 3 teaspoons. You may think your afternoon cup of coffee only has a little sugar, but a 16-ounce Starbucks Frappuccino actually contains 50 grams of sugar, or 10 teaspoons[5]—that's like eating three donuts! Overconsumption of refined sweets and added sugars found in everyday foods has led to an explosion of hypoglycemia and type 2 diabetes.

Many people eating a Western diet struggle with hypoglycemia, which literally means, "low glucose levels in the blood." Glucose is a type of sugar that provides energy to every cell in the body. Our bodies normally maintain blood glucose levels within a narrow range. When this homeostasis is lost, hypoglycemia can result. A poor diet, especially one with an excess of refined sugars, can cause a gradual breakdown in our body's ability to manage blood glucose. When this happens, blood glucose levels may initially spike after a meal (hyperglycemia) and then crash to abnormally low levels several hours after the meal (hypoglycemia). This roller-coaster effect is implicated in the onset of type 2 diabetes. It may take years for hypoglycemia to develop into full-blown diabetes, but the sooner you intervene the better. Symptoms of hypoglycemia include faintness, dizziness, sweating, anxiety and hunger. If you think you have hypoglycemia, you definitely want to reduce the amount of refined sugar in your diet.

Worldwide, more than 371 million people have diabetes. Experts say that by 2030 this number will increase to more than 550 million people. The rates are increasing in every country each year, and it's estimated that about half of the people with diabetes are undiagnosed.[6]

Type 1 diabetes, known as juvenile-onset or insulin-dependent diabetes, typically develops in childhood or early adulthood. With this condition, the pancreas is unable to produce insulin. When a person without diabetes eats something that creates glucose in the blood, the pancreas produces insulin in order to maintain blood sugar balance. Insulin acts as the gatekeeper, allowing the proper amount of glucose into the body's cells to be utilized as fuel. People with type 1 diabetes must rely on daily injections of insulin to keep their blood sugar from getting too high.

Type 2 diabetes usually develops much later in life, though recently it is on the rise among children and adolescents. In fact, type 2 diabetes was commonly referred to as adult-onset diabetes until the rates of children diagnosed with the condition skyrocketed. With type 2 diabetes, the pancreas is still capable of producing insulin, but the cells in the body are less responsive to it. One of the most alarming statistics in medicine right now is the rate at which people are diagnosed with this type of diabetes, which is far more prevalent than type 1. This news is especially heartbreaking when we know that reducing processed sugar and eating a healthy, balanced diet can prevent the condition.

When people lose the ability to maintain a steady blood sugar level, the entire human organism is affected. A healthy body exists in a state of homeostasis, maintaining a steady balance within all systems that ensures smooth functioning for the whole organism. Take body temperature for example. Somehow the body knows how to maintain a temperature of 98.6 degrees. If we get overheated, we perspire to cool down; if we get too cold, we shiver to warm up. Many systems in the body are designed to maintain this status. We know when to urinate, so our bladders don't swell and explode. We know when to stay awake, so we don't drift into slumber while driving and crash. The body maintains these interlinked systems by itself, for itself, without any need for conscious control. Maintenance of blood sugar is controlled by the hormonal system, which is interconnected with many other vital body control systems, including the sexual reproductive system, adrenal glands, thyroid and pineal glands. The breakdown of blood sugar regulation can lead to the breakdown of other systems, until the entire organism is out of whack.

It wasn't until quite recently that the scientific community acknowledged sugar's connection to diabetes. Results from the first large-scale epidemiological study published in 2013 showed that sugar has a direct, independent link to diabetes. California researches looked at data on sugar availability and diabetes rates in 175 countries from the last decade. They found increased sugar in the food supply was linked to increased rates of diabetes.[7]

But sugar isn't the problem. The problem is the vicious, addictive cycle we have created by eating processed sugar, feeling the rush, crashing, and then taking in more sugar to begin the vicious cycle again. If we are on a healthy,

Sugar Alternatives

Agave Nectar

Agave nectar is a natural liquid sweetener made from the juice of the agave cactus. It is 1.4 times sweeter than refined sugar, but does not create a "sugar rush," and is much less disturbing to the body's blood sugar levels than white sugar.

Brown Rice Syrup

This product consists of brown rice that has been ground and cooked, converting the starches to maltose. Brown rice syrup tastes like moderately sweet butterscotch and is quite delicious. In recipes, you may need to use up to 50% more brown rice syrup than the amount of sugar you would normally need, and reduce the amounts of other liquids.

Date Sugar

Date sugar consists of finely ground, dehydrated dates, utilizing this fruit's vitamin, mineral, and fiber content. If you like the taste of dates, this will definitely appeal to you. Date sugar can be used as a direct replacement for sugar, and comes in a granulated form.

Honey

One of the oldest natural sweeteners, honey is sweeter than sugar. Depending on the plant source, honey can have a range of flavors, from dark and strongly flavored to light and mildly flavored. Raw honey contains small amounts of enzymes, minerals and vitamins. Some vegans choose not to eat honey, as it is a byproduct of bees.

Maple Syrup

Maple syrup is made from boiled down maple tree sap and contains many minerals. Forty gallons of sap are needed to make one gallon of maple syrup. It adds a pleasant flavor to foods and is great for baking. Be sure to buy 100% pure maple syrup, and not maple-flavored corn syrup.

Maple Sugar

Maple sugar is created when the sap of the sugar maple is boiled for longer than is needed to create maple syrup. Once most of the water has evaporated, all that is left is the solid sugar. Maple sugar is about twice as sweet as standard granulated sugar, but much less refined.

Molasses

Organic molasses is probably the most nutritious sweetener. It is derived from sugar cane or sugar beet, and is made by a process of clarifying and blending the extracted juices. The longer the juice is boiled, the less sweet, more nutritious, and darker it becomes. Molasses imparts a very distinct flavor to food. Blackstrap molasses, the most nutritious variety, is a good source of iron, calcium, magnesium and potassium.

Stevia

Native South Americans have used this leafy herb for centuries. The extract from stevia is 100 to 300 times sweeter than white sugar. It can be used in cooking, baking and beverages, does not affect blood sugar levels and has zero calories. Stevia is available in a powder or liquid form, but be sure to get the green or brown liquids or powders, because the white and clear versions are highly refined.

Sucanat

Short for Sugar Cane Natural, this brand-name product consists of evaporated organic cane juice made through a mechanical rather than a chemical process; and thus it is less refined, retaining many of sugarcane's original vitamins and minerals. It has a grainy texture and can be used in place of white sugar.

Coconut Sugar

This sugar is made when the sap of coconut palm trees is dried and granulated. It's a very low glycemic sweetener that is light brown in color and exhibits a rich, caramel-like flavor.

Yacon Sugar

This sweetener comes from a root vegetable in Peru that gets extracted to create a slightly sweet syrup. Yacon does not elevate blood glucose levels, making it a safe alternative to sugar, especially for diabetics and people with candida overgrowth. It contains prebiotic qualities that help promote calcium absorption and strengthen the immune system.

balanced diet, nourishing ourselves with milder forms of sweet vegetables, we don't need a big sugar hit from a candy bar or soda to boost our energy levels.

Unfortunately, more research shows that intense sweet flavors are as addictive as drugs like cocaine to our bodies. Sugar and, in particular high fructose corn syrup, are so overused in foods today that we are all left addicted and wanting more.[8]

Increasingly, more people have begun to understand the need to find alternatives to sugar, creating a demand that has led to the creation of artificial sweeteners, like saccharin (Sweet'N Low) and aspartame (Equal, NutraSweet). Although these products have been linked to serious health problems, such as cancer, public demand for sugar alternatives continues to increase.

Research continues to show that these substitutes actually cause weight gain by stimulating your appetite and your body's fat storage capabilities, even though they are touted as "diet" products.[9]

So manufacturers continue to explore other options. Sucralose is the latest to hit the market under the brand name Splenda. It has become the nation's number-one selling artificial sweetener in a remarkably short period of time. Splenda claims to be the perfect sugar substitute, as sweet as sugar with no calories, no surge in insulin and no side effects or long-term health damage. But some health advocates say it is no better than the pesticide, DDT.

Splenda is a synthetic compound discovered in 1976 by British scientists attempting to create a pesticide. Sucralose is made from sugar in a patented five-step process that substitutes three atoms of chlorine for three atoms of hydrogen-oxygen, converting sugar into a fructo-galactose molecule. It is a chlorinated molecule, which is the basis for DDT, and can accumulate in body fat. This type of molecule does not occur in nature, and therefore your body does not possess the ability to properly metabolize it. So although sucralose tastes like sugar and sweetens like sugar, the body does not know how to assimilate it, which is why it has zero calories. Questions about the safety of sucralose have been raised, but it's too early to determine its negative effects. Long-term studies are needed. One can assume it would not enhance health.

From a holistic point of view, it makes more sense to go with naturally occurring sweeteners, rather than artificial products. However, switching from white to brown sugar or coarse turbinado sugar is also not the answer. These alternatives contain 96% sucrose—not much of an improvement on the 99.9% sucrose content in refined white sugar. An easy way to reduce your overall intake is to just use less. If you are baking a recipe that calls for one cup of sugar, try using a 1/2 cup. If you put three tablespoons of sugar in your coffee, try using two and then one until you are ready to try something more natural like coconut sugar. As you slowly decrease your sugar intake, you will notice your palate changing and you will crave fewer sweets.

Dairy

Female mammals in the wild nourish their babies with their own milk and stop after a relatively brief period of growth. After this time, young mammals never again show any interest in milk, nor do they have access to it. Humans are the only mammals who continue to consume milk into adulthood. The plain truth is we don't need dairy.

I am not saying we should stop enjoying the wide range of dairy products available in modern society, but it is worth acknowledging that dairy is not an essential part of the human diet, and, in fact, most adults around the world do not consume it at all. Most of them can't because they are lactose intolerant, which means they lack the digestive enzymes needed to digest dairy.

Even people who can digest dairy typically consume too much. Dairy products, especially cheese and ice cream, are loaded with fat and cholesterol that contribute to clogged arteries and heart disease. The Harvard School of Public Health even cites a possible increased risk of ovarian and prostate cancer in those who consume three cups per day, as the government recommends. In addition, dairy has been cited as a significant contributing cause of the following ailments: menstrual pains, asthma, brain fog, mucus and a wide range of allergies with symptoms such as skin conditions and mood swings. Many people never realize that their problems are caused by dairy sensitivity and take various medications instead of addressing the underlying issue. A brief break from consuming dairy often leads to surprising improvements in many health conditions.

Modern methods of dairy processing are cause for concern. The typical cow produces milk for about 300 days after giving birth.[10] In an attempt to keep daily production levels high throughout this time, the industry began

Calcium Content in Dairy and Non-Dairy Foods*

Dairy

Cow's Milk	291 mg
Yogurt	252 mg
Human Breast Milk	33 mg

Non-Dairy

Sesame Seeds	1160 mg
Sardines	371 mg
Amaranth	267 mg
Collard Greens	250 mg
Kale	249 mg
Almonds	234 mg
Parsley	203 mg
Dandelion Greens	187 mg
Mustard Greens	183 mg
Salmon	167 mg
Watercress	151 mg
Chickpeas	150 mg
Beans	135 mg
Pistachio Nuts	131 mg
Tofu	128 mg
Figs	126 mg
Sunflower Seeds	120 mg
Buckwheat	114 mg
Beet Greens	99 mg
Spinach	93 mg
Swiss Chard	88 mg
Soybeans	60 mg
Leeks	52 mg
Broccoli	48 mg
Cauliflower	42 mg
Brussels Sprouts	36 mg

*Calcium content of foods based on 100-gram or 3.5-ounce portions.

Source: Agricultural Resource Service. Nutrient Database for Standard Reference. Release 17, 2002.

widespread use of bovine growth hormone, or BST, a controversial, genetically engineered growth hormone that is injected into cows to increase milk production. The manufacturers of BST claim the hormone has no adverse side effects on animals or humans, but many experts disagree. Canada and the European Union have banned its use.

In order to maximize milk production, dairy cows are kept pregnant most of their lives on both commercial and organic farms. During pregnancy, female cows' hormones like, estrogen and progesterone, go sky-high, and these hormones are present in their milk. There is both concern and evidence that high hormone content in dairy products is linked to high rates of breast cancer among women in America. I suggest women who regularly consume significant amounts of dairy products consider seeking alternatives, like the ones listed in the Dairy-Free Options, or at least take care to improve the quality and reduce the quantity of dairy they are eating.

If you eat dairy, I strongly encourage eating organic. The organic cow's natural diet contains no added hormones, chemicals or antibiotics. Studies show that organic milk contains higher levels of omega-3 fatty acids, vitamins A and E and antioxidants.[11] Unfortunately, even organic dairies can be controversial. Horizon Organic Dairy, the largest U.S. supplier of organic milk, is owned by Dean Foods, the largest processor and distributor of milk in the United States. Horizon has been accused of not enforcing the standards necessary to be labeled organic. On genuine organic dairy farms, cows are raised on open pastures, fed grass and not given extra hormones. Experts say the cows at Horizon are raised in pens and fed mostly protein and grains.

They have also been accused of manipulating and abusing the organic labeling criteria, misrepresenting their product and misleading health-conscious consumers into buying it. Although the milk from the Horizon farms may not be the best possible quality, it is still better than the milk produced at conventional dairy factories, with thousands of cows pumped up with antibiotics and confined in small spaces. Organic milk costs up to twice as much as regular milk, but I contend that it is worth it. Just make sure you are educated about its source.

Contrary to popular belief, dairy does not prevent osteoporosis or bone fracture by boosting calcium intake. In fact, numerous studies have demonstrated that countries with the highest intake of dairy, such as the United

Dairy-Free Options

Soy

Made from the liquid extract of whole soybeans, soy milk is a popular alternative to milk and has been produced in Asian countries for centuries. Plain, unfortified soy milk is a great source of protein, B vitamins and iron, but does have a strong aftertaste. This alternative is the most processed of the dairy-free options. It's not suitable for infants or anyone with soy allergies.

Rice

Rice milk is made from blending brown rice and water. It contains more carbohydrates than cow's milk and has a lighter taste and texture. Commercial varieties usually add some type of sweetener and fortify the milk with calcium, iron and B vitamins. Rice milk is the base for a popular Latin American and Mexican drink called horchata, which is made with a blend of cinnamon, vanilla and sugar.

Almond

Almond milk is made from ground almonds. It contains no lactose or cholesterol but is high in natural fats. Commercial varieties usually contain added vitamins, vanilla and sweeteners, but unsweetened varieties are also available. You can also make nut milks with other nuts, including hazelnuts, walnuts and Brazil nuts.

Oat

Oat milk has a creamy taste that comes from blending cooked oats and water. It's naturally high in fiber and low in protein.

Coconut

Coconut milk is a naturally sweet, white liquid made from the meat of a mature coconut. This milk is very rich, due to its high oil content. You typically find it canned, usually in the Asian foods section of a grocery store, since it's used as a base for many Thai curries. You can also use it for desserts and making creamy sauces.

> ### Hemp
>
> Made from soaking and grinding hemp seeds with water, this milk is quite creamy. Hemp seeds do not contain THC, the psychoactive substance found in marijuana. But they do have an amazing amount of healthy fats with a three-to-one ratio of omega-6 to omega-3, along with magnesium, calcium, fiber and amino acids—making this drink a great vegan source of protein.

States, Sweden and Holland, have the highest incidence of osteoporosis and fractures, while countries with the lowest dairy intake, such as Japan and South Africa, have the lowest rates of osteoporosis and fractures.[12] Harvard University's landmark Nurses' Health Study followed 78,000 women during a 12-year period and found that those who consumed the most dairy broke more bones than those who rarely consumed dairy. Healthy bones need calcium, magnesium, phosphorus, boron, copper, manganese, zinc and many vitamins. An excess of calcium without these other vitamins and minerals can actually increase the likelihood of fracture. Vegetable foods high in calcium, such as collards, bok choy and sea vegetables, also contain an abundance of magnesium and other minerals. Eating a good amount of green vegetables, whole grains and sea vegetables can provide all the essential calcium needed for the human body, without the added negative side effects of dairy.

For some people, dairy is an emotional issue. It's a food that provokes a lot of feelings and attachment, possibly stemming from early memories of breast-feeding. When I point out the hazards of high dairy consumption at school, many students adamantly refuse to give it up. If you have an emotional response to the idea of reducing or eliminating dairy, it may be helpful to examine the source of these emotions. Perhaps dairy is providing you with nourishment outside of the protein, fat and minerals, nourishment that is not about secondary food nutrition. If so, try to think of other ways you can get this nourishment.

Meat

Excessive meat eating has been implicated in many types of chronic disease. Advertising and high-protein diet books emphasize the need to eat more and more meat. This advice is dangerous. Any kind of mass-produced, factory-farmed, commercially grown meat—whether it is beef, pork or chicken—is loaded with hormones and antibiotics that are designed to generate the maximum amount of meat per animal, and therefore the maximum amount of profit for the producers. When you eat the meat, you eat the hormones and antibiotics. These animals are also subject to life in unnatural and confined environments and are fed processed diets.

Red meat is full of saturated fats and has no fiber and no phytochemicals. Commercially raised chickens are not a good alternative. These animals spend their lives in tiny cages, crammed with thousands of other birds, which leads to major stress and disease outbreaks. These chickens contain excessive levels of antibiotics, steroids and growth hormones, all of which are fed to them in an attempt to keep them healthy and fat while confined in these unnatural conditions. Moreover, the fat levels of commercially raised chickens are more than three times the level of their free-range relatives. Organic, free-range varieties may cost two or three times as much as commercial chickens, but the price is worth it. Remember, too, that animals raised in factory farms suffer, and this suffering is passed on to those who consume their meat. I've already discussed how humans take on the qualities of animals we consume through Cross-Species Transference, and we also take on their pain of being reared in cruel conditions.

For many people, eating meat is a question of ethics. Some vegetarians and vegans are adamant in their belief that eating animals is inhumane. Other people feel as strongly about their need to eat meat to feel healthy. I believe people should choose whatever protein source feels comfortable for them. I pray for the day when all people can thrive on a vegetarian diet. But through my years of experience, I have seen many vegetarian-type people become healthier by incorporating small amounts of organic meat into their diet. I have also seen many heavy meat eaters become healthier after reducing the amount of meat in their diet.

Deconstructing Meat Labels

Organic

According to the USDA, organic meat, poultry, eggs and dairy products come from animals that are given no antibiotics or growth hormones.

Natural

The terms natural and organic are not interchangeable. Only food labeled "organic" has been certified as meeting USDA organic standards.

Free Range

This term implies that animals are raised in an open air or free-roaming environment. The USDA defines "free range" for poultry products only— not for eggs. For poultry, the government requires outdoor access for "an undetermined period each day." No other meat carrying the "free range" label has been regulated by the USDA or any other governing agency. The best way to determine if the meat you are buying is free range is to contact the individual manufacturer.[13]

Grass-fed

The American Grassfed Association defines "grass-fed" cattle, bison, goats and sheep as those that have eaten nothing but their mother's milk and fresh grass or grass-type hay from birth. Pigs and poultry are "grass-fed," if they have had grass as a large part of their diets. The USDA is currently reviewing its guidelines on grass-fed marketing claims.

Pasture-Raised

Recently this term has popped up on labels of meat, milk and egg cartons to describe animals that were raised in open fields in an ecologically friendly manner. Some people consider this designation a step above organic. Always get to know your farmers or sources whenever possible, as this term is not regulated.

Marine Stewardship Council

This label found on seafood products aims to promote sustainable fishing practices. The council is an independent global nonprofit created to "ensure that the catch of marine resources are at the level compatible with long-term sustainable yield, while maintaining the marine environment's bio-diversity, productivity and ecological processes." They work with various fisheries to maintain these standards and label fish accordingly.

A funny thing happens to students at my school. The ones who come in as heavy meat eaters often graduate with a more vegetarian-type diet, and many who enroll as vegans or vegetarians leave as fish or meat eaters. When presented with the opportunity to experiment with food in a nonjudgmental, supportive community, people are able to find balance in their individual needs for protein.

Bearing all this in mind, I generally recommend people limit meat eating to a few times a week and supplement their diets with other protein sources such as eggs, beans, and whole grains. If you are a regular meat eater, choose organic meats whenever possible. Many stores and restaurants now offer meat from small, local farms that have been raised in humane ways without the use of chemicals and antibiotics.

Coffee

Millions of people jump-start their days with a cup of coffee, and then drink another cup or two or three throughout the day. Starbucks stores and others have proliferated throughout the world. More and more people try to move faster and faster to keep pace with the increasing demands of modern society. Not surprisingly, coffee represents 75% of all caffeine consumed in the United States alone. But more than 400 billion cups are consumed each year, making coffee the world's most popular beverage.[14] Caffeine is a drug, and we are a world of caffeine addicts.

Drinking coffee isn't just a matter of personal taste. It has become a cultural habit, an entertainment and a form of comfort. It's warm, it's foamy;

Alternatives to Coffee

Black Tea

Black tea is made from the dried leaves of the Camellia sinensis plant, a perennial evergreen shrub. The leaves of black tea are oxidized and heavily fermented before drying, which gives this tea a strong flavor. Varieties of black tea are named for their growing regions, like Ceylon or Darjeeling. Black tea has about 50 mg of caffeine per 8-ounce cup, as compared to coffee which has anywhere from about 100-190 mg per 8-ounce cup.[12] The amount of caffeine depends on how long the tea has brewed and the quality of the tea.

Dandy Blend

This instant dandelion beverage is an herbal coffee substitute made from dandelion, chicory and sugar beet. Rich in minerals, this alternative provides extra energy without caffeine. Dandelion is known for its detoxifying properties.

Green Tea

Known for its popularity in Japan and powerful antioxidant qualities, green tea has been shown to reduce the risk of certain types of cancer and lower LDL cholesterol. Green, black and oolong teas all come from the leaves of the same plant. What sets green tea apart from black teas is the way it is processed. The leaves are steamed, rather than fermented, as they are for black teas and oolong teas. This steaming process is said to enhance its disease-fighting qualities. Green tea has about 30 mg of caffeine per 8-ounce cup. Many people describe its taste as a grassy or earthy flavor.

Oolong Tea

Oolong tea originated in the Fujian province of China. This tea is semi-oxidized, providing a milder flavor than black or green tea. Oolong is known for having digestive and detoxifying properties. The caffeine level is between the levels of black and green tea.

Pero

This caffeine-free, instant coffee substitute is from Switzerland and is made from malted barley, chicory and rye.

Teechino

A blend of roasted herbs, grains, fruits and nuts make up this caffeine-free coffee alternative. It brews similarly to coffee, can be used in a coffee machine and has a similar aroma and taste to coffee. It has high levels of potassium, which helps to balance acidity. It offers a natural energy boost from the nutrients, not from the stimulants.

White Tea

White tea comes from the same plant as green, black and oolong, but the difference is in the leaves. They are picked earlier in the season when the leaves are young and the buds are covered with white hairs, giving this tea its name. White tea has gone through a minimal amount of processing and is not fermented. This tea has a light, sweet taste and has a small amount of caffeine, about 15 mg per serving.

Yerba Mate

Yerba Mate is a species of holly, native to South America. It is prepared by steeping dried leaves in hot water, rather than boiling hot water, as you would for coffee or tea. The flavor is bitter, herbal, grassy and somewhat similar to green tea. The stimulant in yerba mate is called xanthines, which is similar to caffeine, although many people report fewer side effects. It also contains potassium, magnesium and manganese.

and it tastes good with sugar, chocolate powder or cinnamon on top. It's an enjoyable social moment, a ritual and a symbol of dynamic, busy, working people.

Coffee producers spend a lot of time and money to reassure the American public that drinking coffee isn't bad for their health, including a general statement that up to three cups per day causes no health problems whatsoever, and may in fact even prevent diseases such as cancer and diabetes.[15] Caffeine, the essential ingredient, is said to enhance alertness, concentration and mental and physical performance, and its negative side effects are downplayed. But coffee does have some health risks. It inhibits the absorption of essential minerals, such as iron, magnesium and zinc, as well as B vitamins. Many studies have also linked heavy coffee consumption with higher risks for miscarriages, osteoporosis and heart disease.

Coffee is, essentially, an adrenaline delivery system that jolts the body's central nervous system. In the short term, this jolting action wakes us up and gets us going. In the long term, the constant and unnatural stimulation of our nerves creates stress levels that damage the resilience of the immune system, which protects against disease. Coffee is part of a stress cycle. We need coffee to keep up with the pace of modern life, and coffee itself helps to create the nervous energy of this pace.

People like to talk about the aroma and the flavor of various coffee brands, just as they enthuse about certain vintage wines, and it's true to a point. But if you're knocking back a bottle of cabernet a day, it's not just the taste that's attracting you. It's the same with coffee. If you're drinking three or four cups a day, you have an addiction. Drinking water and healthy snacking throughout the day can help to crowd out coffee, boosting your energy through nutrition rather than adrenaline rushes.

Caffeine should be given up slowly. Caffeine withdrawal is not fun, and people often report headaches and mood swings. I recommend quitting by slowly reducing the number of cups of coffee you drink each day, or by diluting full-strength coffee with decaf. Crowd out coffee by frequently drinking bottled or filtered water throughout the day. Rediscover the delights of drinking tea. Green and white teas contain a much lower amount of caffeine and can be a great way to get over the withdrawal headaches.

If you are a heavy coffee drinker, I urge you to consider what your life would be like without coffee and who you are without coffee. Think about your natural state as a person without all that coffee speed. Maybe you would get to bed earlier, take more time to get places or take a closer look at what foods really help energize you. Have you ever driven, ridden your bike or walked through the same block in your neighborhood? Wasn't each experience completely different? I often compare slowing down in life to riding a bike instead of driving or even walking instead of riding a bike. In each action we become more connected to our surroundings and we see things with a new perspective. If you still can't imagine a life without coffee, I urge you to find the highest quality available and drink it in moderation.

PROFILE

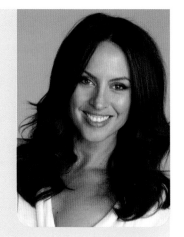

Sarah Wilson, Sydney, New South Wales, Australia
www.sarahwilson.com.au

"I had to heal myself, from the inside out."

Four years ago my body came to a screeching halt. I was the editor of *Cosmopolitan* magazine, the biggest magazine in Australia. I was sleeping 5 hours a night, running every day, underweight, exhausted and stressed beyond belief. Then I collapsed with adrenal fatigue and an autoimmune disease—Hashimoto's. I couldn't walk and was told I was infertile. I had to reevaluate my life. I believe my body stopped me in my tracks because I was long overdue for a "regroup and refocus". Our bodies are great like that!

I soon learned that my illness was something that couldn't be fixed by traditional medicine overnight. I had to heal myself, from the inside out. I decided to turn my search for wellness—whole, true, fundamental wellness—into a career. I launched a column in the national weekend newspaper magazine on "how to make life better" and hosted two television series on food. One of which, MasterChef, went on to be the biggest show in Australian history. I also blog daily on my discoveries, helping people heal themselves, predominantly with food.

This is how I came to study at Integrative Nutrition. I was in search of a course that I could follow as a path for my own healing, but that also qualified me to help others and to give what I was doing in the media cache and legitimacy. I was after a course that discussed wellness as a way of being, that wasn't didactic or prescriptive, but inspiring. My experience has shown me that rules and regulations ordained from above don't work (ergo, diets don't work!).

I applied many of the principles learned through my studies—"crowding out," preserving my digestive enzymes by soaking and sprouting, and most importantly, working out the rhythms and systems that work for me. The big change came when I quit sugar, as inspired by the course. I wrote about my journey to eliminate all fructose from my diet and have inspired hundreds—possibly thousands—to do the same.

Since completing my studies at Integrative Nutrition, I've been called upon to do keynote speaking on wellness and to be an ambassador for various organizations and brands. The messages I learned in the course are now part of my "brand" and my career has truly evolved into the wellness sphere.

Unhealthy Fats

Starting in 1975, government recommendations, food advertisers, medical doctors and nutrition experts advocated a diet low in fat. What this fad failed to address was the difference between low-quality fats contained in junk foods and naturally occurring high-quality fats that can be beneficial to health.

In the early 1990s a low-fat craze swept the U.S. Every cookie, cracker and cake variety came in a low-fat version. Yet, Americans continued to get fat. We became a nation of fat fearers, believing that eating fat made us fat. The truth is that our bodies need fat, and knowing what kinds of fats to consume and what kinds to avoid is not complicated.

Isn't it funny that the word we use to describe people who are overweight is the same word for this food group? I think this connotation perpetuates the idea that fats makes you fat, but it's not true. Your body needs fat to nourish your heart, brain, nerves, hormones and every cell. Fat is good for the health of your hair, skin and nails too. Studies conducted in the 1970s of the native Greenland Eskimo population showed that despite their high intake of fats—about 70% of their diet—they had very low rates of heart disease, diabetes and cancer. The main source of fats in their diet came from wild, marine foods—a far cry from what's on most supermarket shelves.

Your body's fat storage is not necessarily related to the fat you consume. When eating the wrong kinds of fats, your body lacks the ability to create healthy cells, leading to nutritional deprivation. You could be overweight and still undernourished, especially if you are eating chemicalized, artificial junk foods. Many people on low-fat diets feel hungry all the time and as a consequence, overeat. Did you ever set out to have a few low-fat or fat-free cookies and end up eating the whole box? That's because there is nothing in them that makes you feel satiated. The brain doesn't get the "stop eating" message. You actually need the fat to feel full. Fat also makes food taste good. It carries flavors and smells more than carbohydrates or protein do. Cooks combine spices with a fat or oil, such as butter or olive oil for this very reason. They know it makes their food taste great.

The four basic types of fat found in food are *saturated*, *monounsaturated*, *polyunsaturated* and *trans fats*. All fats, or lipids, are composed of fatty acids, which are chains of carbon atoms with hydrogen atoms filling the bonds.

The chemical composition of the fatty acid chains determines the type of fat. *Saturated* fats are found mainly in animal foods and tropical oils, like coconut and palm oils. The fatty acid chain is highly stable and straight-shaped, so these fats are solid or semi-solid at room temperature. *Monounsaturated* fats have a double bond, making them more flexible, so they tend to be liquid at room temperature and solid when refrigerated. Examples of monounsaturated fats include olive, sesame and avocado oils. *Polyunsaturated* fats are considered essential because the body cannot make them and must rely on food sources to get them. The two polyunsaturated fatty acids found most frequently in food are omega-6 and omega-3. These fats have two or more double bonds, which makes them more reactive and unstable, especially at high temperatures. They also remain liquid even when refrigerated and can form free radicals when they are heated during extraction and processing or when used for cooking. These free radicals can initiate disease. Examples include corn, soy, safflower and sunflower oils. So although some of these oils seem healthy, they quickly become unhealthy when heated.

Trans fats are found in many processed junk foods, frozen foods, margarines, French fries, donuts and other baked goods. On labels these fats are listed as hydrogenated and partially hydrogenated oils. Trans fats are artificially produced by combining hydrogen with polyunsaturated oils—a process called hydrogenation. Consuming hydrogenated oil can interfere with your body's natural processes, leading to many health problems including increased risk of coronary death.

As mentioned in chapter 1, the FDA now requires all packaged foods to list trans fats on their labels. But many people are unknowingly consuming trans fats when they eat out. Integrative Nutrition became personally involved with the issue of trans fats at the end of 2006, when the New York City Department of Health called for a public hearing to potentially limit the amount of trans fats in all New York restaurants. As buzz built in the city, we saw an opportunity to get involved. I spoke both at the hearing in support of the ban on trans fats and at a rally across from the health department, which Integrative Nutrition organized with vendors, music and speakers including Anne Lappé, Dr. Walter Willett and Michael Jacobson, executive director of the Center for Science in the Public Interest.

Our voices were heard. New York City became the first major U.S. city to ban trans fats in restaurants and fast-food chains in 2007. Other cities and local governments have since followed suit. Worldwide, there's a movement to ban or label trans fats. Many large chains are now voluntarily switching their cooking oils, including Denny's, Burger King, KFC, T.G.I. Friday's, and Starbucks. Even the Walt Disney Company introduced new food guidelines in 2006 that would eliminate trans fats from food served at its parks by the end of 2007.

To beat the overall fat-fearing mentality, work on substituting good fats for bad fats. Choosing healthy portions of good fats can actually help you lose weight, increase your energy, boost your immunity and optimize digestion. Even saturated fats are needed to keep the body functioning. Coconut oil is one example of a good saturated fat source. It can help you lose weight, because the body converts it quickly to energy. It also contains lauric acid, a medium-chain fatty acid found in only one other naturally occurring place: human breast milk. Coconut oil is also more stable than other oils and can stand up to heat, which makes it a great choice for cooking. Other natural sources of good fats include avocados, olive oil, raw nuts, sesame and hemp seeds and cold-water fatty fish such as salmon, mackerel and tuna.

Salt

Salt is not inherently bad. Throughout history, people have used salt to season and preserve their food. A good quality sea salt can contain up to 92 minerals and can be considered a dietary supplement. Sodium acts as an electrolyte and assists in regulating cell function, while chloride supports potassium absorption and helps regulate body fluids. The health problems associated with overconsumption of salt are from the refined, processed, white sparkly salt found in prepared foods and in the table salts so many Americans use at home.

The World Health Organization now recommends that adults consume less than 2,000 mg of sodium per day, along with at least 3,500 mg of potassium.[16] With just one teaspoon of salt containing about 2,300 mg of sodium, the average adult American consumes nearly double the WHO recommended amount each day.[17,18] Most medical experts agree that diets high in sodium are a major cause of high blood pressure as well as pre-hypertension, both of which significantly increase the risk of having a heart attack or stroke. Today, raised blood pressure causes about 7.5 million deaths or about 12.8% of the total of all deaths, according to WHO.[19] While excessive salt intake is not the only reason for these alarming statistics, it is a significant contributing factor. A 2005 study reports that high-salt diets cause 150,000 premature deaths a year in the United States.[20]

Restaurant foods, fast foods and processed, packaged junk foods contribute to the majority of sodium in our diets. One serving (half a cup) of Campbell's Chicken noodle soup has 890 mg of sodium and one slice of cheese pizza, from a Pizza Hut 12-inch pan pizza, contains 570 mg. If you have a full cup of canned soup, you've already reached your recommended daily sodium intake and you're almost half way there with two slices of cheese pizza. Healthier versions are not much better.

Public health advocates claim that if we could reduce the sodium in processed and restaurant foods by half, we could save thousands of lives. My solution is simpler and immediate: Master the art of home cooking. The next chapter will discuss how to get started or improve your current routine.

I strongly recommend using a high-quality sea salt for home cooking. High-quality, natural sea salt is a better choice than poor quality, refined table salt. For the most part, people today use processed, sparkling white salt that is stripped of the trace elements and minerals in high-quality sea salt. Food companies also put additives—such as sugar and potassium iodide—into refined salt. Potassium iodide is added to reduce iron deficiency and thyroid disease, but it's actually been linked to the increased incidence of hyperthyroidism. All this processing takes place to make salt less expensive and a prettier color, as natural sea salt has a brownish tint.

Using high-quality sea salt in limited quantities is a healthier and tastier way to get minerals and satisfy your body's cravings for salty flavor. Watch out for highly processed sea salts, which usually list magnesium carbonate as an ingredient. Look for sea salts that are free of coloring, additives, chemicals or bleaching. They should have a reddish or brown tint.

Chocolate

I don't think I've ever met a person who doesn't like chocolate. Whether dark or light, sweet or bitter, chocolate has a widespread appeal in our culture. Europeans account for almost half of the chocolate consumed in the world.[21] Americans consume almost 12 pounds of chocolate per person each year. The Swiss consume the most chocolate worldwide at about 22 pounds per person. Chocolate comprises a number of raw and processed foods that originate from the seed of the tropical cacao tree. The beans have an intense bitter taste. Cacao is high in iron, calcium, potassium and vitamins A, B, C and D and E. It can also provide protection against cancer, heart disease and high blood pressure. The Mayan, Aztec and Olmec civilizations in Mexico and Central America first took these beans and mixed them with chili powder, honey or vanilla to make a drink, creating chocolate. They considered chocolate a divine food. In Steve Gagne's book, *Energetics of Food*, he writes that both the Mayans and Aztecs referred to cacao as a "food of the gods." Other research shows medicinal uses for chocolate, using it primarily as a means to deliver medicine. Cacao flowers were also used to treat fatigue and cacao paste was used to treat poor appetite.

Of course, commercially produced chocolate does not contain many of these natural nutrients, nor does it have the same spiritual connection, although some people do create daily rituals around Hershey's or Godiva. One of the reasons chocolate has a bad rap is because most chocolate sold in supermarkets has high amounts of added sugar, fat, trans fats and preservatives. Long regarded as a sinful, addictive and fattening temptation, chocolate provides a natural feel-good high.

Part of why we love chocolate is that it helps release serotonin in the brain, which produces feelings of pleasure. This pleasure may also help explain intense chocolate cravings. Its melting point is also slightly below our body temperatures, so it really does melt in our mouths. I recommend finding an organic brand with a high percentage of cacao. In a world that is becoming increasingly contracted and stressful, chocolate gives people a sense of lightness, expansiveness, comfort and relaxation. In some ways, it's a really good food for people who are trying to gain weight. I have helped clients who were looking to gain weight add more chocolate to their diet with much success.

The issue of whether chocolate is good or bad really comes back to bio-individuality. Remember one person's food is another person's poison. Some people are so addicted to chocolate that they may need to reduce or eliminate this food. For others, indulging in a small amount of high-quality organic chocolate every now and again can really be an enjoyable part of life.

Exercises

1. Reduce One Food

Choose one food from this chapter—sugar, dairy, meat, coffee, unhealthy fat, salt or chocolate—that you feel would be useful to reduce.

Which one did you choose and why?

For one week, gently decrease your consumption of this one food and write down the results.

What is difficult about reducing this food?

What is easy about reducing this food?

Does your body feel different? Healthier? More energized? Clearer? How did reducing this food impact your cravings for other foods?

Are you going to continue to minimize this food in your diet?

2. Be Bad

Now that I've covered foods that can lead to health problems when over-consumed, I want to introduce you to the joy and freedom of throwing away the rules and being bad. Over the next week I invite you to do something bad every single day. When I say "bad," I mean something you feel you shouldn't do or feel is irresponsible. Obviously, I'm not asking you to rob a bank or hurt another human being. Perhaps you'll delete unread emails, play hooky from work, or tell someone what you really think. Start slowly. Gradually build your "being bad" muscles.

The purpose behind this exercise is to put you back in charge of your life. Many of us feel like being good is what makes us worthwhile. We put pleasing others above pleasing ourselves. Learning to put yourself first and find your voice is priceless. If people like you—great. If they don't, know that you are still a very good person. This way, you remain true to you. There's nothing more health promoting than that.

Now write down three things you want to do this week to practice being bad.

Examples:

1. Leave early from work to get a massage.

2. Order the expensive dessert at my favorite restaurant.

3. Schedule a playdate for me, instead of the kids.

CHAPTER 11

Cooking Like Your Life Depends on It

tell people to cook like their life depends on it, because it does. The food we take into our mouth goes into our stomach, where it gets digested and eventually assimilated into the bloodstream. Our blood is what creates our cells, our tissues, our organs, our skin, our hair, our brains and even our thoughts and feelings. We are, at our most basic level, walking food. Learning to cook high-quality foods for yourself and those you love changes everything. The three most important aspects of cooking are that the food be homemade, freshly made and lovingly made.

For me, there's nothing like when I am home and in my own kitchen. I get up, make some quinoa and vegetables and a cup of tea. When I'm home it's, "La-ti-da. Maybe I'll add some ginger." It's so peaceful and so nurturing. It's strange to me that restaurant food has become the rage today, minimizing the beauty and the value of home-cooked food. With restaurant food, people get caught up in the décor, the atmosphere and even the menu. The food itself is often very flamboyant with lots of salt and flavoring. But it's all show. I love eating out on occasion, but the environment can be very hectic. If I was at home and 30 people were moving around and talking in my kitchen, I would freak out. I don't want to put down restaurants, but sometimes when I'm traveling, I fantasize about homemade vegetables. I long for my simple routine and making food on my own time.

Homemade

Cooking nourishes our bodies on a variety of levels. When we put our own energy into the food, we ultimately put that energy back into ourselves.

When we cook, we have control over the quality and quantity of ingredients we are eating. Our body's natural intelligence will fine-tune our cooking style to create meals that are just what we need. When we are in a restaurant, we relinquish that control. We do not know where the food came from, how much salt or spices were added, what kind of oil was used, or the health and cleanliness of the various people who touched our food along the way. By cooking our own food, we ultimately create more love for ourselves, more love for our lives, and therefore, more health.

As we have evolved from living together in tribal societies to living together in our extended families and living in nuclear families, meals have mostly been eaten together in groups. Not long ago, dinner was at 6 p.m. every night with few exceptions. Mom made the meal, and the rest of the family members would all come home from work or school, and sit around the table together. The food would be served and everyone would eat while talking about the various events of the day. This ritual bonded people, and the family that ate together stayed together.

Today everything has changed. People increasingly eat most of their meals out, in restaurants, delis, fast-food chains or snacking along the way. Home is often like a hotel, serving only as a place for people to sleep at night. Parents, teenagers and children wake up at different times, go in different directions, eat separately and have little communication throughout the day. It's rare that everyone gets to have a home-cooked meal together. This schedule creates distance in family relationships, and the lack of quality, home-cooked food leads to a deficiency of primary nourishment.

Women's important roles in the home have more often than not been underappreciated in society, and are changing a lot, too. It is important to recognize how traditional, motherly nourishment supports the whole family. It keeps everyone healthy and happy in many ways. I am not suggesting that women go back to the typical role of homemaker, but I am a big believer in people eating homemade food as often as possible. When families are dealing with two careers, longer working hours and children with multiple extracurricular activities, it is unrealistic and unfair for the woman to be responsible for feeding the entire family. Men and children can also participate in shopping, preparing, cooking and cleaning. Just as sitting and eating together strengthens family bonds, so too can preparing a delicious meal together.

Children can wash and peel vegetables, set and clear the table, and when they get older even help chop and cook. A good policy in the kitchen is that whoever cooks is free from doing the dishes. Each household will be different, so please find a routine and system that works for yours. Be sure to utilize everyone and appreciate everyone's contributions.

Freshly Made

Food that is fresh affects us differently than food that's been sitting out for days. Think about the times you've been in a restaurant and a waiter passed by who was carrying a hissing tray of freshly cooked food, piled on a hot plate. The platter has so much energy that the whole restaurant turns around to see what is happening. We take in that same kind of energy when we eat food that's just been made.

Getting produce from farm to table is a complicated business. In chapter 3, I talked about food miles, or the distance food travels to get to your plate. Many fruits and vegetables don't arrive in the store until weeks after they were harvested, then they sit on the store shelf for a few days and spend a few more days in the fridge at home. For many restaurants there's a similar delay, and food sourcing has become a big issue. Many restaurants have moved to work closer with local farms to create farm-to-table or farm-to-fork restaurants. These restaurants locally source produce, meats and seafood and put a bigger emphasis on fresh, slowly cooked foods, prepared simply. Some even grow herbs and produce in the backyard or on the roof of their restaurants. When you don't have time to make your own food, I recommend finding a farm-to-table restaurant to enjoy fresh, simple food.

Because of practical convenience, we often eat food that has been canned, frozen, sitting in a freezer or made hours earlier. Sometimes we have to do this, and I'm not against it. Canned and flash frozen vegetables can be quite fresh since they're often packaged just after being harvested, and many stores now carry organic varieties. These foods are also a great transition for people looking to add more vegetables into their diets.

In countries where fresh food has traditionally been valued, many people go shopping and cook vegetables on the same day. Most modern consumers prefer the convenience of shopping only once a week. Wherever you live, I would like to point you in the direction of your local farmers. It wasn't that long ago that all food was grown locally. In the U.S. about 80 percent of the almost 2 million farms are small and family-owned businesses. Many farmers now sell their products directly to the public through farmers' markets, food coops, CSAs, farm stands and more. At farmers' markets the food is grown nearby, probably in the same county or at least in the same region or state. It's more alive, and this aliveness will transfer to your body.

Another way to have regular access to fresh, local food is to join a Community Supported Agriculture group. A CSA is when a group of people pledges to support a nearby farm in an economic partnership. The farm share model began in the 1960s in Europe and Japan in response to the rise of imported foods and urbanization of farmland.[1] Typically, members of the farm or garden pledge in advance to cover the anticipated costs of the farm operation and farmer's salary. In return, they receive shares of the farm's harvest throughout the growing season and the satisfaction of reconnecting to the land and participating directly in food production. Members also share in the risks of farming, including poor harvests from unfavorable weather or pests. Through this partnership, farmers receive better prices for their crops and gain some financial security. More than 12,500 CSA farms are in America today.[2]

Lovingly Made

After many years of personal observation, I've noticed that food prepared at home by a loving person has a different nutritional effect than the exact same food prepared in a restaurant. When we eat our mother's or grandmother's cooking, there's love in the food and care in its preparation, which creates a higher quality of love and energy. Invisible forces are at work, and they have an alchemical effect on the food itself. It tastes differently. It feels differently in the body. It affects us differently.

Foods made by someone you love contain a vital nutrient, something I call vitamin L, for love. Food that is cooked by someone who loves you, who is happy to be cooking and nourishing you, can be some of the best tasting food in the world. The energy of love is passed into the food and nourishes you in ways that go beyond micronutrients.

Have you ever been in a restaurant kitchen? It has a lot of crazy energy. Having been in the restaurant business, I know there are huge discrepancies between what goes on in the front and the back. In the front, everyone is nicey, nicey. "Oh Mr. Rosenthal, good to see you," they say. In the back, people are throwing knives. Do you really think that energy doesn't affect the energy of your food? The people preparing most restaurant food are underpaid kitchen workers, living on minimum wage without basic health- care. I may be wrong, but I'm guessing most of these people are not in love with their jobs. This fact alone is bound to make the quality of the food we eat at restaurants very different from that of home-cooked food. In addition to the hectic energy, restaurant managers and cooks are pressured into reducing costs, maximizing profits and getting food out on a very tight timeline. Their priority is to sell food, not to promote your health. Of course, in today's demanding world, we all need to eat out sometimes, we all want to eat out and enjoy a new atmosphere. Just remember that eating out every night of the week can have an impact on your health.

I feel privileged that I can make food at home that is so much better than restaurant food. It's a myth that preparing food is a complicated thing or that it has to look like Martha Stewart prepared it. When I'm at home, I use three to four ingredients, but when guests eat my food, they're like "Oh my God. What's in this?"

Rituals can increase your awareness around cooking at home. You might simply wash your hands, put on an apron or take a moment to close your eyes, take a breath in and set an intention for the meal you are about to create. You may also want to light a candle or put on some gentle music—anything that helps you be more present.

The last few minutes of cooking are usually the most stressful. Everything has to be done at the same time: final flavoring, transferring from cooking pot to serving dish, getting the dining area ready. It's helpful to have a ritual at the end of cooking too, before you dash to the table, sit down and start eating. Here are a couple of suggestions:

1. Pour yourself a glass of water and drink it slowly, to help you calm down and rehydrate. Cooks tend to become very tight—contracted and single-focused—and this simple act of drinking water helps ease you into a mellow, relaxed state of mind.

2. Serve yourself a small portion first and take a moment to smell the food and appreciate your gift of love through food.

When serving the food you've just cooked, please resist the temptation to apologize for imperfections. This habit will only focus your guests' attention on the limitations that you mention, rather than on their appreciation for your efforts. Instead, you want them to think, "Wow! Someone actually took the time to prepare a meal for me." If you are proud of your food, your family will enjoy it and appreciate you more, and it will help them remember the value of a homemade, freshly made and lovingly made meal.

Cooking with the Seasons

In many parts of the world when we buy food at the supermarket, we are not buying what's really in season. In the U.S. we find mangoes and bananas in the middle of winter and winter squash in the middle of summer. When I pick up an apple at the store during the fall, I'm always amazed at how much better it tastes than in the winter. By following the natural harvest of fruits and vegetables, we can strengthen our connection to our surroundings. Cooking with locally grown produce is a great way to honor the natural environment in which you live. It helps you feel more at home where you are, and supports your body in adapting to changes in season. Of course, seasons are different throughout the world, but start to notice how you feel during each season and what kind of foods make you feel the best. For me, I know when it's warm I'm drawn to more fruit and raw foods. When the weather starts to cool, I look for more hardy vegetables and whole grains. In the coldest months, I eat protein and fat to help my body stay warm, and as the weather warms again, I eat more greens to help lighten my body.

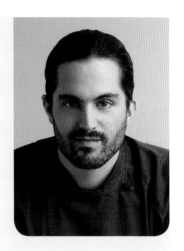

Frank Giglio, East Waterboro, ME, USA

www.frankgiglio.com

"True health is measured from happiness in all areas of life."

At the time I heard of Integrative Nutrition, I was running a small vegetarian kitchen in a local health food store in Connecticut. As a classically trained chef, this was a major departure from the fast paced world of working in restaurants. This new position allowed me to have a direct relationship with my customers and proved to be invaluable. Although I was motivated to help others, I wasn't thriving in my own environment. My life was incredibly out of balance in a number of ways. I was overweight, lacking proper exercise, inconsistent with my diet, and missing deep connections with friends and family. I was in a funk and looking for a way out of it.

A great friend approached me and offered a free health consultation. She was enrolled at Integrative Nutrition and was very motivated to help me out. After my consult, I decided that I needed to be a part of IIN and see what the school was all about. Instantly, I saw the light at the end of the tunnel and enrolled. My life began to click, and I was finally figuring out how to love myself and take my health to new heights.

By the time I actually began the program, I was nearly 25 pounds lighter and began living the life I was truly meant to live. I had taken up running, and within 6 months, I completed my first marathon. Just a few years later, I would go on to complete a 100-mile race in Vermont.

The ability to share with others allowed me to open up and express my true self. IIN helped me to find my passion in leading classes and workshops. Through my teachings, I have stressed the idea that we are all unique, and we require different foods for different times in our lives. Learning so many dietary theories has allowed me to improve my work with clients and support them in achieving their goals. Since graduating, I have led several workshops around the country, and most recently conducted demonstrations at events hosting over 1000 people.

The idea of finding balance is what has resonated with me the most from my training at Integrative Nutrition. True health is measured from happiness in all areas of life. I appreciate Joshua and all the staff at Integrative Nutrition for stressing that.

Eating foods out of season can make you more susceptible to colds, flu and other illnesses.

You can also adjust your cooking methods for the time of year. During the colder months, put more heat into your food and cook your food longer. Try roasting, baking, using a Crock-Pot and making stews to keep warm. When springtime comes, allow your food preparation to become a little simpler. You can start to incorporate more raw foods, quick high-temperature sautés and steamed dishes. Or notice how your body naturally craves more fruit, salad and lighter foods during warmer months.

You may also want to consider how your lifestyle reflects seasonal changes. In the spring months, people feel refreshed, get their gardens going, start new projects or pursue new romantic interests. When it's warm, people enjoy outdoor sports, play at the beach, go on vacation and engage in other high-energy activities, which are appropriate for the season. With fall, children return to school and people get into a kind of organizing mode. People tend to become very busy in September and October, running around, getting ready for winter. I notice during the fall that many animals also scurry around in preparation for winter. Until recently, humans did the same thing, scurrying to see if we had enough food or wood to keep us warm. No one has alerted our DNA that we now have heating in our homes or that we can drive to the store anytime we need food; we are preprogrammed to act this way. We still tap into our ancestral, cellular memories of the harvest season.

All that preparation comes to a head with an extended holiday season that lasts from the end of October through the beginning of January. Come Halloween, children scour the neighborhood and gather as much candy as they possibly can. Next come the holidays, and our actions fall out of pace, as we engage in the extreme sports of holiday shopping, partying and eating. At Thanksgiving, Americans nationwide congregate and overeat. The next day everyone complains about how stuffed they are and goes shopping. Then we're into December, with office parties, family get- togethers and social events that usually involve lots of drinking. This season leads to Christmas and more overeating, with a final blowout on New Year's Eve that entails even more eating and drinking. Other countries have your version of this cycle at this time of the year and others.

In North America, all this partying is happening when the normal, natural rhythms of life—colder weather, darker evenings, the end of the growing season—indicate this is the right time to turn inward. Humans are mammals, and mammals have a tendency to hibernate during the winter. They are not really sleeping; they are in a kind of battery saving mode, a state not unlike meditation. But, oddly, Americans do the opposite. Instead of going inward, slowing down and replenishing our energy for springtime, society is set up to keep us burning the candle at both ends. Then, in January and February, people feel exhausted and depressed, and the country has a widespread outbreak of colds and flu. People's exhausted immune systems cannot cope with the demands of winter, often combined with the inappropriate food consumption mentioned above.

Doctors have given a special name to the exhaustion and depression experienced during colder, darker months. They call it Seasonal Affective Disorder or SAD, and attribute it to people not getting enough sunlight. If you have been diagnosed with SAD, I encourage you to go more slowly, respecting the seasons and eating and drinking more moderately. I also recommend finding ways to get more sunlight into your life at this time. You'll likely feel much different by the end of the season; these seasonal blues will be a thing of the past.

If you want to go to holiday parties, enjoy yourself, but be moderate with food and alcohol, and strive to get enough down time. Remember to keep up your own cooking with seasonal, locally grown ingredients and share with others during this season. If the majority of your food is healthy and homemade, the occasional party or indulgence won't affect you. In addition, your immune system will become stronger and you'll avoid getting sick in the wintertime.

Simplicity

One of the main reasons people don't cook is because they think they don't have the time. It looks too complicated, and they don't know where to start. From the very beginning, they feel overwhelmed. They may open a cookbook and see a recipe for lasagna that looks delicious, but calls for a lot of ingredients and hours of labor. So they lose their initial enthusiasm, close the book and forget cooking. Don't confuse taste with function. If you want a fancy, tasty meal, go out to a restaurant. You don't need to be a gourmet chef at home; you need to be able to feed yourself and those you love in a nourishing, convenient way.

Occasionally, you may enjoy making a complex recipe, but for daily diet, you probably want to have simple, down-to-earth meals that can be prepared quickly and easily. It takes about five minutes to prepare a piece of fish or meat, another five minutes to prepare greens and less than 20 minutes of cooking time to get your meal on the table. If you decide to make a more complicated meal, make your main ingredients, like grains and vegetables, from scratch, and complement them with canned or frozen foods. With a little planning, you can soak beans overnight and reduce their cooking time for the next meal. Or if you're crunched for time, use canned beans. Cooking simple meals on a regular basis will lead you step by step to a simpler, more relaxed and enjoyable lifestyle.

Home cooking also saves you money. Many people unconsciously spend a lot of their income on food. People eat most of their meals in cafes, snack bars and restaurants, and these outings can run about $30 a day—that's almost $1,000 a month. Although organic produce and meats are more expensive, I think you'll find they are still cheaper than eating out. Look for local produce markets with reasonable prices and shop for seasonal fruits and vegetables, which naturally have lower prices. Get familiar with your local health food store and the bulk foods section, where you can find many staples including rice, pasta, beans, nuts and even herbs. The bulk section not only saves money, but also reduces the amount of packaging waste.

Cooking Tips

Use a Timer

Just because a recipe takes 40 minutes to cook doesn't mean it takes 40 minutes of your time. Using timers helps you know what's due to be taken off the stove and frees you for other activities. People think if they make their own food, they have to follow a recipe and be in the kitchen for an hour or more.

This thinking creates a negative attitude toward cooking. Maybe we don't really have much else to do, but the idea of waiting around the kitchen seems torturous. Timers allow people to eat in a healthy way without big demands on their schedules.

Burn the Rice

Try to keep your cooking simple. In the beginning, let yourself experiment and make mistakes. It's okay to burn the rice. Remember, everything in life has a learning curve. In the beginning, it will take time and may seem difficult, and you'll likely burn some foods and maybe some pots. But as you stay with it, cooking will become easier, more enjoyable and hugely rewarding. Once you become confident, you will have a lifetime of delicious, home-cooked food for yourself, your family and friends, save thousands of dollars, and increase health, vitality and family relatedness.

Add Flavor

One of the keys to an easy life in the kitchen is to cook food in a simple way, and then use condiments, spices and other dressings at the table. Make a wide variety of flavorings available so everyone can personalize the meal to their own taste. Your best companion in this regard is a condiment tray or lazy Susan, a circular dish that sits in the middle of the table on a swivel and rotates with the touch of your hand. Stock it with your favorite condiments. Some love garlic, some love ginger and spices, others prefer more salt, less salt, more oil or less oil. A lazy Susan can hold all of these, plus other standards like nut butters, salsa and salad dressings. People love to personalize their food, and this method makes it much easier for the cook. A list of readily available condiments is at the end of this chapter.

Cook Once, Eat Two or Three Times

You don't have to start from scratch at each meal. I'm a big fan of cooking once and eating twice to increase the amount of homemade food in the diet without spending too much time in the kitchen. I always try to incorporate something fresh into my leftovers, by heating them with a little water, olive oil and some fresh herbs, or sautéing carrots and onions and adding them to the dish. This gives my old food new energy and new flavor.

Whenever you cook, make extra. Take grains as an example. You can cook your favorite grain in the morning and use some for a hot breakfast cereal, perhaps adding some sweet flavor, like fresh fruit or raisins, and something hearty, like tahini or nut butter. Then you can add some different flavor to the leftover grains, or put them into a soup and take it to work for lunch. In the evening, you can add vegetables and protein, and stir-fry the remainder with oil to give it some extra sizzle. You can also put leftover food into the fridge in small containers for a great, healthy, wholesome snack in between meals. Cooking once and eating two or three times makes you feel like your investments of money on groceries and time in the kitchen were well worth it.

Notice the Effects of Your Cooking

Cooking for yourself is the best way to understand how you are affected by food. Since you know what you are putting into the meal, you can understand the food's effects on your body more directly. Maybe you feel sleepy after a meal and want to take a nap, or maybe you feel more active and have the urge to go somewhere and do something in order to generate energy to digest the meal. You will know if your cooking was too much for your body to handle, or if you feel unsatisfied and need more—an extra flavor perhaps or one more ingredient. I encourage you to explore, experiment, and learn to distinguish the foods and quantities that support your health from those that do not.

Healthy Restaurant Eating

Regardless of how hungry we are, we often find ourselves at restaurants ordering and eating large quantities of rich and heavy foods that we would never have at home. Most people don't realize it, but professional menus are designed to draw your eye to the most expensive food, or foods that are most profitable for the establishment. You need to sharpen your awareness to know clearly what you really want to eat, what you habitually eat if you don't stop to think about it, and what the restaurant owners would like you to eat.

When eating out, pause for a moment, keeping the menu closed, and take a moment to check in with yourself. What do you feel like eating right now? How hungry are you? What are the appropriate foods for you to be eating? The restaurant menu is not designed to answer such questions. It makes food sound so tantalizing, you start thinking, "Oh my God, fudge brownie with drizzled chocolate and a few added twists of sugar-crystallized tangerine topped with whipped cream. That sounds incredible!" Your mouth is watering so much that you develop complete amnesia and forget your intention to be aware about what you are eating.

One way to avoid a few common pitfalls of eating out is to not read the menu. If you are out with friends, enjoying a social connection, it ensures you don't suddenly cut off from each other and bury yourselves in the menus, destroying the convivial atmosphere. It also invites a direct dialogue with the waiter, as you inquire, "What do you recommend that has some vegetables and some protein, either fish or chicken?" When the waiter comes up with a couple of recommendations, you can ask, "What does it come with?"

Keep in mind that restaurants have a lot of vegetables in the kitchen that are not necessarily on the menu. Ask the waiter what vegetables are available and if the kitchen can make a side dish of steamed, sautéed vegetables in olive oil and garlic, or any way you prefer. This kind of request will help you get accustomed to building vegetables into all your meals.

Flexitarian

Although I strongly encourage home cooking, I am not saying we must cook all our food or never eat out. It is important to have balance and a flexible attitude. Become a flexitarian. Sometimes, it is healthier to go to a restaurant rather than stress out about preparing a meal, especially for people who work and have children. During busy times, I encourage eating at restaurants with healthy options and enjoying the food without guilt. Also, when dining at someone else's house, eating what has been prepared for all the guests can be extremely healthy and healing, even if it is something we would never eat on our own. It can be healthier to just have that piece of pizza, fried chicken or ice cream cake, and not be singled out as the "healthy" one who always rejects other people's food.

Being a health food addict can be isolating. People tend to cook alone, eat alone and feel alienated from society. Sometimes we just want to go out, eat whatever we want and have a great time. And sometimes this flexibility can be healthier than staying home alone and eating high-quality healthy foods and chewing well. People can become overly obsessed with eating the "right" food, something known as Orthorexia Nervosa. This condition can impede other important elements of life, including relationships, creativity and just feeling part of a community. Either we avoid others because we don't want to see what they are eating, or they avoid us because they know we will disapprove of their undisciplined eating habits. We want to relate with people as a friend, not as a preacher, and projecting our own food concerns onto others is a great way to lose friends fast. Let others eat as they wish, and learn to accept and enjoy their company, regardless of how many spoonfuls of sugar they stir into their coffee.

Exercises

1. Condiment List

Go to the store and pick up a bunch of condiments. Keep them on the table at mealtimes so everyone can flavor and personalize the food to their liking. Getting a lazy Susan to keep on your table and store your condiments in is an option. Here are some condiments to try, plus you can add your own favorites.

basic spices

garlic

ginger

turmeric

oregano

cinnamon

peppers

cayenne

chili powder

chili flakes

white pepper

black pepper in a grinder

curry powder

salts

sea salt

gomasio

nuts and seeds

tahini

nut butters: peanut, cashew, almond

nuts: pine, brazil, cashews, walnuts, almonds, pistachios raw or toasted

pumpkin seeds

sunflower seeds

sesame seeds

sweeteners

honey

maple syrup

rice syrup

barley malt

stevia

agave nectar

natural fructose sweetener

oils, vinegars, and sauces

extra virgin olive oil

toasted sesame oil

coconut oil

chili sesame oil

umeboshi paste

umeboshi vinegar

balsamic vinegar

apple cider vinegar

Bragg's amino acids

tamari soy sauce

hot sauces

salad dressings

sea vegetables

dulse flakes

nori flakes

other

nutritional yeast

sprouts: alfalfa, sunflower, mung

grated daikon radish

sliced red cabbage

sliced cucumbers or scallions

fresh limes or lemons

ketchup

mustard

2. Try a New Recipe

Now that you've read all about the benefits of cooking homemade, freshly made, lovingly made food, it's time to try a new recipe. The back of this book has many to choose from, so pick one and cook it for your family or friends. Be sure to get fresh ingredients and to cook with love, thinking about what a pleasure it is to nourish those closest to you.

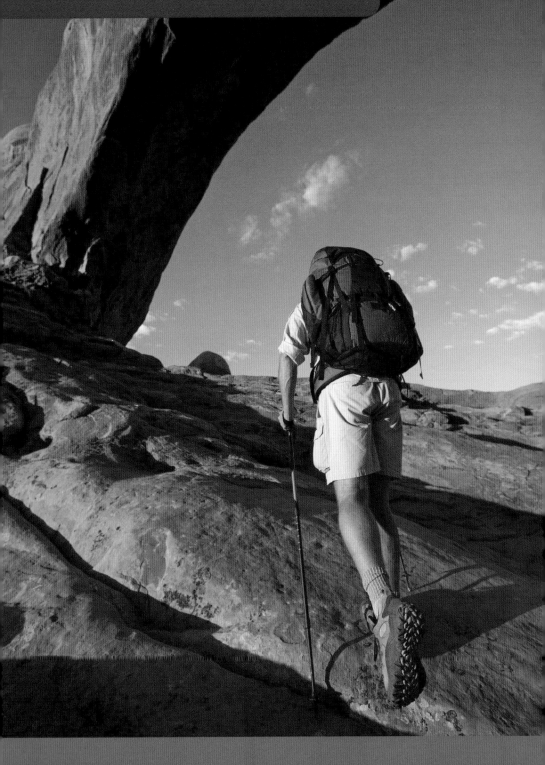

CHAPTER 12

Why Be Healthy?

ealth is a vehicle, not a destination. Excellent health is about more than just feeling good. Normally, when you are feeling low, dealing with a medical problem or trying to lose weight, you think of health as something to achieve. Of course, good physical health is an important goal, but if you simply stop there, you will miss out on so much more. Robust health allows us to be active in the world and achieve more than we can when we are tired or sick.

Ask yourself, "Why be healthy?" What would you do with your life if you became healthy? How would you use this gift to enhance your life and the lives of those around you? What would happen if you experienced high-level wellness most of the time? Imagine what your life would be like if strength, flexibility, endurance and clear thinking were part of your everyday life. Sadly, most people are missing it. They eat chemicalized, artificial junk food, don't move their bodies and don't think about their health until they are diagnosed with illness. They deal with health concerns, such as allergies, headaches, constipation, sugar crashes and low energy as recurring parts of their lives. They are caught up in a matrix mentality concerned with keeping up, fitting in and looking good.

When you switch to a natural-foods diet and lifestyle you begin dancing to the beat of a different drummer. You start to think and feel quite differently than others. As your daily diet changes, your blood quality also changes. Slowly but surely you notice that you don't fit in like you used to. You naturally see the world from a different perspective than those who are eating fast foods and junk foods. You become clearer, calmer and more aware.

As this transition occurs, you may feel like you are on the periphery of society, looking in. And you may be inclined to disguise how differently you feel from others. You may even develop chameleon-like behavior that allows you to fit into a wide range of environments without standing out. As this trend devel- ops, you may look around, scratch your head and wonder, why me? Why am I so unusual? Why am I so unlike my brothers and sisters, old friends, parents and neighbors?

Each of us comes to Earth with a different agenda. As we get older, we continually make choices that individuate us from others and keep us on track with our destinies. And for some of us, the path is focused on personal growth and development, which frequently leads to a curiosity about food, diet and lifestyle. In my experience, natural-food eaters tend to be smarter, clearer and more in touch with themselves and the natural rhythms of life than people who eat junk food. Trying to fit in has little value. Rather than pretending that you are like everyone else, you might as well take a deep breath, be authentic and be yourself. As a health-conscious person, you have added potential to step out and create change in the world.

The first step is to shift away from a fitting-in mentality. By continuing to expend large amounts of your energy and intelligence just to fit in, you'll have less strength to focus on the more important aspects of yourself and your life. You may even create health problems for yourself, if you are not being openly expressive. You are hiding your inner light, concealing your unique beauty and shying away from your deeper destiny. I believe you have the capability to become an element for change. Think about people through- out history who have had a profound impact on society. Mahatma Gandhi, Nelson Mandela, Martin Luther King Jr., Mother Teresa and Amelia Earhart come to my mind. Unconcerned with the status quo, they pushed their own potential and expanded the realities of the their times. They remind me of a German expression, "zeitgeist," which means the spirit of the time. In 1491, the zeitgeist was that the world was flat, and it took extraordinary courage for anyone to think outside that box and propose a different way of seeing the world—but that's exactly what happened. I see the people who are eat- ing natural foods today in the same way as those who believed the world was round—they have a better capacity to see a healthy future than those fueled by artificial junk food.

Authentic Self-Expression

As your diet and lifestyle improve, you will feel a greater sense of balance, and through this process become more fully present. You will probably notice your breath more fully, feel the breeze on your face and really listen to what other people are saying. You will be more fresh and alert to new situations with access to a wider choice of behaviors at any given moment. This consciousness makes you more likely to steer away from foods and people that are detrimental to your health.

Our personalities are not fixed or rigid. The more we slow down and understand ourselves, the more flexible and present we become. Authentic self-expression means being the person we truly are at this point in time. Too many people live life based on events that happened a long time ago: a difficult relationship with a parent, a humiliating situation at school or a challenging relationship that ended in an unsatisfying way. Many others live life as though they are constantly in preparation for something in the future, blind-sighted to the beauty of the present moment. It's time to snap out of this mentality. The past is over. The future never arrives. All you have is the present. The present is a gift, yours to treasure every moment, every day, in every way. You may have had a difficult childhood, challenges with your parents, and all kinds of things that happened to you that never should have happened. But that was then and this is now. Today, you are an adult who has a wonderful life. I urge you to let go of the past, forgive it, and know that, in some magnificent way, whatever happened was meant to happen. It is exactly those events that have made you who you are today.

Don't forget that authentic self-expression can apply to both primary and secondary foods. You don't need to hide what new foods you are eating, and you don't have to dial down your energy to make others feel better. It may feel hard at first to let go of certain friendships that drain you or to make the time to get to the gym, but I urge you to pay just as much attention to your primary foods and treat them with the same importance as eating greens. People might tell you it's selfish, but there's nothing wrong with prioritizing you. Think of it like when you are on an airplane. You have to put your oxygen mask on first before you can help others. When you start to prioritize the elements of your primary food circle including career, relationships, exercise and spirituality, you will enjoy an even higher level of health.

Unpredictable Futures

I want to tell you the story of the frog in the grasshopper jar. It goes like this:

> A man had a grasshopper, which he kept in a glass jar so that he could admire it. A grasshopper, being a grasshopper, will jump. One day the grasshopper jumped and escaped from the glass jar. The man discovered that the grasshopper had gone missing and went looking for it. Fortunately, he found the grasshopper and placed it back in the glass jar. However, the man wanted to make sure the grasshopper wouldn't escape this time. So he placed a glass lid on the glass jar. When the grasshopper awoke the next morning, he saw that the sun was shining and the sky was blue. The grasshopper, being a grasshopper, jumped again. This time, the glass lid greeted the grasshopper. He didn't know what hit him. He jumped and jumped and jumped. The man was annoyed by the grasshopper's antics, so he lowered the glass lid to try to prevent the grasshopper from jumping. The next morning the cycle began again. This time the lid was so low that the grasshopper could only move forward and back, so he gave up and stopped jumping. When he woke again, he didn't jump. He didn't even try. He didn't notice that the man had removed the glass lid the night before. Freedom was staring him in the face and he didn't attempt to make it his.

Many people behave like the grasshopper, afraid to jump. They are so accustomed to their own limited views of life that they don't bother to try other ways of being. There are so many ways to live life and countless opportunities for each of us every single day.

Everyone has a predictable future, a future that would automatically occur by continuing to fit in, following the rules and moving along in the expected way. I had a predictable future. I was raised in an Orthodox Jewish household in Canada. I could have stayed there, followed my parents' religious belief system and worked as a lawyer in a corporate setting. Instead, I decided to travel and explore other life paths, which eventually brought me

PROFILE

Melanie Albert, Phoenix, AZ, USA
www.experiencenutritiongroup.com

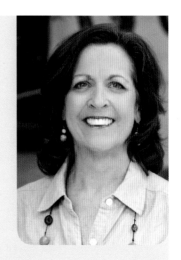

"I am living the life of my dreams!"

For nearly two decades, I was a successful, award-winning corporate marketing, branding, advertising, and public relations executive in Fortune 500 companies. Immediately prior to enrolling at Integrative Nutrition, I was a marketing consultant to Weil Lifestyle/Andrew Weil, M.D. I knew that Dr. Weil was a guest speaker at Integrative Nutrition, so I asked him about the program. Based on his positive recommendation that I'd thoroughly enjoy the program, I immediately enrolled.

Reflecting on Integrative Nutrition, one of the most important areas of learning was actually implementing the nutrition theories taught to us in the curriculum to determine my own healthy eating bio-individuality. These personal experiences have been the foundation for the education that I share in books, blogs, videos and speaking engagements.

The school is life changing. My experience at Integrative Nutrition has totally transformed my life, especially in the business area. The school has given me the credentials and voice to be a leader, expert, and author in the integrative nutrition world.

My passions are healthy food and football. My personal and business mission is to educate current and former professional athletes, beginning with former NFL players, and the sports fan community to enjoy foods and enjoy life. After three years of focus, persistence, relationship building, and massive action, I am proud and honored that my company, Experience Nutrition is the first Official Health and Wellness Partner of the NFL Alumni. Experience Nutrition positively impacts the obesity, heart disease, and diabetes epidemics in the United States today, alongside former professional athletes, beginning with the NFL Alumni, with sound nutrition experiences and healthy food products.

I am living the life of my dreams! I love working experientially alongside my clients, especially the former NFL players, to guide them to learn what to eat, why to eat, and how to cook simple healthy foods. I also love my interactive speaking engagements for the sports and corporate world, and our youth. Plus, I love writing about good nutrition. My second book, *Experience Nutrition,* was published as an e-book in 2012 and my third book with companion video series will be published in 2013. I'm doing the work I love everyday!

into the health food industry. I moved to New York and began health coaching. I didn't care about the security of a regular paycheck; I had a passion for helping people and wanted to put my skills and education to use. I couldn't believe I was there, in my jeans, working with people to get well. When I decided to start a nutrition school that would cover all dietary theories, some people thought I was crazy. I was trying something that no one had done before. For years, I slept on friend's couches or in the school's offices, while I was building something I truly believed was possible. If I can do it, so can you.

Food has a powerful effect on our future. Avoiding junk food reduces brain fog and allows you to see opportunities that others can't. It's like when an animal realizes the electrical fence isn't working or the grasshopper discovers the glass jar has no lid; suddenly a world of new options opens and all types of unimaginable things become possible. Natural-food eaters have a freedom and openness that most people can't fully understand. They are more able to step away from their limited, predictable futures and take advantage of the limitless openings of life. These people often move in unexpected directions. Family and friends sometimes find their choices odd, unwise or threatening, but these are some of the happiest, healthiest, most alive people in the world. They have the capacity and curiosity to start fresh, to explore more creative careers, begin new relationships, relocate to another area or travel to distant lands. It's your life, and doors of opportunity are opening and closing at every moment. It's okay to take risks. The world is a safe place. It's a powerful experience to know you are strong enough and clear enough to survive and thrive through major life changes.

In Western thinking, we get very isolated and think, "I've got to make it happen for myself." We push and push to achieve success. Eastern thinking says everything is going to work out for itself. In India, they have a saying, "Let go and let God." I think we have to find balance between these two ideologies and pay attention to both parts of the equation. You want to be aware of barriers and obstructions to progress and be willful about the future. But with one eye on barriers to progress, you must keep the other on how to surrender to them. One perspective is very yin and the other is very yang.

The more you live in balance, respecting nature and yourself, the more likely you will be in the right place at the right time, all the time. When you have that balance, you're one with nature and more connected to the system. You'll see synchronicity incessantly. You'll be thinking of an old girlfriend and right at that moment, she'll call you. You'll start planning a vacation to Spain and the next day you'll meet someone who just got back and offers tons of appealing advice. You'll be looking for a new job and run into an old family friend who just so happens to have an opening in your field. You'll meet a significant other who complements you beautifully; you'll find a career aligned with your personal values. People will call you lucky and you may think it's simply coincidence, but the truth is that you are aligning yourself with the natural order of everything. How are all those planets in the right place at the right time? How do the leaves all turn color in the fall and the birds know to fly south? Human beings are part of the same order. What looks after all these aspects of life will look after us too, the more we are in harmony with nature.

Building Your Future

As you learn to nurture yourself, space opens up for you to create your future. Whatever you dream is possible. The universe wants you to fulfill your dreams and achieve all your desires. The difficult part is getting clear about what you want and then having the faith and perseverance to make it happen. Allow yourself to put time and energy into understanding what you would like your life to look like and feel like. What do you want to accomplish in your life? Where would you like to go? Who would you like to be with? The clearer your intentions, the more you can build your future according to your hopes and dreams. What do you really want to get done in this lifetime? You are free to create whatever you want in this world.

Stephen Hawking, the British theoretical physicist and author of *A Brief History of Time*, has a theory that the past and the future is a continuum, which means the future has already happened. When I first heard this concept, it completely fascinated me and really changed my life. When I ask my students who their fourth grade teacher was, they are able to trace back relatively quickly to remember that person. But when I ask them what they want their lives to look like in a year, I get that deer-in-the-headlights look. We have the ability to see the future too. It's a muscle that you have to train, just as you would for any sport. You can start by writing weekly, monthly and annual goals. When you get clear about these goals, lo and behold, you see the future. You can create the future because you know it's your destiny.

Whether your goal is to have more energy, heal a health concern or just to be the best version of your true self each day, relish every moment of that journey. Being healthy is about moving beyond a limited philosophy of nutrition and creating your own larger vision for your health and happiness. In my experience, people who adopt a well-balanced diet and lifestyle and avoid junk foods develop a higher degree of creativity, flexibility and aliveness.

Spiritual Beings

As you begin to eat more intelligently, you stop medicating yourself by unconsciously using extreme foods as mood-altering drugs. When you stope-ating extreme foods that bounce you around on a pinball diet, you naturally become more still. With this stillness, you are bound to disentangle yourself from the mundane attitudes that you received from the school system, society and the media. This stillness offers benefits to your body as well. Your body will not have to work as hard to maintain homeostasis. Your blood sugar, temperature and heartbeat will all operate at optimum levels. When our bodies slow down, we slow down. When we slow down, we increasingly come to experience "nothing to do and nowhere to go"—the sensation that life is just perfectly okay the way it is.

Despite this exquisite experience, you may find yourself noticing that most people are operating from a confused state, constantly looking for things outside of themselves to fill the void. You'll notice people who have everything and yet complain constantly. You'll notice people who feel that nothing is ever enough. You may fall into self-doubt and try to blend in, throwing yourself back into constant rushing and grasping for external sources of gratification—such as material goods, more money or superficial relationships with others—since that's what everyone else is doing. Materialistic things can only get you so far. Yes, a better house or a better car can make life more enjoyable, but it's not happiness. When I was in India I saw people living on the street that were smiling and cheerful any time of the day. Kids who didn't have shoes on their feet were playing and laughing. Nothing outside of yourself can ever truly fulfill you. Contentment and true joy come from within and are available to us at any moment.

I do understand the pleasure of being engaged by a strong mission. After all, I've invested a great deal of time in the development of Integrative Nutrition, so I'm well aware of the gratification that comes from using one's creative energies to contribute to the world. Remember, though, that you are a spiritual being in a material world. Spirit is your essential reality, and nothing you achieve or possess on a material level is ever going to fulfill you for long.

Please don't be in a hurry to dismiss or disturb the clear spaces when they come. When the tranquility hits, try to notice and resist the temptation to overeat, argue or busy yourself for the sake of being busy. Allow yourself to live in this relaxed, unoccupied dimension of your being. Give it space. You are a human being, not a human doing. Enjoy the luxury of non-doing. It is an essential part of nature.

This Is Your Life

My father has a bumper sticker on his car that says, "This is your life, not a dress rehearsal." Now is the time to take action toward accomplishing whatever dreams, ideas or aspirations may be lingering in the back of your mind. One of the easiest and most effective ways of making change in your life is to change what you eat. The foods you put into your mouth, together with primary food, create the fuel for your body, mind and spirit. Health and happiness are inextricably linked. The better you feed yourself, the better you feel and the bigger impact you will have on the world.

Don't let yourself get stuck. A lot of holistic people are trying to get themselves healthier, but they're already healthier than 90% of the population. I propose that rather than working on getting yourself to a higher level, why not work on getting the rest of the world to move up? By sharing what you already know with others, you may achieve a higher level of health than if you go to another yoga class or eat more broccoli. Get involved with your community, your kids' schools, your church or your family.

It is my genuine hope and desire that we can all make a difference by bringing the message of Integrative Nutrition into the mainstream. Imagine this world educated on whole foods, holistic practices and alternatives to medicine and surgery. What we eat breaks down in our bodies and changes our whole way of thinking. It's hard to find something as significant as that. The future of nutrition is a world where primary foods and secondary foods are balanced and aligned for all. So the question really isn't, "Are you healthy enough?" The question is, "What are you going to do with your health?"

Exercise

Future-Building Exercise

What do you really want to get done in this lifetime? You are free to create whatever you want in this world. The more specific you are, the easier it is to plan. Your hopes and dreams must be thought through and planned to make them happen.

You may want to do this in a journal. Consider this exercise as a personal trainer for the muscle that sees and creates your future. You are not going to show this list to anyone, so just write without self-consciousness.

Write down all the things you need to get done or want to get done by:

1. the end of the day tomorrow

2. the end of the week

3. the end of this month

4. the end of next month

5. New Year's Day

    a. what's the year?

    b. how old will you be?

    c. how old will your loved ones be?

    d. what are all the things you want to have done by that time?

6. New Year's Day, two years from now. Again write down the following:

    a. what's the year?

    b. how old will you be?

    c. how old will your loved ones be?

    d. what are all the things you want to have done by that time?

7. New Year's Day, five years from now. Again write down the following:

   a. what's the year?

   b. how old will you be?

   c. how old will your loved ones be?

   d. what are all the things you want to have done by that time?

8. in 10 years

9. in 20 years

Now remember: This is your life. Make it happen!

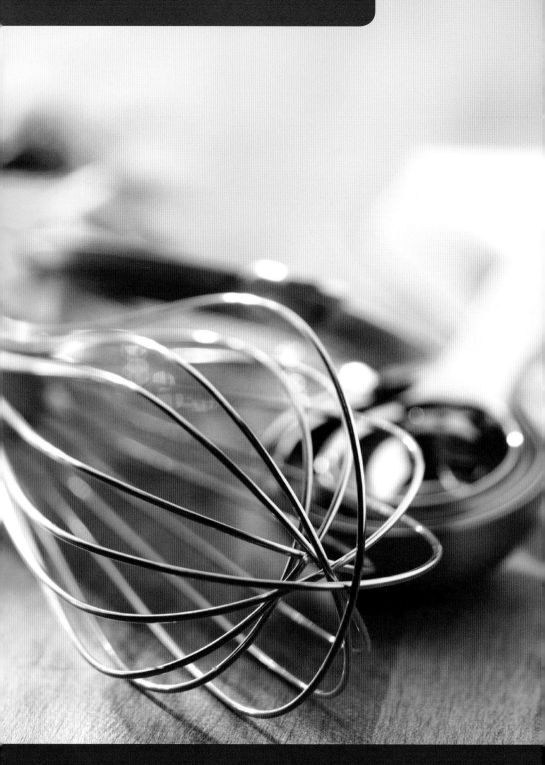

RECIPES

Recipes

Hunger is the best sauce in the world.

—Cervantes

breakfast

If you did the breakfast experiment in chapter 2, you now have a better sense of the importance of breakfast. Starting your day with the fuel that works best in your body can set the tone for your whole day. Many people feel like they are too busy to eat breakfast, but once you get into the breakfast habit, you will see the benefits and a healthy morning meal will naturally become part of your day.

Try expanding your idea of what breakfast should look like. It doesn't have to be fruit and cereal or waffles and eggs. Vegetables, whole grains, fish and other highly nutritious foods can be eaten at any time of day, including in the morning. These breakfast recipes are simple to prepare and will help broaden your breakfast palette.

Warm Gingery Oatmeal

Prep time: 5 minutes
Cooking time: 15 minutes
Serves 3

> 1 cup rolled oats
> 2 cups water
> ¼ cup raisins
> ¼ cup goji berries
> ¼ cup sunflower seeds
> 2 teaspoons grated ginger
> 1 tablespoon agave syrup

- Bring water to a boil.
- Add oats, raisins, goji berries, ginger and a pinch of salt.
- Reduce heat to low.
- Continue cooking until water is absorbed and oats become nice and creamy, about 7 minutes.
- Add sunflower seeds and agave.

TIP: *Try using rice, soy or nut milk instead of water to make it even creamier.*

Muesli

Prep time: 5 minutes
Cooking time: none!
Serves 3

> 1 cup rolled oats
> 2 cups almond or soy milk
> 5 to 6 dates, chopped
> ½ cup sunflower seeds

- Soak all ingredients overnight covered, and it will be done by the morning. Without cooking!

TIP: *Add shredded coconut, raisins or a tablespoon of brown rice syrup before eating.*

Amaranth and Polenta Porridge

Prep Time: 5 minutes
Cooking time: 40 minutes
Serves 4

> ½ cup polenta
> ½ cup amaranth
> 3 cups water
> ½ teaspoon sea salt
> ½ cup dried cranberries
> ½ cup pine nuts
> 1-2 tablespoons honey
> ¼ cup milk (or non-dairy milk)

- Heat water with salt to boil.
- Add polenta and amaranth.
- Reduce heat and simmer, covered about 30 minutes, stirring occasionally.
- After 20 minutes, stir in cranberries.
- Taste to see if it's done. It should be soft and creamy.
- Add pine nuts, honey and milk and enjoy!

Rice Porridge with Apples

Prep Time: 5 minutes
Cooking Time: 15 minutes
Serves 3

2 cups leftover brown rice

1 apple

¼ cup water, rice milk or coconut water

1 tablespoon brown rice syrup

1 teaspoon maple syrup

1 teaspoon ground cinnamon

pinch of sea salt

- Add rice, liquid, sweeteners, cinnamon and salt to a pan and begin cooking over medium low heat.
- Peel and dice the apple, and add to the pot.
- Stir to mix everything well.
- Bring to a boil, then reduce heat to low and simmer.
- Continue cooking about 10 minutes, until the apple has become a little soft
- Enjoy hot!

Tofu Scramble

Prep Time: 5 minutes
Cooking Time: 20 minutes
Serves 2

1 block firm tofu

2 to 3 tablespoons olive oil

½ teaspoon tamari soy sauce

⅛ teaspoon turmeric

1 red onion

½ red bell pepper

⅛ teaspoon paprika

1 tablespoon umeboshi vinegar

dash of black pepper

- Press tofu to remove excess water and then crumble into small pieces.
- Chop onion and pepper.
- Heat oil.

- Add tofu, tamari and turmeric.
- Sauté for a few minutes.
- Add vegetables, paprika, umeboshi vinegar and black pepper to tofu.
- Cook for 5 minutes or until mixture thoroughly heats and flavors blend.

TIP: *Use alfalfa sprouts or fresh parsley to garnish.*

Japanese Style Breakfast

Prep Time: 5 minutes
Cooking Time: 10 minutes
Serves 1

    4 big bok choy leaves

    1 teaspoon toasted sesame oil

    1 tablespoon brown rice vinegar

    1 tablespoon tamari

    ½ cup cooked brown rice

- Wash bok choy and chop into bite-sized pieces.
- Heat sesame oil in a sauté pan.
- Add bok choy and stir fry for one minute.
- Add vinegar, tamari and rice.
- Stir gently and continue cooking about 3 minutes, until everything is warm.
- Transfer to a bowl to eat.

TIP: *Garnish with sesame seeds.*

TIP: *If you want some extra protein with your breakfast, add 4 ounces cooked salmon or other fish.*

Morning Sausage and Kale

Prep Time: 5 minutes
Cooking time: 10 minutes
Serves 2

    1 teaspoon olive oil

    ½ small yellow onion

    1 precooked chicken apple sausage

    ½ bunch kale

    1 tablespoon balsamic vinegar

- Slice onion into half moons (long, thin slivers)
- Heat oil in a frying pan and sauté onion for 5 minutes
- Meanwhile, slice sausage into ½ inch rounds and chop the kale into 1-inch pieces.
- Add sausage and kale to the frying pan and cook for 5 minutes, or until sausage is hot and kale has become soft.
- Remove from heat and sprinkle with balsamic vinegar before eating.

TIP: *If you are a vegetarian, try substituting marinated tempeh for the sausage.*

Scrambled Eggs and Greens

Prep Time: 10 minutes
Cooking Time: 12 minutes
Serves 1-2

    1 tablespoon olive oil
    1 leek, chopped into small pieces
    1 clove garlic, minced
    2 eggs
    1 carrot, diced
    1 cup chopped spinach, dandelion, watercress or chard

- Beat the eggs in a small bowl.
- Heat the oil in a frying pan.
- Sauté leek for 3 minutes. Add garlic and sauté another minute.
- Add carrots, cover and cook 5 minutes on low heat, until carrots are softened.
- Remove veggies and put on a plate.
- Add a little oil to the pan if it's dry, add the eggs, and cook over medium heat for 3 minutes until eggs are mostly cooked.
- Add greens and other veggies and stir everything together, scrambling the eggs.
- Add salt and pepper to taste and serve.

simple grains

Top 10 Secrets to Cooking the Best Grains

1. Use organic, unrefined whole grains. Quality matters.
2. Store your grains in an airtight container.

Before cooking:

3. Gently wash your grains in cold water. This reawakens dormant energy.
4. Soak them anywhere from 1 to 12 hours. This will eliminate phytic acid and help with digestion.
5. Dry-toast grains in a skillet over medium heat until they smell nutty. This enhances their natural flavor, allows them to cook more evenly and decreases bitterness.

During cooking:

6. Use a pinch of sea salt or add pieces of sea vegetables. This adds flavor and nutritional value.
7. Add a splash of olive oil to help prevent grains from sticking together.
8. Do not stir, as this makes them mushy and lets cooking water evaporate too quickly.
9. When grains hit boiling point, reduce heat to low, cover and let simmer for the suggested time.

After cooking:

10. Mix grains in the pot, allowing them to gently steam. Cover for 10 minutes.

The 11th secret: Your energy as a cook is just as important as the quality of the ingredients that you are using. Keep your energy positive and joyful around food. What you put into the food will come back when you eat it.

Basic Brown Rice

Soaking Time: 1 to 12 hours
Prep time: 5 minutes
Cooking time: 45 minutes to 60 minutes
Serves 4

> 1 cup brown rice
> 2 cups water
> pinch of sea salt

- Presoak rice. Gently rinse rice.
- Add water and salt. Bring to boil.
- Cover. Reduce heat to low.
- Simmer for 50 minutes if it is short grain, and 35 minutes if it is long grain basmati rice.
- When it is done, pull from heat and let stand covered for 10 more minutes.
- Fluff rice with fork before serving.

TIP: *For extra fluffy rice, put your water on to boil. Then put the rinsed grains in a dry skillet. Cook over medium low heat, stirring until the grains are dry. Add the hot, dry rice to the boiling water, add salt and continue cooking.*

Wild Rice

Prep time: 5 minutes
Cooking time: 60 minutes
Serves 4

> 1 cup wild rice
> 4 cups water
> pinch of sea salt

- Wash and drain rice.
- Bring rice and water to a boil.
- Add salt
- Turn heat to low, cover and simmer for 45 to 50 minutes.
- Your grain is ready when black seeds are opened up.
- Mix and serve.

TIP: *Try half wild rice and half long grain brown rice.*

Very Easy Fried Rice

Prep time: 10 minutes
Cooking time: 20 minutes (if using leftover rice)
Serves 8

1 tablespoon olive oil

1 small onion

2 cloves garlic

1 carrot, diced

½ bunch scallion

1 tablespoon grated ginger

4 cups cooked long grain brown rice

2 tablespoons tamari soy sauce

1 teaspoon toasted sesame oil

- Sauté onion in olive oil for 5 minutes.
- Mince garlic and add to onion.
- Add carrot and sauté for 4 minutes.
- Add scallion and ginger.
- Sauté for about 4 more minutes so flavors can melt into each other.
- Add rice and sprinkle with water. Water gives extra steam to the dish.
- Add tamari soy sauce and toasted sesame oil.
- Lower heat and cook for 5 more minutes, stirring occasionally.

TIP: *Beat an egg together with the tamari and sesame oil. Pour this mixture into the pan and move it around quickly with a fork to spread the egg as it cooks.*

Gypsies' Singing Rice Salad

Prep time: 10 minutes
Cooking time: 15 minutes (if using leftover rice)
Serves 8

1 cup cooked brown basmati rice

1 cup cooked white basmati rice

1 red bell pepper

1 medium red onion

2 stalks celery

1 cup parsley

½ cup white sesame seeds

½ cup pumpkin seeds

2 tablespoons olive oil

¼ teaspoon black pepper

- If you use leftover rice, put it in the steaming basket to re-energize it and steam for 10 minutes. Otherwise, cook according to basic rice preparation method.
- Chop bell pepper and onion.
- Dice celery.
- Chop parsley.
- Toast sesame and pumpkin seeds together. Make sure you don't let them get dark brown.
- Combine all ingredients in a big bowl, adding olive oil and black pepper.

TIP: *Add zest to it by squeezing ½ a lemon and adding ⅓ cup chopped mint leaves.*

Buckwheat with Carrot and Arame

Prep time: 5 minutes
Cooking time: 25 minutes
Serves 4

¼ cup arame

1 large carrot, shredded

1 cup raw buckwheat

1⅔ cups water

- Soak arame.
- Shred carrot.
- Dry-toast grains until nutty and golden brown.
- Bring water to boil.
- Slowly add buckwheat, bring back to a boil, reduce heat and cover. Simmer for 15 minutes.
- Remove from heat and let sit for 5 minutes.
- Rinse arame and mix with shredded carrot and buckwheat

TIP: *Add toasted sesame oil and sprinkle with fresh scallion.*

Millet with Roasted Sunflower Seeds

Prep time: 5 minutes
Cooking time: 45 minutes
Serves 4

> 1 cup millet
> ½ cup sunflower seeds
> 3 cups water
> pinch of sea salt

- Wash and drain millet
- Dry-toast sunflower seeds in a skillet over medium heat until they smell nutty, approximately 4 minutes.
- Bring water to boil.
- Add millet and seeds.
- Cover and simmer for 30 minutes.
- When done, fluff and let sit for 10 minutes. Mix, serve and enjoy.

TIP: *If millet is too dry for you, add more water when cooking. Or add a tablespoon of olive oil when it is done.*

Millet–Carrot–Hijiki–Burdock

Prep time: 5 minutes
Cooking time: 45 minutes
Serves 6

> 2 stalks scallion, sliced
> 2 tablespoons olive oil, divided
> 2 shredded carrots
> 3-inch piece thinly sliced burdock root
> 1 cup millet
> ¼ cup soaked, rinsed hijiki
> 6 cups water
> gomasio to garnish

- Sauté scallion in 1 tablespoon of olive oil. Add carrots and sauté for 4 minutes.
- Add sliced burdock, millet and hijiki and sauté for about 3 minutes.
- Add water and bring to a boil. Cover and cook over low heat for 30 minutes.
- Mix and let sit covered for 5 minutes.
- Add remaining olive oil, sprinkle with gomasio and serve.

Millet Mashed "Potatoes"

Prep time: 5 minutes
Cooking time: 30 minutes
Serves 6

1 cup millet
2¼ cups water
½ medium cauliflower, sliced
½ teaspoon sea salt
2 cloves garlic, sliced
1 tablespoon extra virgin olive oil
1 teaspoon umeboshi vinegar
salt and pepper to taste
handful of chopped parsley

- Wash grains. Bring water to a boil.
- Add grains, cauliflower, garlic and salt.
- Reduce heat to low and simmer covered for 20 minutes or until grains are cooked and water is absorbed.
- Turn the heat off and let sit, covered for 5-10 minutes.
- Add other ingredients and mash with a potato masher, or mix in a blender or food processor.
- Garnish with chopped parsley and serve.

TIP: *For extra rich and delicious mash, roast the garlic cloves in olive oil over low heat while the grains are cooking.*

Spring Out Quinoa

Prep time: 2 minutes
Cooking time: 30 minutes
Serves 8

2 cups quinoa
3½ cups water
1 bag peppermint tea
1 tablespoon olive oil
fresh mint, basil and cilantro

- Wash grains. Place them in water and add peppermint tea bag.
- Bring to a boil. Cover and simmer for 15 to 20 minutes, then remove from heat and let stand for 5 minutes.

- When it is done, add olive oil and fluff.
- Garnish with chopped fresh herbs and serve.

Quinoa Tabouleh

Prep time: 5 minutes
Cooking time: 35 minutes
Serves 6

    1 cup quinoa
    2¼ cups water
    1 cucumber
    1 tomato
    1 bunch mint
    ½ bunch parsley
    2 tablespoons lemon juice
    3 tablespoons extra virgin olive oil
    sea salt to taste

- Wash quinoa and add to boiling water with a pinch of sea salt.
- Reduce heat to low and simmer covered for 20 minutes or until grains are fluffy and water is absorbed.
- Fluff with a fork, cover and let sit for 10 minutes.
- Prepare the veggies while the quinoa is cooking.
- Seed and dice the cucumber and tomato.
- Mince the mint and parsley. (You can also chiffonade the mint, meaning roll up the leaves and slice in very thin strips.)
- Transfer the quinoa into a large bowl and combine all ingredients.
- Mix gently and taste, adjusting the lemon juice, olive oil and salt to your taste.

Hearty Winter Grain Salad

Prep time: 5 minutes
Cooking time: 55 minutes
Serves 6

    1 cup kamut or wheat berries (or ½ cup of each)
    3 cups vegetable or chicken stock
    ½ teaspoon sea salt
    1 small yellow onion
    ½ boiled yam
    ¼ cup chopped walnuts

½ bunch kale

2 tablespoons balsamic vinegar

3 tablespoons extra virgin olive oil

- Wash grains. Bring stock to boil.
- Add grains and salt.
- Reduce heat to low and simmer covered for 45 minutes or until grains are cooked and water is absorbed.
- Fluff with a fork and let sit covered for 10 minutes.
- While the grains are cooking, prepare other ingredients.
- Dice the onion and sauté in olive oil until translucent, about 7 minutes.
- Dice the yam.
- Cook the walnuts on the stove in a dry pan over medium heat until toasted, about 5 minutes, stirring frequently.
- Chop the kale into small pieces, bring a small pot of water to a boil and blanch.
- Transfer grains to a large bowl, add all of the ingredients and mix gently.
- Add vinegar and olive oil to your taste. Enjoy!

Basic Polenta

Prep time: 2 minutes
Cooking time: 30 minutes
Serves 3

1 cup polenta

3 cups water or stock

½ teaspoon salt

- Bring water or stock to boil.
- Add polenta and salt, stirring gently.
- Reduce heat to low and simmer covered for about 30 minutes, stirring occasionally to assure that the polenta isn't sticking to the bottom of the pot.
- It is finished when the grains are soft to taste and most of the water is absorbed.

TIP: *You can also grill or fry polenta. Pour it into a baking dish, and let it chill in the refrigerator for an hour. When it has solidified, slice it into triangles and fry in a hot pan with a little olive oil, or brush with oil and grill for 2 minutes on each side. Try it topped with pesto!*

vegetables

Basic Cooking Methods for Vegetables

Steaming

Steaming is a simple way to cook vegetables, allowing you to experience their simple flavors in a pure form. Steaming takes 5 to 10 minutes for leafy, green vegetables and 10 to 25 minutes for root vegetables. All you need is a steaming basket, a pot with about 2 inches of water at the bottom and a lid.

Stir-Frying

Stir-frying is another quick and nutritious way to prepare vegetables. This method highlights their natural flavors. It takes just 5 to 10 minutes. You can stir-fry in oil or water. All you need is a skillet with a lid. If you choose to use oil, heat a skillet and add 3 to 5 tablespoons. Add vegetables and sprinkle them with a pinch of sea salt to enhance their flavor. To reduce fat but keep the flavor, you can use 2 to 3 tablespoons of water and 1 tablespoon of oil. This is called a wet sauté. After stir-frying the veggies for a few minutes in the oil, add the water and cover to give the vegetables extra steam and heat. Another option is a pure water sauté. Place 1 inch of water in your skillet and add garlic, ginger or spices if desired. Bring to boil, add thinly sliced vegetables, cover and simmer for 5 to 10 minutes.

Baking

Many vegetables taste best baked. Baking brings out the very essence of the vegetables, especially squashes and roots. You need a baking pan or sheet, vegetables, an oven heated between 375 and 450 degrees, and 50 to 60 minutes of cooking time. Be sure to use a nonstick pan or oil the vegetables so they don't stick.

Quick Boiling

When quick boiling vegetables, put them in boiling water and leave for 3 to 5 minutes. This method removes their raw flavor, makes them more digestible and brightens their color. When you're done boiling, rinse vegetables with cold water to stop additional cooking and to preserve the color. You can save the boiled water and use it for drinking, cooking grains, watering your plants or adding to soups.

How to Make Plain, Steamed Vegetables More Exciting

- After cooking, add 1 tablespoon olive oil or toasted sesame oil to every 2 cups of veggies.
- Add 2 bay leaves or 1 teaspoon cumin seeds to the cooking water.
- Sprinkle cooked veggies with toasted pumpkin, sesame, flax or sunflower seeds. Or sprinkle with almonds, walnuts or dried shredded coconut.
- Sprinkle greens with fresh herbs: mint, dill, basil, parsley, cilantro or scallion.
- Use tamari soy sauce or umeboshi vinegar to add extra flavor to cooked veggies.
- Squeeze fresh lemon or lime juice over steamed vegetables.
- After steaming, quickly stir-fry with a pinch of sea salt, olive oil and garlic.

Steamed Kale

Prep time: 5 minutes
Cooking Time: 15 minutes
Serves 4

> 1 bunch of kale
> 2 cups water
> pinch sea salt

- Put water, salt and a steamer basket in a medium-size pot and heat on high.
- Wash kale.
- Remove leaves from stems and cut or tear leaves in any size you like.
- Chop the stems into ½-inch pieces, discarding the bottom as it tends to be tough.
- When the water is boiling, add the stems to the pot, cover, and cook for one minute.
- Now add the leaves, cover, lower the heat, and steam for another 2-4 minutes. Leaves should be wilted, yet bright green.
- Carefully remove the steamer basket and transfer kale to a serving dish.

TIP: *Enjoy the kale plain, or add a little tamari or lemon juice.*

TIP: *Try this same technique with collard greens, bok choy and mustard greens.*

Basic Blanched Greens

Prep Time: 5 minutes
Cooking Time: 15 minutes
Serves 4

> 1 bunch any leafy green (kale, collards, bok choy, chard etc.)
> ½ inch water in a pot
> umeboshi vinegar
> tamari
> flax oil

- Heat water in a large pot.
- Chop or tear greens into bite-size pieces, removing stems.
- Chop stems into small pieces.
- When water boils, add stems and cook 1 minute.
- Add leaves and cook another 3 minutes.
- Strain through a colander and transfer to serving dish.
- Add a bit of umeboshi, tamari and flax to taste.

Brazilian Style Collards

Prep Time: 5 minutes
Cooking Time: 5 minutes
Serves 6

> 2 tablespoons olive oil
> 3 cloves garlic
> 2 bunches collard greens
> salt and pepper to taste

- Wash collards.
- Remove leaves from stems, tear leaves in half, and stack into piles 4 leaves thick.
- Roll the stack tightly, turn to the side, and cut carefully into very thin strips. Repeat with all of the collards. The effect is that the leaves will be shredded.
- Mince the garlic.
- Heat oil in a frying pan and sauté garlic until golden brown, about 30 seconds.
- Add collards, salt and pepper and toss quickly for about 3 minutes with tongs or a fork, making sure all greens get cooked.
- Remove from heat and transfer to a serving dish.

Sautéed Greens with Pine Nuts and Raisins

Prep Time: 10 minutes
Cooking Time: 10 minutes
Serves 6

½ bunch mustard greens
½ bunch kale
½ bunch dandelion greens
1 tablespoon olive oil
½ teaspoons sea salt
¼ cup pine nuts
⅓ cup raisins

- Toast pine nuts on a cookie sheet in a 325 degree oven for 5 minutes. Set aside.
- Wash and chop greens.
- Heat olive oil.
- Add greens, sea salt and raisins. Stir and cook 5 minutes.
- Turn off heat, add in pine nuts and transfer to serving dish.

TIP: *Sprinkle with lemon juice before serving.*

Baby Bok Choy and Shiitakes

Prep Time: 8 minutes
Cooking Time: 8 minutes
Serves 6

1 small yellow onion
4 heads baby bok choy
6 fresh shiitake mushrooms
1 tablespoon toasted sesame oil
3 tablespoons mirin
1 tablespoon tamari

- Peel onion and slice into long, thin strips.
- Heat oil in a frying pan.
- Add onions, turn heat down and cook 5 minutes, stirring occasionally.
- Meanwhile, wash bok choy and slice each leaf in half.
- Thinly slice shiitakes.

- Add shiitakes, bok choy, mirin and tamari to pan. Cover and cook 3 minutes.
- Spread on a flat surface to cool and stop greens from cooking.

TIP: *Garnish with toasted sesame seeds.*

Oh So Delicious Green Cleanser

This dish has got all of the five tastes: sweet, sour, bitter, salty and pungent. It can be helpful in bringing balance to the system after a period of not so healthy eating.

Prep Time: 8 minutes
Cooking Time: 5 minutes
Serves 4

1 bunch lacinato kale
½ medium daikon radish
1 tablespoon tamari
1 teaspoon toasted sesame oil
1 tablespoon brown rice vinegar
1 tablespoon agave syrup
1 tablespoon nutritional yeast flakes

- Heat a medium sized pot with 2 inches of water.
- Chop the kale into 2-inch pieces (stems can stay on).
- Chop the daikon into 1-inch chunks.
- When the water boils add veggies and blanch 2 minutes.
- Remove to a colander to drain and transfer to a large mixing bowl.
- Add all other ingredients and mix well, tasting to adjust amounts to your desire.

TIP: *It is even more amazing if you add some dulse flakes and sesame seeds.*

TIP: *Also try adding other vegetables as you like, such as cauliflower, broccoli, string beans, asparagus, etc.*

Gayatri Greens

These Indian-style greens bear the name of a powerful Hindu Goddess, and also a beautiful mantra (prayer) that is said to represent the divine awakening of the mind and soul.

Prep Time: 8 minutes
Cooking Time: 10 minutes
Serves 4

2 tablespoons coconut oil
1 teaspoon black mustard seeds
1 teaspoon ground cumin
1 teaspoon ground coriander
1 bunch swiss chard
½ cup organic plain yogurt
½ teaspoon sea salt

- Wash chard, cut out stems, and chop leaves into 1-inch pieces.
- Prepare spices and place them next to the stove.
- Heat oil in a frying pan on medium high.
- When the oil is hot add mustard seeds and cook, stirring for 1 minute.
- Add cumin and coriander and cook for another 30 seconds, stirring.
- Add chard and salt, mix well and cook 3-5 minutes, until chard is wilted.
- Turn off heat, stir in yogurt, and enjoy.

Lemon Broccoli with Avocado

Prep Time: 5 minutes
Cooking Time: 15 minutes
Serves 8

2 bunches broccoli
1 avocado
1 lemon
1 tablespoon olive oil
¼ teaspoon sea salt

- Chop broccoli into bite-size pieces, keeping stems separate from crowns.
- Fill a pot with 1 inch of water, place a steamer basket inside, cover and heat to boiling.

- Add stem pieces, and steam for 2 minutes.
- Add crown pieces, cover and steam for 5 minutes while you prepare the other ingredients.
- In a mixing bowl, combine the juice of the lemon, the olive oil and salt.
- Chop the avocado into chunks and add to the bowl.
- Add the warm broccoli to the bowl, mix gently and serve.

Bitter Greens with Walnuts

Prep Time: 10 minutes
Cooking Time: 15 minutes
Serves 8

   1 bunch dandelion greens
   1 bunch mustard greens
   1 bunch collard greens
   1 tablespoon olive oil
   4 cloves garlic
   ½ cup walnut pieces
   sea salt to taste

- Toast the walnuts in a 350-degree oven for 5-10 minutes, until they release a fragrant odor.
- Wash the greens and remove any coarse stems (especially from collards and mustard greens).
- Bring 3 inches of salted water to boil, add the greens and boil for 5 minutes uncovered.
- Drain the greens, lay on a flat surface to cool, and then chop roughly.
- Heat the oil in a large sauté pan, add the garlic and cook for 1 minute, stirring so the garlic doesn't burn.
- Add the greens, walnuts, and salt to taste and sauté for another minute.
- Enjoy!

Quick Daikon Pickles

Prep Time: 8 minutes
Cooking Time: none!
Serves 15

> 1 large daikon radish
> ¼ cup mirin
> ⅛ cup umeboshi vinegar
> water

- Wash and peel daikon and slice into half circles that are ½-inch thick.
- Place daikon in a container.
- Add mirin, umeboshi and just enough water to cover the daikon.
- Cover, shake and store in the fridge.
- The pickles will be ready in 30 minutes and will
  stay good in the fridge for weeks.

TIP: *Use a few pieces as a condiment to go along with any other vegetable, grain, salad or protein dish.*

Beet-Carrot-Parsnip-Fennel Extravaganza

Prep Time: 10 minutes
Cooking Time: 45 minutes
Serves 6

> 5 small beets
> 3 big carrots
> 2 parsnips
> 1 fennel bulb
> 2 tablespoons olive oil
> ½ teaspoon sea salt

- Preheat oven to 425 degrees.
- Scrub all your vegetables.
- Chop vegetables into 2-inch pieces and finely chop fennel bulb.
- Mix vegetables with oil and sea salt. Transfer them to a baking dish.
- Bake covered for 30 minutes.
- Uncover and bake for 15 minutes.

Roasted Rutabaga with Celery Root

Prep Time: 8 minutes
Cooking Time: 40 minutes
Serves 6

> 1 rutabaga
> 1 celery root
> 2 tablespoons olive oil
> ½ teaspoon sea salt
> 1 teaspoon fresh rosemary

- Preheat oven to 400 degrees.
- Wash and scrub vegetables. Cut them into 1-inch-thick rounds.
- Mix with oil, salt and rosemary.
- Cover and bake for 30 minutes. Turn vegetables over and bake uncovered for 10 more minutes.

Carrot Burdock Strengthener

Prep Time: 10 minutes
Cooking Time: 20 minutes
Serves 6

> 1 onion
> 1 large burdock root
> 1 large carrot
> 1 teaspoon olive oil
> pinch of sea salt

- Wash and chop the vegetables into odd shapes.
- Heat oil in a skillet.
- Sauté veggies together with a pinch of salt on medium heat for 5 minutes.
- Add ½ inch of water to the skillet, cover and simmer for 10-15 minutes on low heat.

TIP: *Try serving with a sprinkle of toasted sesame seeds or fresh parsley for variety.*

Baked Caraway Sweet Potato with Rosemary

Prep Time: 10 minutes
Cooking time: 50 minutes
Serves 6

> 3 medium sweet potatoes
> 2 tablespoons olive oil
> ½ cup fresh rosemary
> ½ tablespoon caraway seeds

- Preheat oven to 400 degrees.
- Scrub sweet potatoes under running water and cut them into big chunks.
- Sprinkle baking dish with oil, place the sweet potatoes into the dish, and add rosemary and caraway seeds.
- Mix all ingredients together.
- Cover and bake for 50 minutes.

TIP: *Rosemary and caraway seeds can be substituted with cinnamon and 2 tablespoons of maple syrup or 1 tablespoon of ground cumin and a couple dashes of cayenne.*

Veggie Bake

Prep Time: 20 minutes
Cooking Time: 50 minutes
Serves 4 or more

> all the leftover veggies in your fridge that need to be used up
> 1 large can chopped tomatoes
> 1 can chickpeas
> 1-2 large yams, slices into ⅛-inch-thick sheets
> extra virgin olive oil

- Preheat the oven to 350 degrees.
- Chop veggies (not yams) and sauté in a bit of oil until soft, 5-10 minutes.
- Add can of tomatoes and drained can of chickpeas. Mix well and remove from heat.
- Slice yams into thin sheets.
- Spread a little olive oil on the bottom of a casserole dish and cover with a layer of yam sheets (as you would with lasagna noodles).
- Spoon out veggie-tomato-chick pea mixture and spread evenly on top of yams.

- Finish with a layer of yams.
- Lightly drizzle olive oil on top.
- Bake, covered, for 30 minutes.
- Take off the cover and turn up temperature to 450 degrees for 10 minutes to crisp up the top later.

TIP: *Add your favorite spices, like basil, oregano, fennel, cumin, chili pepper or sea salt when adding tomatoes and chickpeas.*

Spaghetti Squash Marinara

Prep Time: 10 minutes
Cooking Time: 45 minutes
Serves 4

> 1 spaghetti squash
> olive oil
> 1 small onion
> 1 carrot
> 5 button mushrooms
> 2 fresh tomatoes
> 2 tablespoons minced fresh herbs (basil, oregano, or thyme)

- Preheat the oven to 425 degrees.
- Carefully cut the squash in half, lengthwise and remove the seeds.
- Rub the inside with olive oil, and place open side down in a baking dish with ½ inch of water.
- Bake 45 minutes, or until a fork pierces easily through the squash.
- While squash is baking, prepare the sauce.
- Dice the onion, carrot and tomatoes. Slice the mushrooms. Mince the herbs.
- Sauté the onions for 5 minutes in 1 tablespoon olive oil.
- Add the carrot and tomatoes and cook another 5 minutes.
- Add the mushrooms, herbs and salt and continue cooking another 5-10 minutes.
- When the squash is cooked and cooled a little, use a fork to scrape the meat into spaghetti-like strands.
- Mix sauce and squash together in a bowl and serve.

TIP: *Add garlic, other veggies or cooked chicken pieces to the sauce.*

Satisfying Sesame Burdock

Prep Time: 5 minutes
Cooking Time: 10 minutes
Serves 3

> 1 large burdock root
> 2 teaspoons toasted sesame oil
> 1 teaspoon Bragg liquid aminos
> 1 teaspoon tahini
> a few squirts of umeboshi vinegar

- Heat the sesame oil in a sauté pan.
- Slice the burdock in ½-inch rounds and add to the hot oil.
- Sauté for 5 minutes, stirring frequently.
- Add a little water, cover and steam for 5 minutes.
- Meanwhile, add the other ingredients to a bowl and mix well.
- Add the burdock to the bowl and mix to coat with the sauce.

TIP: *Chop fresh spinach or dandelion greens and add during the last 2 minutes of cooking.*

beans

Soaking Beans

If you are new to beans, introduce them slowly, allowing your digestive system time to adjust and learn how to break them down. Soaking will make beans more digestible by reducing complex sugars.

Quick soak: Boil the beans in water for 5 minutes, remove from heat, cover and allow them to soak for 2 to 4 hours (soaking longer does not damage). Drain, rinse, add to fresh water and proceed with cooking.

Overnight soak: Soak beans 8 to 12 hours, drain, rinse, add to fresh water and proceed with cooking.

A simple way to tell if you have soaked your beans enough is to slice a bean in half; if the center is still opaque, soak more.

Basic Bean Cooking Guide

- Wash and clean beans.
- Soak beans using either of the two methods above.
- Do not cook beans in water they were soaked in.
- Place beans in heavy pot with suggested amount of water.
- Bring to boil.
- Skim off the foam.
- Cook beans with a 1- to 3-inch strip of kombu (a sea vegetable), which makes them more digestible and adds flavor and minerals.
- Spices that aid digestion are bay leaf, cumin, anise and fennel. These can be added to the water while cooking.
- Cover, reduce heat and simmer for the suggested time.
- Only add salt at the end of cooking, about 10 minutes before beans are done. Otherwise, it will interfere with thorough cooking.

Pressure Cooking Guide for Beans

- Wash and clean beans.
- Soak beans using either of the two methods above.
- Add beans to pressure cooker.
- Also add soaked 1- to 3-inch strip of kombu with beans.
- Cover and bring to pressure.
- Reduce heat and cook for the suggested time.
- Remove cover, season and cook uncovered until water evaporates.

Canned Beans

A busy lifestyle does not always allow time for soaking and cooking dried beans. Having canned beans on hand provides a quick meal option. Some people even find canned beans easier to digest than dried, soaked beans. When buying canned beans, consider these few tips:

- Buy canned beans that do not contain added salt or preservatives.
- Look for beans that have been cooked with kombu, which aids digestion.
- Rinse beans once removed from the can.

Basic Aduki Beans

Prep Time: 10 minutes
Cooking Time: 70 minutes
Serves 4

> 1 cup aduki beans
> 5-inch piece kombu
> 4 cups water
> 2 bay leaves
> 1 teaspoon sea salt

- Wash beans.
- Place kombu and aduki beans in a pot.
- Cover with water, 2 inches above the level of the beans.
- Bring to a boil.

- Add bay leaves.
- Cover and simmer for 1 hour.
- Check periodically, adding extra water if necessary so beans do not dry out or stick to the pot.
- Allow beans to cook until they are soft enough for your taste. Add salt.
- Drain excess water if necessary.

TIP: *To check for softness, take a couple of beans out from your pot and squeeze them between your thumb and pointer finger. If beans press easily, they are finished. If they feel hard in the middle, they need more time.*

Red Lentil Stew

Prep Time: 10 minutes
Cooking Time: 30 minutes
Serves 4

1 cup red lentils
4-5 cups water or stock
1 tablespoon olive oil
½ small onion, diced
1 carrot, rustic cut
1 burdock root, rustic cut
½ teaspoon cumin powder
a few splashes umeboshi vinegar

- Heat oil in a frying pan.
- Add spices and cook, stirring, for 30 seconds.
- Add onion and cook 5 minutes.
- Add carrot and burdock and sauté another 3 minutes.
- Add lentils and water or stock and cook 20 minutes, until lentils and roots are soft.
- Add a few splashes of umeboshi vinegar, stir, and taste. Add more ume or salt if necessary.

TIP: *For a rustic style cut, chop the vegetables in asymmetrical shapes that are roughly the same size. Notice if a different style cut creates a different mood when you eat the food.*

Basic Chickpeas in a Pressure Cooker

Prep Time: 5 minutes
Cooking Time: 60 minutes
Serves 4

> 1 cup chickpeas
> 2 cups water
> 5-inch piece kombu
> Pinch of sea salt

- Wash beans.
- Place them in pressure cooker with water and kombu. Cover.
- Bring to pressure.
- Reduce heat and cook for 1 hour.

TIP: *You can make delicious salads by adding chopped vegetables, sea vegetables (hijiki, arame), onions, scallion, fresh rosemary and sage and a little olive oil.*

Hummus

Prep Time: 15 minutes
Cooking Time: none!
Serves 8

> 2 cups chickpeas precooked in pressure cooker
> ⅓ cup chickpea water left over from pressure cooker
> 3 tablespoons tahini
> 3 cloves garlic
> ½ teaspoon sea salt
> 2 tablespoons fresh lemon juice
> ⅛ teaspoon cumin

- Combine all ingredients in a food processor or blender. It's easier to do it in several smaller batches.
- Once it's all blended, stir in a mixing bowl and taste.
- Use your taste buds to determine if you need more lemon juice, tahini, garlic, cumin or salt.
- Spread on a serving platter and sprinkle paprika or chili powder and a little olive oil over the whole plate.

TIP: *Try the same recipe with different kinds of beans such as navy beans or black turtle beans.*

Vegetarian Chili

Prep Time: 15 minutes
Cooking Time: 30 minutes
Serves 8

>   1 tablespoon olive oil
>   1 chopped onion
>   3 cloves minced garlic
>   2 tomatoes, diced, (or one can organic diced tomatoes)
>   1 carrot, cut into quarter moons
>   1 tablespoon chili powder
>   1 teaspoon ground cumin
>   3 cups cooked or canned red, black or kidney beans
>   1 cup water
>   2 tablespoons organic tomato paste
>   1 teaspoon sea salt

- Heat oil in a large heavy pan.
- Add onions and garlic and sauté 5 minutes.
- Add the rest of the vegetables, chili powder and cumin.
- Sauté for 5 minutes.
- Add the rest of the ingredients.
- Cook on low to medium heat for 20 minutes.

TIP: *Add as many veggies as you like such as bell peppers, zucchini and corn kernels.*

TIP: *Serve topped with cashew sour cream. (See sauces and dressings section.)*

Mexican Style Pinto Beans

Bean Soaking Time: 2–4 hours
Prep Time: 5 minutes
Cooking Time: 1 hour
Serves 4

>   1 cup dried pinto beans
>   4 cups water
>   3 cloves garlic, minced
>   1 jalapeno pepper, minced
>   ½ teaspoon cumin
>   ½ teaspoon chili powder
>   juice of one lime
>   salt to taste

- First, quickly soak the beans by boiling for 3 minutes in water.
- Remove from heat and let sit for 2-4 hours.
- Drain and rinse beans.
- Add to a large pot with 4 cups fresh water and bring to a boil.
- Add garlic and jalapeno and cook for 1 hour, until beans are soft.
- Add cumin, chili, lime and salt to taste.

Kitchari

Kitchari, a combination of rice and mung beans, is used in Ayurveda for cleansing the system.

Bean Soaking Time: 2 hours
Prep Time: 10 minutes
Cooking Time: 1 hour
Serves 6

> 1 cup basmati rice
> ½ cup mung beans
> 2 tablespoons ghee or olive oil
> 1 teaspoon mustard seeds
> 1 teaspoon cumin seeds
> ½ teaspoon turmeric powder
> ½ teaspoon salt
> 4 cups water

- Soak the beans in a bowl with water for 2 hours, then drain and rinse.
- Cook the beans in 4 cups of water for 30 minutes and drain excess liquid.
- Heat the ghee or oil in a deep pan over medium heat.
- Add mustard and cumin seeds and stir until they pop, about 2 minutes.
- Add the rice, beans, turmeric and salt and stir.
- Add the water, and bring to a boil.
- Reduce heat, cover most of the way, and simmer 25 minutes, until rice and beans are cooked.

TIP: *Add any vegetables you like to the pot while the rice and beans are cooking.*

Tofu and Tempeh

Tofu and other soybean products are versatile vegetarian protein options. Tempeh is a fermented soybean product made from whole soybeans. It's high in protein, fiber and vitamins.

Tofu Stir-Fry
Tofu Press Time: 1 hour
Marinade Time: at least 30 minutes
Prep Time: 10 minutes
Cooking Time: 15 minutes
Serves 4

1 block firm tofu
2 to 3 tablespoons olive oil
2 tablespoons sesame oil

Marinade:
1 tablespoon ginger juice
½ tablespoon tamari soy sauce
½ cup brown rice vinegar
½ cup toasted sesame oil
½ cup chopped fresh cilantro
2 cloves shredded garlic

- Drain liquid from tofu.
- Press excess water from tofu by placing it in a strainer over a bowl.
- Cover tofu with plate and place a heavy object on top, pressing the tofu. Leave for 1 hour.
- Cut tofu into 1-inch squares after draining.
- Set tofu aside and prepare marinade by mixing all ingredients.
- Marinate tofu for at least 30 minutes or overnight.
- Heat olive oil and sesame oil in a skillet.
- Add tofu and quick stir-fry until tofu becomes golden brown.

TIP: *To make ginger juice, grate about 2 inches of ginger into a piece of cheesecloth or a dishtowel. Then wrap the cloth or towel around the ginger and squeeze into a bowl, and you'll get the juice!*

Marinated Baked Tofu

Prep Time: 10 minutes
Marinade Time: 1 hour
Cooking Time: 30 minutes
Serves 4

    1 block firm tofu
    apple cider
    tamari
    brown rice vinegar
    honey
    olive oil

- Cut tofu into ½-inch thick slabs.
- Prepare marinade by mixing all ingredients. Trust your intuition to tell you how much of each ingredient to use. You want to end up with enough marinade to cover tofu in a container.
- Add tofu and marinate in the refrigerator for 1 hour.
- Preheat oven to 375 degrees.
- Place marinated tofu on a baking sheet and bake 15 minutes.
- Flip each piece over and continue to bake 15 more minutes.
- Marinade should dry up and tofu should turn a little brown and crispy.

TIP: *Serve over brown rice with some leafy greens on the side.*

The Chicken Way

This vegan dish is popular with adults and kids, and particularly with people who don't think they like tofu.

Prep Time: 15 minutes
Cooking Time: 40 minutes
Serves 4

    1 pound firm tofu
    ½ cup nutritional yeast flakes
    ½ cup powdered "unchicken" broth
    2 tablespoons fresh parsley, minced
    olive oil
    1 lemon, sliced into thin quarter moons

- Preheat oven to 350 degrees.
- Slice tofu into 9 slabs.
- Pour olive oil into a soup bowl.
- Mix yeast and broth in another soup bowl.
- Make an assembly line from left to right, in this order: tofu, olive oil bowl, yeast-broth bowl, cookie sheet.
- Dip a slab first in the oil.
- Then drop into the yeast-broth and coat well. (Use the hand that is dry, not oily.)
- Then lay the slab on the cookie sheet.
- Repeat with the other slices.
- Bake on 350 degrees for 30-40 minutes, until the tofu looks golden brown.
- Garnish each slab with parsley and a lemon slice.

Marinated Tempeh

Prep Time: 5 minutes
Marinade Time: 30 minutes
Cooking Time: 10 minutes
Serves 2

> 1 8-ounce package tempeh
> 1 tablespoon olive oil
> 3 tablespoons honey
> 2 teaspoons tamari
> 3 tablespoons your favorite mustard
> 2 teaspoons curry powder

- Mix ingredients (except olive oil) for marinade.
- Cut tempeh into large triangles.
- Marinate tempeh for 30 minutes.
- Heat skillet, add a tablespoon of olive oil and quickly stir-fry tempeh until it is golden brown, about 5 minutes each side.

Tempeh Reuben Sandwich

Prep Time: 10 minutes
Cooking Time: 10 minutes
Serves 2

4 slices whole grain bread

1 recipe marinated tempeh (see above)

3 tablespoons sauerkraut

2 slices Swiss cheese

2 tablespoons Russian dressing (see sauces and dressings section)

2 teaspoons olive oil

- Spread Russian dressing on two slices of bread.
- Top each slice with half of the tempeh, sauerkraut, cheese and then another slice of bread.
- Heat olive oil in a large pan and fry sandwich on each side for 2 or 3 minutes, until the cheese melts and the bread is a little browned.

Tempeh Croutons

Prep Time: 10 minutes
Cooking Time: 30 minutes
Serves 4

1 package tempeh

2 cloves garlic

¼ cup tamari

2 tablespoons brown rice vinegar

½ cup water

1 tablespoon olive oil

1 teaspoon dried oregano

- Slice tempeh into bite-size cubes.
- In a saucepan, mix together garlic, tamari, vinegar and water.
- Bring to a simmer over medium heat.
- Add tempeh and cook 15 minutes.
- Drain and cool tempeh.
- Heat oil in a skillet, add tempeh and sauté until golden brown, flipping tempeh to brown all sides.
- Add oregano and cook another 2 minutes.
- Serve in your favorite salad.

meat & fish

When choosing meat and fish for cooking, always look for the best quality available. With meats, try organic, grass-fed meats that are leaner and full of more nutrients than meats from large factory farms. With fish, try wild varieties with vibrant colors and pick fish that smells fresh, like the ocean. If you are unsure about the quality of meat and fish available at your local store, ask the butcher or fishmonger for assistance in making the best choice.

Salmon Cakes

Prep Time: 10 minutes
Cooking Time: 10 minutes
Serves 4

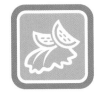

4 ounces cooked salmon

6 rice crackers

½ onion, minced

2 cloves minced garlic

1 tablespoon fresh lemon juice

dash of black pepper

dash of coriander

1 tablespoon olive oil

- Break salmon and rice crackers into small pieces.
- Mix all ingredients together.
- Create several small patties.
- Refrigerate for 1 hour.
- In a skillet, heat oil on high.
- Quickly fry both sides of each patty for 3-4 minutes.

TIP: *Serve with brown rice and lemon slices.*

Ideal Dill Fish

Prep Time: 5 minutes
Cooking Time: 10 minutes
Serves 4

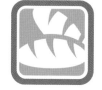

> 1 pound cod fish fillet
> dash of sea salt
> dash of black pepper
> ½ cup fresh dill
> 1 tablespoon fresh lemon juice

- Rinse fish.
- Season with salt and pepper.
- Finely chop dill.
- Fill skillet with about ½ inch of water and heat till steaming.
- Drop in fish, cover top with dill and cook until it is soft, about 5 to 7 minutes.
- Serve immediately.

Honey-Macadamia Halibut

Prep Time: 10 minutes
Cooking Time: 10 minutes
Serves 4

> 4 4-ounce halibut fillets (1-inch thick)
> ¼ cup macadamia nuts
> 3 tablespoons honey
> 1 tablespoons coconut oil

- Chop nuts, spread on a cookie sheet, and toast in the oven or in a toaster on 350 degrees until golden brown, about 5-7 minutes. Check every minute or two and stir or spin tray around to toast evenly.
- Heat oil in a skillet.
- Sprinkle salt and pepper on both sides of each fish fillet, and cook first side over medium heat for 4 minutes.
- Flip each fillet and cook for 3 minutes on the other side.
- While fish is in the pan, spread a layer of honey on each fillet and add a layer of nuts on top.
- Flip over and cook for 2 minutes, while you add honey and nuts to the other side.
- Flip again and cook 2 minutes.

- Halibut is cooked when the meat is no longer translucent.
- Remove from heat and serve.

Moroccan Chicken Tagine with Prunes

Prep Time: 15 minutes
Cooking Time: 45 minutes
Serves 4

 2 chicken breasts cut into 2-inch chunks
 1 yellow onion, sliced into strips
 ½ teaspoons turmeric
 2 cloves minced garlic
 ½ teaspoon powdered ginger
 ½ teaspoon powdered cinnamon
 10 pitted prunes

- Heat 1 tablespoon of olive oil in a deep pan and sauté onions on low heat until translucent, 10 minutes or so.
- Add everything else except prunes and mix well.
- Add ½ cup water, cover, and cook over medium heat 30 minutes. Chicken should be cooked all the way through but should not be dried out. (Cut a piece open to check.)
- Add prunes and cook another 5 minutes, until they get soft and saturated with juice.

TIP: *Top with toasted sesame seeds and chopped parsley.*

Chai Chicken

Chai is the Indian way of drinking tea. You can buy chai tea bags, or make it yourself by putting shredded ginger, cinnamon powder and ground cardamom seeds in a pot with 2 cups of water and bringing it to a boil. Cook for 2 to 3 minutes to bring flavor out of the spices, then add tea and stir.

Prep Time: 10 minutes
Cooking Time: 45 minutes
Serves 4

 4 chicken legs
 4 to 5 sliced carrots
 1 cup coconut milk
 2 cups chai tea

- Preheat oven to 350 degrees.
- Place chicken and carrots in a casserole dish.
  Sprinkle with a pinch of salt and pepper.
- In a pot, combine coconut milk and tea and bring to a boil.
- Pour over the chicken in the casserole dish.
- Cover with lid and bake in the oven at 350 degrees for
  45 minutes, or until chicken is cooked through.
- Serve with brown basmati rice and greens. Use
  coconut milk mixture as a sauce.

Smoked Turkey with Kale

Prep Time: 10 minutes
Cooking Time: 20 minutes
Serves 4

> 2 teaspoons olive oil
> 1 red onion, sliced into thin strips
> 1 bunch curly kale, sliced into thin ribbons
> ½ pound smoked turkey breast, sliced into bite-size chunks
> 1 tablespoon balsamic vinegar
> salt and pepper to taste

- Slowly sauté the onions over medium low heat for 15 minutes, until they start to turn a little brown.
- Add kale and stir until wilted, about 3 minutes.
- Add turkey and cook another 2 minutes until it is warm.
- Transfer to a serving dish and add balsamic vinegar, salt and pepper to taste.

Beef and Arugula Stir-Fry

Prep Time: 15 minutes
Cooking Time: 15 minutes
Serves 3

> ½ pound sirloin, cut into thin strips
> 2 teaspoons olive oil
> 1 tablespoon minced fresh ginger
> 1 clove minced garlic

2 red bell peppers, cut into very thin strips

1 to 2 bunches well-washed arugula

2 teaspoons kuzu

2 teaspoons tamari

2 teaspoons brown rice or apple cider vinegar

¼ cup water

- Stir-fry the beef in a pan with 2 teaspoons of oil over medium-high heat for about 2 minutes or until browned.
- Remove beef with tongs or fork, allowing excess oil to drip off, and set side.
- In same pan in remaining oil, stir-fry ginger and garlic for 2 to 3 minutes, and then add the bell pepper. Cook for another 2 to 3 minutes.
- Mix together fresh arugula and bell pepper mixture in a serving bowl.
- In a small bowl, combine kuzu, tamari, vinegar and water.
- Place kuzu mixture into skillet and cook over medium heat until sauce starts to thicken.
- Return the beef to the skillet and cook for 1 minute, just enough to warm up the beef.
- Add the beef to the serving bowl with arugula and bell peppers.
- Mix and serve warm.

soup

Everyone craves comfort food. When we are busy and stressed, we tend to reach for our favorite convenience foods to get a soothing effect. Soup is the ultimate comfort food and a healthier choice. Remember eating soup as a child, when you were sick? As adults, eating soup can still give us that cozy, nurtured feeling.

Soups are highly nutritious. Almost any vegetable can go into a soup; it is a great way to use leftover vegetables in your fridge. Cooking soup from scratch may sound like a big project, but in fact soups are incredibly quick and easy to make. The active prep time for all these soups is 10 minutes. You can prepare other components of your meal while you wait, or kick back with a magazine until your soup is done and ready to be enjoyed.

Roasted Vegetable Stock
Prep Time: 10 minutes
Cooking Time: 1 hour and 45 minutes

1 onion
1 parsnip
1 carrot
5 cloves garlic
4 mushrooms
1 bunch parsley
olive oil
sea salt and black pepper

- Preheat oven to 400 degrees.
- Peel and wash veggies, cut into chunks (you can leave garlic cloves whole) and spread on a cookie sheet.
- Drizzle a little olive oil over veggies and sprinkle with salt and pepper.
- Roast in the oven for 45 minutes, turning veggies occasionally until everything gets a little brown.

- Remove veggies from oven and place in a large
  soup pot with 10 cups of water.
- Bring to a boil, reduce heat to low and simmer for at least one hour.
- Strain stock and it's ready to go!

TIP: *After you strain the stock put it back on the stove on low heat for another hour or more. It will reduce to become more of a concentrate. To store it, pour it into an ice cube tray and freeze it. Then the next time you need some stock, just pop out a cube or two to flavor your rice or soup.*

Mighty Miso Soup

Prep Time: 10 minutes
Cooking Time: 15 minutes
Serves 4

8-inch piece wakame
1 medium onion
1 medium daikon radish
½ block tofu
5 cups water
1 to 2 tablespoons miso paste
2 green onions

- Wash wakame, soak for 5 minutes or until softened, and cut into 1-inch pieces.
- Cut onion into long, thin strips.
- Cut daikon into half moons.
- Cut tofu into ½-inch cubes.
- Add veggies, wakame and tofu to water and bring to boil.
- Reduce heat to low, and simmer for 10 minutes.
- Meanwhile, remove 1/2 cup of liquid from the pot and stir in the miso to dissolve.
- Return miso mixture to pot, reduce heat to very low and cook for 2 to 3 more minutes. Do not boil.
- Garnish with chopped scallion.

Easy Breezy Soup

Prep Time: 10 minutes
Cooking Time: 20-30 minutes
Serves 4

Try any of these vegetable combinations to create a simply delicious soup: carrot, parsnip, celery, winter squash, yam ginger, broccoli, onion, cauliflower, daikon radish, leek, carrot, mustard greens, shiitakes, onion, kale, cabbage, rutabaga.

- Use one of each vegetable.
- Cut all veggies to roughly the same size, around 2-inch chunks.
- Place cut veggies in a pot with water just covering them.
- Bring to a boil then lower to simmer.
- Cook until a fork inserts smoothly into each vegetable, probably about 20 minutes.
- Add your favorite condiments.
- Eat like this, or puree in a food processor, blender or with a hand mixer.

TIP: *Garnish with parsley and scallion.*

TIP: *To add richness to soup, sauté one medium onion and add to water before cooking.*

Carrot Ginger Soup

Prep Time: 10 minutes
Cooking Time: 30 minutes
Serves 4

6 carrots
1 medium onion
1 teaspoon sea salt
4 cups water
6-inch piece fresh ginger
Fresh parsley to garnish

- Wash, peel and cut carrots and onion into chunks.
- Place vegetables and salt in a pot.
- Add water. Bring to a boil. Cover with a lid.

- Simmer on low heat for 25 minutes.
- Transfer soup into blender, adding water if necessary to achieve desired consistency.
- When blending is done, squeeze juice from grated ginger and add to soup.
- Garnish with parsley.

TIP: *For extra flavor, sauté vegetables before cooking.*

TIP: *Substitute carrots with squash, parsnip or beets. Squash and beets need 35 to 40 minutes to cook.*

Creamy Broccoli Soup

Prep Time: 10 minutes
Cooking Time: 30 minutes
Serves 4

1 bunch broccoli
5 cups water
1 small onion
2 cloves garlic
2 tablespoons barley miso
1 cup cooked brown rice

- Wash broccoli and separate stems from florets.
- Chop onion.
- In a pot, bring water to a boil.
- Add broccoli stems and onion.
- Mince the garlic and add to the pot.
- Reduce heat and simmer for 15 minutes.
- Meanwhile, remove 2 cups of liquid from the pot, dissolve miso paste in the liquid, add brown rice and return to the pot.
- Put soup in the blender and blend. When it is smooth, return to the pot.
- Add broccoli florets and cook 10 more minutes.

Garlic Lover's Soup

They say that garlic is as good as ten mothers due to its incredible healing properties. Try this soup when you are feeling a cold coming on.

Prep Time: 10 minutes
Cooking Time: 1 hour
Serves 4

>   2 heads garlic
>   2 teaspoons olive oil
>   5 cups vegetable stock
>   2 bunches spinach, chopped

- Preheat oven to 425 degrees.
- Slice off the top of each head of garlic, exposing the top of each clove.
- Pour a teaspoon of oil on each head.
- Place in a casserole dish with a lid or wrap in foil.
- Roast for 45 minutes or until cloves are completely soft.
- Let the garlic cool for a few minutes and squeeze cloves into a pot.
- Add stock and stir to break up the garlic and combine.
- Bring to boil, reduce heat and simmer for 10 minutes.
- Just at the end, add in the spinach to wilt, stir well, and serve right away.

Cool Cucumber and Avocado Soup

Prep Time: 10 minutes
Cooking Time: none!
Serves 4

>   1 cucumber, peeled
>   1 avocado
>   2 green onions
>   juice of 1 lime
>   1 cup plain yogurt or soy yogurt
>   1 cup water
>   salt and pepper to taste

- Roughly chop the cucumber, avocado and green onions and toss in the blender.
- Add other ingredients and process until smooth.

TIP: *Garnish with chopped fresh cilantro and a dash of cayenne pepper.*

salads

Ideas for Green Salads

Sometimes it's nice to get your greens from a good 'ole salad of mixed greens. Here are some ways to put a new twist on an old favorite.

For the greens themselves, try a mixture using any of these:

- Romaine, red leaf, green leaf, butter lettuce, mesclun mix, spinach, blanched dark leafy greens, any cabbage, endive, radicchio, arugula, frisee or whatever organic greens look fabulous at your market today.
- Add some veggies: use any that look and sound good to you. Try green beans, radishes, roasted winter squash, sugar snaps, corn from the cob or root veggies.
- Add some fruits: fresh or dried berries, apples, tangerines, avocados, melons, figs, goji berries or cucumbers.
- And don't leave out the nuts, seeds and beans: sunflower seeds, pumpkin seeds, sprouts of all kinds, toasted nuts, sesame seeds or coconut flakes.
- Be experimental! Add anything else you can imagine—dulse flakes, leftover grains, tofu, fish, toasted nori—just go for it!
- Then top it off with a delicious dressing (see dressings section) and enjoy!

Quinoa Salad

Prep Time: 15 minutes
Cooking Time: none!
Serves 8

> 2 cups cooked quinoa
> ½ cup chopped radishes
> ½ cup chopped cucumber
> ½ cup chopped celery
> ½ cup chopped red onion
> ½ cup chopped fresh parsley
> ½ cup chopped red bell pepper
> 1 tablespoon olive oil
> 2 teaspoons balsamic vinegar

- Combine all ingredients together in a big bowl.
- Mix well.

TIP: *Garnish with cherry tomatoes and shredded garlic cloves and chill before serving.*

Carrot Raisin Salad

Prep Time: 10 minutes
Cooking Time: none!
Serves 6

> 2 carrots
> handful of raisins
> umeboshi vinegar
> tamari
> flax oil

- Grate carrots by hand or in a food processor.
- Place carrots and raisins in a mixing bowl.
- Dress with the other ingredients, to taste.

TIP: *This is a quick and easy salad to make when you get home from work, starving, and you want to devour everything in your fridge. Make this salad, sit down and relax for few minutes, and then move on to making dinner or whatever your evening entails.*

Barley Sun Salad

Prep Time: 20 minutes
Cooking Time: 1 hour
Serves 8

> 1 cup hulled barley
> 2¼ cups water
> 2 bunches arugula
> ½ cup sunflower seeds
> 1 carrot
> ½ bunch scallions
> 2 tablespoons olive oil
> juice of 1 or 2 lemons

- Place barley water and ¼ teaspoons sea salt in a pot.
- Bring to a boil, reduce heat to low, and simmer, covered for 45 minutes.
- Meanwhile, wash arugula and chop into small pieces.
- Place sunflower seeds on a cookie sheet and toast for 5 minutes in a 350-degree oven, being careful not to burn them.
- Wash and chop the carrot into a small dice.
- Wash and finely chop the scallions.
- When the barley is cooked, transfer to a large mixing bowl, add all ingredients, and mix well.
- Add salt, pepper, oil or lemon juice to meet your taste preference.

Cold Soba Noodle Salad

Prep Time: 20 minutes
Cooking Time: 15 minutes
Serves 4

8 ounces soba noodles
6 cups water
1 bunch chopped sunflower sprouts or pea shoots
½ cup chopped red radishes
½ cup chopped celery
½ cup chopped cucumber

- Put soba noodles into a pot of 6 cups boiling water.
- Cook until tender, no more than 8 minutes.
- Rinse with cold water when finished cooking.
- Mix all vegetables and noodles.

Dressing:
½ cup finely chopped fresh basil
1 tablespoon toasted sesame oil
$1/4$ cup tahini
2 tablespoons tamari soy sauce
2-inch piece grated fresh ginger
juice of ½ lemon

- Mix all these ingredients and pour over noodles.

Beet Salad with Fennel and Mint

This salad is famous for converting non-beet eaters into beet lovers!

Prep Time: 20 minutes
Cooking Time: 30 minutes
Serves 6

2 beets
1 small fennel bulb
1 bunch mint leaves
2 oranges
¼ cup balsamic vinegar

- Place beets in a pot, cover with 1 inch with water, and boil for 20-30 minutes, until a fork pierces easily through the middle of each beet.
- While beets are cooking, wash fennel and slice very thin.
- Chop mint into thin ribbons.
- Zest oranges and juice them into a bowl.
- When beets are cooked, drain them in the sink.
- Cool them by rinsing under cold water, and peel the skin off with your hands. (It should slide right off.)
- Chop the beets into ¼-inch thick, quarter rounds.
- Add all ingredients into a large bowl and mix well.

Late Summer Corn Salad

Prep Time: 20 minutes
Cooking Time: 10 minutes
Server 6

4 ears corn
½ small red onion
½ small green bell pepper
½ small red bell pepper
½ bunch cilantro
1 tablespoon olive oil
juice of 1 lemon
sea salt and pepper to taste

- Boil corn in a large pot for 5-10 minutes.
- Remove from pot and cool by running under cold water.

- Cut kernels from the cobs and place in a large mixing bowl.
- Finely dice the onion and peppers, mince the cilantro and add them all to the corn.
- Add oil, lemon, salt and pepper and mix well.
- Taste and adjust seasonings.

Raw, Nutty, Not Tuna Salad

Soaking Time: 8 hours or more
Prep Time: 15 minutes
Cooking Time: none!
Serves 4

1 cup almonds
1 cup sunflower seeds
1-2 stalks celery, finely chopped
1 tablespoon minced dill
½ small red onion, finely chopped
1 teaspoon kelp granules
juice of 1 lemon
½ teaspoons sea salt

- Place almonds in a bowl, cover with water and let soak overnight.
- Do the same with the sunflower seeds.
- Discard most of the soaking water and combine nuts and seeds in a food processor or blender.
- Process until almost smooth.
- Combine with other ingredients in a bowl and mix well.

TIP: *Serve on a bed of mixed greens with a vinaigrette, as a sandwich filling or roll in a sheet of nori.*

sauces & dressings

Tahini Lemon Dressing

Prep Time: 5 minutes
Serves 6

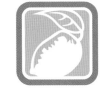

> 2 tablespoons tahini
> juice of 1 lemon
> ½ cup water
> ¼ tablespoon tamari soy sauce

- Mix with a fork in small bowl.
- Adjust the amounts of each ingredient to meet your taste preference.

TIP: *Try adding a little miso paste too!*

Ginger Parsley Garlic Dressing

Prep Time: 8 minutes
Serves 8

> 4-inch piece fresh ginger
> 1 bunch fresh parsley
> 2 cloves garlic
> juice of ½ lemon
> ½ tablespoon sesame oil
> ¼ tablespoon tamari soy sauce

- Dice ginger root. Put all ingredients in blender and blend until smooth.

Pumpkin Seed Dressing

Prep Time: 5 minutes
Serves 8

> 1 cup toasted pumpkin seeds
> 2 tablespoons brown rice vinegar
> 1 tablespoon umeboshi vinegar
> 1 teaspoon tamari soy sauce
> 1 cup water

- Mix in a bowl. Great on cooked greens!

Green Goddess Dressing

Prep Time: 5 minutes

½ pound silken tofu
1 bunch scallions
juice of 2 lemons
½ bunch flat leaf parsley
1 clove garlic
salt to taste

- Add all ingredients to blender and blend until creamy.
- Taste and adjust to your preference.

Maple Dijon Vinaigrette

Prep Time: 5 minutes

1 tablespoon Dijon mustard
½ cup balsamic vinegar
½ cup maple syrup
a couple pinches of sea salt and pepper
1 cup olive oil

- Blend first 4 ingredients in a food processor or with a whisk.
- Slowly add oil while mixing to emulsify.

Vegan Caesar Dressing

Prep Time: 15 minutes
Serves 8

¼ cup almonds
3 cloves garlic
3 tablespoons nutritional yeast flakes
2 tablespoons tamari
juice of 1 lemon
3 tablespoons Dijon mustard
1 tablespoon olive oil or flax oil

- Blanch the almonds by putting them in a bowl, pouring boiling water to cover them, and letting them sit for 1 minute.
- Drain and pat dry.
- Slip the skins off between your finger and thumb.
- Add all ingredients to a blender or food processor and blend until smooth.

TIP: *Serve with the classic combo of chopped romaine hearts and tempeh croutons.*

Simple Pesto

Prep Time: 5 minutes
Serves 8

¼ cup olive oil
1 cup basil leaves
1 cup pine nuts or walnuts
2 cloves garlic
2 tablespoons white miso
2 teaspoons umeboshi vinegar
1 teaspoon brown rice syrup
water

- Warm the oil over very low heat for 3 minutes.
- Combine all ingredients in a blender, except water.
- Blend together, adding as much water as necessary to get the consistency you desire.

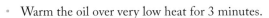

Soothing Shiitake Gravy

Prep Time: 5 minutes
Cooking Time: 15 minutes
Serves 15

10 fresh shiitake mushrooms
1 heaping tablespoon kuzu root
1 teaspoon tamari
water

- Remove stems from shiitakes and slice caps thinly.
- Add to a pot with 2 quarts water.
- Bring to a boil, reduce heat and simmer for 10 minutes.
- Add tamari.
- Dissolve kuzu root in ¼ cup cool water. It's nice to mash it up with your hand.
- Slowly add kuzu mixture to the pot, stirring as you pour it in.
- Stir for another minute, until the gravy thickens.
- Taste to see if you need to add more tamari, and serve.

Russian Dressing

Prep Time: 15 minutes
Serves 10

> ½ pound soft tofu
> 1 tablespoon lemon juice
> 3 tablespoons brown rice syrup
> 1 tablespoon olive oil
> 1 teaspoon mustard
> 1 tablespoon minced red onion
> ⅔ cup sun-dried tomatoes, soft and finely chopped
> ⅓ cup minced dill pickles
> ½ teaspoons sea salt

- Place sun-dried tomatoes in a bowl and cover with boiling water.
- Combine tofu, lemon juice, rice syrup, oil and mustard in a food processor and puree until creamy.
- Chop and add tomatoes.
- Add pickles, onion and salt.
- Pulse a few times to combine.

TIP: *Serve as part of a Reuben sandwich with baked tempeh, sauerkraut and cheese on sprouted bread.*

sea vegetables

Sea vegetables are one of the most nutrient-packed foods on the earth. They are a highly concentrated source of minerals and contain a range of vitamins, all of which nourish you, beautify your skin, hair and nails and help you feel grounded. They are very versatile, and can be added to soups, salads, stir-fries and desserts. Sea vegetables have many health benefits including, reducing blood cholesterol, improving digestion, counteracting obesity, strengthening bones and teeth, and they contain antibiotic properties. Sea vegetables grown wild and harvested from the ocean are top quality. You can also find high-quality brands in your local health food store. Commercially harvested seaweeds are easily found in Asian markets.

Arame Mild, semisweet flavor and thin but firm texture. Great as a side dish, but especially yummy with buckwheat.

Hijiki Robust in flavor and black in color. A great side dish.

Kombu Light in flavor and chewy. Expands and softens when soaked. Excellent food tenderizer and helps with the digestibility of beans. Adds a sweet flavor to root vegetables. Creates wonderful stocks and soups.

Nori Paper-thin, dark green sheets made from pressed sea vegetables. Nori has a flavor similar to tuna. Originally used as sushi wrap. Nori flakes may be used as a condiment.

Dulse Savory-tasting, brownish-green-colored stalks. Wonderful for roasting with seeds and as a condiment.

Wakame Delicate, long, green strips. Has a sweet flavor. When soaked, wakame expands a great deal, so cut it into small pieces. Wakame loves the company of carrots and parsnips and adds a sweet taste to all legumes.

Soaking Sea Vegetables

Soaking will help with sea vegetables' digestibility, cooking time and taste.

1. Put sea vegetables in a bowl filled with cold water.
2. Move fingers through the stems as if you were shampooing.
3. Discard this "first wash" water.
4. Rinse through again.
5. Fill the bowl with cold water again.
6. Add sea vegetables and let stand for 15 to 20 minutes. Arame requires less time to soak than hijiki.

TIP: *Use the water to add to your houseplants or rinse your hair with it and watch them grow!*

Kung-Fu Hijiki Salad

Prep Time: 15 minutes
Cooking Time: 10 minutes
Serves 6

1 cup hijiki
5 cups water
1 teaspoon sesame oil
2 teaspoons umeboshi vinegar
1 yellow or red pepper
4 stalks scallions
1 carrot
½ cup corn kernels, fresh off the cob
5 to 6 cherry tomatoes chopped in half (optional)
2 cloves shredded garlic
1 tablespoon fresh ginger juice

- Rinse and soak hijiki according to directions above.
- Cook hijiki in water for 10 minutes.
- Drain from water and allow to cool.
- Chop and mix remaining ingredients in a bowl.
- Add hijiki.

TIP: *This was Bruce Lee's favorite meal.*

Wakame with Greens

Prep Time: 5 minutes
Cooking Time: 15 minutes
Serves 4

½ cup wakame, soaked and chopped
1 bunch leafy green vegetables (collards, kale or mustard greens)
1 tablespoon olive oil
dash of sea salt
juice of ½ lemon
2 tablespoons gomasio

- Wash, soak and chop wakame into small pieces.
- Wash and chop greens into bite-size pieces.
- Cook wakame in a small amount of water until it becomes tender, about 5 minutes.
- In a skillet, heat oil, add greens and sauté for 5 to 7 minutes until leaves wilt.
- Add a dash of salt to sauté.
- Add soaked wakame and lemon juice.
- Sauté together for 3 to 5 more minutes.
- Sprinkle with gomasio and serve.

Arame Sauté

Prep Time: 15 minutes
Cooking Time: 30 minutes
Serves 4

½ cup arame
1 teaspoon sesame oil
1 onion, sliced in long, thin strips
1 carrot, sliced into matchstick-shape pieces
apple juice
1 tablespoon tamari
water

- Soak arame in water for 10 minutes.
- Sauté onion in oil, over medium heat for 10 minutes.
- Add carrots and sauté another 3-4 minutes.
- Add arame, plus tamari and enough apple juice and water to cover the

veggies. (Use half juice and half water.)

- Simmer for 15 minutes or until liquid has evaporated.

Seaweed Salad

Prep Time: 5 minutes
Marinade Time: 30 minutes
Serves 4

> ¾ ounce combined 3 varieties of seaweed
> 1 teaspoon agave syrup
> 2 tablespoons brown rice vinegar
> 1 teaspoon sesame oil
> 1 teaspoon sesame seeds

- Combine all ingredients in a bowl.
- Marinate for at least 30 minutes before serving.

Veggie Nori Rolls

Prep Time: 10 minutes
Assembly: 5 minutes
Serves 5

> 1 cup cooked brown rice
> 2 tablespoons brown rice vinegar
> 1 tablespoon brown rice syrup
> ½ teaspoon sea salt
> 5 sheets toasted sushi nori
> fillings of your choice*

- Lay rice out on a cookie sheet.
- Top with vinegar, rice syrup and sea salt.
- Mix well and transfer to a bowl.
- Lay a sheet of nori on a dry cutting board or sushi rolling mat.
- Put down a thin layer of rice covering the half of the nori sheet that is closest to you.
- Layer 2-3 rows of toppings on the rice, on the end that is closest to you.
- Roll the nori away from you, starting with the end closest to you.
- As you roll, make sure to keep tucking the roll under so it's pretty tight, much like you would roll a sleeping bag.

- When you get to the end, wet your finger with a little water, and wet the edge of the nori to make sure it stays sealed.
- Wet the edge of a very sharp knife and cut the roll in half.
- Wet the knife again and cut each piece in half again.
- Enjoy your professional style sushi.

*Sushi filling ideas:
- avocado, cucumber, carrot
- daikon, cucumber, umeboshi paste, sesame seeds
- mango, avocado
- shiitake mushrooms marinated in tamari and rice vinegar, blanched kale ribbons
- cashew butter, sauerkraut (really, it's amazing!)
- baked tofu, spinach, almonds
- salmon, avocado

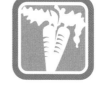

Kelp Cucumber Salad

The word "kelp" refers to any of the brown seaweeds including alaria, wakame and kombu. I have made this salad with wakame and it is very tasty, but feel free to experiment with other varieties too!

Prep Time: 20 minutes
Serves 6

> 1 cucumber
> ¼ pound kelp
> 4 tablespoons rice vinegar
> 1 tablespoon maple syrup
> 3 tablespoons tamari
> 2 tablespoons sesame seeds

- Put kelp in a bowl and cover with water.
- Let sit for 15 minutes.
- Slice into bite-size pieces.
- Peel cucumber and slice into thin rounds.
- Whisk together vinegar, maple syrup and tamari in a bowl.
- Add cucumber and kelp and mix well
- Garnish with sesame seeds and serve.

savory snacks

We are a snack foods culture. Grab them on the go. Dip into a treat at that 3 p.m. to 4 p.m. energy slump. Many health-supportive alternatives can help you avoid processed, quick snack foods. They are tasty, simple and easy to throw in your bag for those days on the go.

Snack Ideas:

- **baked yam chips:** slice the yam and place on a baking sheet, bake for 20 to 25 minutes at 350 degrees
- **carrot sticks with hummus:** a perfect blend of crunchiness and smoothness; make your own hummus or find spiced varieties made without preservatives at your natural food market
- **edamame in a pod:** edible soybean found in frozen food section, defrost and sprinkle with sea salt
- **fresh fruit:** an apple a day . . . so many different kinds, one day a granny smith the next a gala; or pick from what is in season: pears, plums, peaches, cherries, berries or bananas
- **granola:** a baked, crunchy mixture of rolled oats, nuts, dried fruit and honey or maple syrup; eat on its own or with yogurt or nut milk
- **mochi:** a traditional Japanese treat like puff pastry without wheat or flour, made from cooked, puréed rice and can be found in the refrigerator section of your health food store in savory and sweet flavors
- **nori sheets:** found in the seaweed section of your health food store or Asian market, try nori with leftover brown rice or use it as a wrap for veggies
- **rice cakes with nut butter:** spread any nut butter (try almond, peanut or cashew) on these light crispy cakes
- **trail mix:** a custom blend of nuts, seeds and dried fruit, which offers a great protein boost

- **various nuts and seeds:** cashews, peanuts, walnuts, tamari almonds, dry-roasted pumpkin or sunflower seeds
- **yogurt:** try cow, goat, sheep or soy; buy plain and add your own topping like jam, fresh fruit, granola or maple syrup.

Afternoon Pick-Me-Up

Prep Time: 5 minutes
Cooking Time: none!
Serves 1

3 carrots or 12 ounces carrot juice
1 tablespoon spirulina or chlorella powder

- If you have a juicer, juice 3 carrots.
- If you don't have a juicer, buy some fresh or bottled organic carrot juice.
- Put green powder into the juice and shake well.
- Drink slowly, and enjoy your energy.

TIP: *Try different types of green, superfoods to see how they affect you differently. I find this combination helps when I'm crashing in the afternoon.*

Ball-O-Nuts

Soaking Time: a few hours
Prep Time: 10 minutes
Serves 10

6 dates
½ cup rolled oats
¾ cup almonds
½ cup sesame seeds
½ cup apple juice
½ cup brown rice syrup
¾ cup poppy seeds

- Soak dates with oats in water for a few hours, then drain excess water.
- Add all remaining ingredients except poppy seeds into a blender and blend until chunks become very small, but are still apparent.
- Form little balls with the mixture, then roll in poppy seeds

TIP: *You can also squeeze lemon or ginger juice into the mixture.*

Kale Chips

Prep Time: 10 minutes
Cooking Time: 10 minutes
Serves 10 or more

1 to 2 bunches kale
olive oil

- Preheat oven to 425 degrees.
- Remove kale from stalk, leaving the greens in large pieces.
- Place a little olive oil in a bowl, dip your fingers and rub a very light coat of oil over the kale.
- Put kale on a baking sheet and bake for 5 minutes or until it starts to turn a bit brown. Keep an eye on it as it can burn quickly.
- Turn the kale over and bake with the other side up. Remove and serve.

TIP: *For added flavor sprinkle with a little salt or spice, such as curry or cumin after rubbing on olive oil.*

Plantain Chips

Prep Time: 20 minutes
Cooking Time: 10 minutes
Serves 12

6 green plantains
juice of 6 limes
2 tablespoons coconut oil

- Peel and slice the plantains diagonally and very thin.
- Soak the slices in lime juice for 10 to 15 minutes.
- Dry thoroughly.
- Heat broiler.
- Toss plantains with coconut oil in a bowl. Make sure oil covers slices. (You may have to heat the oil just a bit so that it is not in solid form.)
- Place on a baking sheet and put under broiler for 3 to 5 minutes or until golden brown.
- Flip to the other side, and repeat.
- Store refrigerated in an airtight container once cooled down.
- They will keep for 1 week.

Veggie Muffins

Prep Time: 15 minutes
Cooking Time: 15 minutes
Serves 8

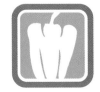

2 cups spelt flour
½ cup finely chopped fresh parsley
pinch of sea salt
2 beaten eggs
1 cup grated or finely chopped veggies
1 cup soy or rice milk

- Preheat oven to 325 degrees.
- Mix flour, parsley and salt in a bowl.
- Make a well, add eggs and veggies.
- Mix lightly, gradually adding milk. This is supposed to be lumpy so don't work too hard!
- Scrape into muffin tray that is lightly oiled.
- Bake for 12 to 15 minutes.
- Remove and allow to sit for 10 minutes, then serve.

Ants on a Log

Prep Time: 10 minutes
Serves 1

2 tablespoons almond butter
2 stalks celery
handful dried blueberries

- Wash celery.
- Spread nut butter inside each stalk.
- Dot with blueberries or "ants".

TIP: *Try with any nut butter and any dried fruit that you like.*

Mixed Spicy Nuts

Prep Time: 5 minutes
Cooking Time: 15 minutes
Serves 8

2 cups mixed, raw nuts—almonds, cashews, pecans
1 teaspoon coconut oil
1 tablespoon garam masala
1 teaspoon maple syrup
1 teaspoon sea salt

- Preheat oven to 300 degrees.
- In a bowl mix together nuts, oil and maple syrup.
- Lay nuts on a cookie sheet and roast in the oven until lightly browned all over, about 15 minutes.
- Remove from heat and toss with garam masala and salt.

Guacamole with Jicama Sticks

Prep Time: 20 minutes
Serves 4

2 avocados
½ small red onion
1 small tomato
1 jalapeno pepper
¼ bunch cilantro
juice of one lime
½ teaspoon sea salt
1 large jicama

- Carefully cut open each avocado, remove the seed and scoop out the meat into a mixing bowl.
- Finely dice the onion and tomato.
- Mince the jalapeno. Be careful, the seeds are hot!
- Mince the cilantro.
- Combine all ingredients by mashing and mixing with a fork in a mixing bowl.
- Peel the jicama and slice into sticks.
- Dip one into the guacamole to taste and adjust seasonings as necessary.
- Enjoy!

Sautéed Edamame

Prep Time: 5 minutes
Cooking Time: 30 minutes
Serves 4

> 2 cups shelled edamame beans
> (get them pre-shelled in the frozen section)
> 1 tablespoon olive oil
> ½ teaspoons sea salt
> juice of 1 lemon
> 2 tablespoons chopped cilantro
> black pepper to taste

- Cook edamame in boiling water for 10 minutes.
- Drain beans and chill in the fridge for 10 minutes.
- Heat oil in a large sauté pan and sauté beans with salt for 5 minutes.
- Add lemon juice, cilantro and salt to taste.
- Mix well and serve hot.

Honey Sesame Treats

Prep Time: 5 minutes
Cooking Time: 10 minutes
Serves 8

> ¾ cup sesame seeds
> 1½ tablespoons raw honey

- Grind ½ cup sesame seeds in a coffee grinder or suribachi. Grind them well, but not so much that they become nut butter.
- Place in a bowl, add honey and combine with a fork until it becomes a unified paste.
- Toast the rest of the seeds in a sauté pan for 5 minutes, stirring constantly until they turn golden brown.
- Transfer to a bowl.
- Make ½-inch balls out of the sesame paste and roll each ball in the toasted sesame seeds to coat.
- Eat warm or refrigerate.

desserts

Rice Pudding

Prep Time: 5 minutes
Cooking Time: 25 minutes
Serves 6

> 2 cups leftover, cooked rice
> 1-2 cups coconut water,* rice milk or water
> 1 cinnamon stick or 1 teaspoon ground cinnamon
> 10 cardamom pods or ½ teaspoon ground cardamom
> ½ cup raisins
> ½ cup shredded coconut
> 2 tablespoons raw honey or maple syrup

- Place all ingredients in a pot and bring to a boil.
- Reduce heat and simmer, stirring occasionally.
- Continue cooking until raisins are plump, coconut is soft and most of the liquid has evaporated.
- Taste and add more sweetener if necessary.

*Coconut water is simply the liquid inside a coconut. You can find it in the refrigerated drink section of the health food store. Also, you can often find fresh young coconuts in the health food store or in Asian markets.

Baked Bananas

Prep Time: 5 minutes
Cooking Time 15 minutes
Serves 4

> 4 firm bananas
> 1 teaspoon olive oil
> 1-inch piece grated fresh ginger
> 1 tablespoon cinnamon
> ½ tablespoon nutmeg
> ½ cup raisins

- Preheat oven to 375 degrees.
- Peel and cut bananas in half, lengthwise.
- Oil a baking pan and arrange bananas.
- Sprinkle with spices and raisins, cover, and bake for 10 to 15 minutes.

Mango Blueberry Sorbet

Prep Time: 5 minutes
Serves 6

1 bag frozen mango
1 bag frozen cherries
1 tablespoon agave syrup or honey
¼ cup apple juice

- Put all ingredients into a blender or vita-mix.
- Blend until creamy, about one minute. You may have to scrape the sides of the machine down a few times if using a regular blender.
- Serve immediately.
- Put the rest in a Tupperware in the freezer to enjoy later.

TIP: *You can use any frozen fruits you like or freeze fresh fruits such as bananas and strawberries.*

Melon, Avocados and Figs

Prep Time: 15 minutes
Serves 4

½ your favorite summer melon (cantaloupe, galia, ambrosia)
½ avocado
4 fresh ripe figs of your choice
2 tablespoons flax oil
1 tablespoon rice vinegar
1 teaspoon agave syrup
pinch of salt
1 tablespoon fresh mint, sliced into thin ribbons

- Slice fruit and arrange on a platter any way you like.
- Whisk together other ingredients.
- Pour sauce evenly over fruit.

TIP: *So delicious at the end of the summer when melons and figs are both available!*

Tropical Breeze

Prep Time: 10 minutes
Serves 4

    ½ pineapple
    1 cup plain yogurt
    ¼ cup dried coconut flakes

- Cut pineapple into bite-size chunks.
- Mix all ingredients together in a bowl and enjoy!

TIP: *This is the most simple and refreshing dessert to enjoy in warm weather. Depending on the sweetness of the pineapple, you may want to add a little honey.*

Kuzu: The Magic Sauce Thickener

Kuzu is a plant, originally from Japan. The white root is made into a powder that dissolves in cold water and becomes thick in hot water. It is all natural, with no bitter or sweet aftertaste. It has tremendous healing benefits in that it is alkalinizing, soothing, relieves stomachaches, controls diarrhea, helps relieve colds and flu and restores overall strength.

Raisin Pudding

Prep Time: 5 minutes
Cooking Time: 25 minutes
Serves 4

    1 cup raisins
    2 cups water
    1 teaspoon cinnamon
    2 tablespoons kuzu

- In a saucepan, cook raisins in ½ cup water for 15 minutes.
- Add cinnamon.
- When finished cooking, blend in blender.
- Meanwhile dissolve kuzu in 1½ cups water and mix in with blended raisins.
- Bring mixture back to saucepan and cook over medium heat for 5 more minutes.
- Dash with additional cinnamon and serve.

Almond Cherry Chocolate Pudding

Prep Time: 5 minutes
Cooking Time: 5 minutes
Serves 4

1 pint chocolate amazake
1 teaspoons almond extract
¼ cup chopped almonds, toasted
16 cherries, seeded and chopped
1 tablespoon kuzu root mixed with ¼ cup water

- Heat the amazake to just under boiling.
- Lower the heat, add vanilla, and stir in kuzu root. The amazake should thicken to the consistency of pudding.
- Pour the amazake into 4 pudding cups or small bowls.
- Sprinkle chopped nuts and cherries on top of each cup.
- Chill in the refrigerator for at least 30 minutes before serving.

For many more free recipes, please check out our website:
www.integrativenutrition.com

Notes

CHAPTER 1

[1] Full-Year and Fourth Quarter 2012 Results, The Coca-Cola Company, February 12, 2013.

[2] "Adult Obesity Facts," Centers for Disease Control and Prevention, August 2012.

[3] Debra Bruno, "In China, Obesity Becomes a Problem That's Foreign to Survivors of Its Great Famine," *The Washington Post*, December 31, 2012.

[4] World Disasters Report 2011, International Federation of Red Cross and Red Crescent Societies.

[5] Cardiovascular Diseases Fact Sheet, no. 317, World Health Organization.

[6] Diabetes Factsheet, no. 312, World Health Organization.

[7] *Confronting Costs*, The Commonwealth Fund, January 10, 2013.

[8] *Health Systems Financing: The Path to Universal Coverage*," World Health Organization, World Health Report 2010.

[9] Briefing Note USA, The Organization for Economic Co-operation and Development, 2012.

[10] *Dying for Coverage: The Deadly Consequences of Being Uninsured*, Families USA, June 2012.11 2012 Employer Health Benefits Survey, The Henry J. Kaiser Family Foundation.

[12] *National Scorecard on U.S. Health System Performance*, The Commonwealth Fund, 2011.

[13] Marion Nestle, *Food Politics: How the Food Industry Influences Nutrition and Health* (University of California Press, 2003).

[14] *Food and Drink Weekly*, April 25, 2005.

[15] Fortune 500, 2012, Industry: Food Consumer Products.

[16] McDonald's Corporation, 2012 Annual Report, February 2013.

[17] Opensecrets.org, the website for The Center for Responsive Politics.

[18] D. M. Finkelstein, E. L. Hill, and R. C. Whitaker, "School Food Environments and Policies in US Public Schools." Pediatrics, vol. 122, no. 1, July 1, 2008, e251–e259.

[19] Mary Story, Karen M. Kaphingst, and Simone French, "The Role of Schools in Obesity Prevention," *The Future of Children*, vol. 16, no. 1, Spring 2006.

[20] Jennifer Peltz, "NYC Soda Ban Sued by Businesses, Beverage Groups Including National Restaurant Association," *Huffington Post*, October 12, 2012.

[21] Duff Wilson and Janet Roberts, "Special Report: How Washington Went Soft on Childhood Obesity," Reuters, April 2012.

[22] Alexander Besant, "Pepsi Launches High-Fiber, Fat-Burning Soda in Japan," *GlobalPost*, November 12, 2012.

[23] Press release, McDonald's Corporation, July 26, 2011.

[24] Bruce L. Gardner, *American Agriculture in the Twentieth Century: How It Flourished and What It Cost* (Cambridge: Harvard University Press, 2002).

[25] United States Senate Committee on Agriculture, Nutrition & Forestry, Agriculture Reform, Food and Jobs Act of 2013.

[26] Patrick Leahy, S. 3240 (2012).

[27] Frank D. Lucas, www.opensecrets.org.

[28] *The Use of Medicines in the United States: Review of 2010*, IMS Institute for Healthcare Informatics, April 2011.

[29] NCHS Data Brief, no. 81, Centers for Disease Control and Prevention, December 2011.

[30] Youyoung Lee, "Celebrity Overdoses: Deaths Highlight Prescription Drug Epidemic," *Huffington Post*, August 28, 2012.

[31] Michele Simon, *And Now A Word from Our Sponsors: Are America's Nutrition Professionals in the Pocket of Big Food?*, January 2013.

[32] Sheldon Rampton and John Stauber, "Who Is the Dairy Coalition?" PR Watch, 4th Quarter 2000.

[33] Pamela A. Popper, "Dietician Licensure Protects Dieticians and Not the Public," Buckey Insitiute.

[34] "2011 Organic Industry Survey," Organic Trade Association.

CHAPTER 2

[1] American Society for Microbiology, "Men And Women Have Different Eating Habits, Study Shows," *ScienceDaily*, March 21, 2008.

[2] "U.S. Weight Loss Market Forecast to Hit $66 Billion in 2013," PRweb, December 2012.

[3] Adapted from *The Self-Healing Cookbook* by Kristen Turner.

CHAPTER 3

[1] "Phytochemicals: The Cancer Fighters in the Foods We Eat," American Institute for Cancer Research, 2013.

[2] "Industry Statistics and Projected Growth," Organic Trade Association, June 2011.

[3] *Journal of Agricultural and Food Chemistry*, February 26, 2003, originally published on American Chemical Society's website on January 25, 2003.

[4] "Prop 37 Cheat Sheet: Labeling Genetically Engineered Foods," KCET.

[5] "Genetically Engineered Foods," Whole Foods Market.

[6] "Amazon Destruction: Why Is the Rainforest Being Destroyed in Brazil?" www.mongabay.com.

[7] "Zero Net Deforestation by 2020," WWF Global Climate Policy.

CHAPTER 4

[1] Rupert Wheldon, *No Animal Food* (The Health Culture Company, 1910), 11–12.

[2] Claire Suddath, "A Brief History of Veganism," *Time*, October 30, 2008.

[3] Press release, National Institutes of Health, National Institute on Aging, August 29, 2012.

CHAPTER 5

[1] Dan Buettner, "The Island Where People Forget to Die," *New York Times*, October 24, 2012.

[2] Daphne Miller, *The Jungle Effect* (HarperCollins, 2009).

[3] Fernando Martínez, *Why Did McDonald's Bolivia Go Bankrupt?*, 2011.

[4] "Bolivia—McDonald's Is Melted by Public Disinterest and Closes All Its Premises," *El Polvorin*, December 19, 2011.

[5] "Global and Regional Food Consumption Patterns and Trends," World Health Organization, 2013.

[6] Ewen Callaway, "Pottery Shards Put a Date on Africa's Dairying," *Nature*, June 22, 2012.

[7] Singhal Arvind, "India's Growing Appetite for Meat Challenges Traditional Values," AFP.

[8] Eliza Barclay, "Nordic Diet Could Be Local Alternative to Mediterranean Diet," NPR, *The Salt* (blog), May 31, 2013.

[9] Steve Inskeep and Maria Godoy, "Za'atar: A Spice Mix with Biblical Roots and Brain Food Reputation," NPR, *The Salt* (blog), June 11, 2013.

[10] Candido Astrologo Jr., "Statistical Indicators on Philippine Development," National Statistics Coordination Board (NSCB), 2008 Survey.

[11] "Health Benefits of Thai Soup Under Study," January 3, 2001.

[12] "10 Reasons to Add Bee Pollen to Your Diet," *The Fresh Network Blog*, January 17, 2013.

[13] Sophie D. Coe and Michael D. Coe, *The True History of Chocolate* (Thames & Hudson, 2013).

[14] Teya Skae, "Examining the Properties of Chocolate and Cacao for Health," *Natural News*, February 7, 2008.

[15] Lindsey Duncan, "Chia: Ancient Super-Seed Secret," www.droz.com.

[16] David Wolfe, *Superfoods: The Food and Medicine of the Future* (North Atlantic Books, 2009).

[17] Ibid.18 "Plant Cultures: Hemp," www.kew.org.

[19] Gero Leson and Walter Russell, "The Amazing Benefits of Hemp Seeds: Too Bad the DEA Is Curtailing the Industry," alternet.org, October 26, 2012.

[20] "Quinoa," The World's Healthiest Foods, www.whfoods.com.

[21] "Manuka Honey," WebMD, www.webmd.com.

[22] "Moringa: The Next Big Superfood?" Duck News, June 10, 2013.

[23] "Superfoods for 2012," www.drlindsey.com.

CHAPTER 6

[1] Sanjay Basu, Paula Yoffe, Nancy Hills, and Robert H. Lustig, "The Relationship of Sugar to Population-Level Diabetes Prevalence: An Econometric Analysis of Repeated Cross-Sectional Data," *PLOS ONE*, vol. 8, no. 2, 2013.

CHAPTER 7

[1] "Depression is a Common Illness and People Suffering from Depression Need Support and Treatment," World Health Organization, October 9, 2012.

[2] National Institute of Mental Health.

[3] James Vlahos, "Is Sitting a Lethal Activity?" *New York Times*, April 14, 2011.

[4] Niels Bosma, Sander Wennekers, and José Ernesto Amorós, "Global Entrepreneurship Monitor 2011 Extended Report."

[5] Kerry Hannon, "Are Senior Start-Ups The Answer?" Forbes.com, September 9, 2012.

CHAPTER 8

[1] Alyssa Oursler, "The Best-Selling Candy Brands of 2012," InvestorPlace.com, September 18, 2012.

[2] "Childhood Obesity Facts," Centers for Disease Control and Prevention, 2013.

[3] "BLS American Time Use Survey," A.C. Nielsen Co.

[4] Amanda Bruce, Rebecca Lepping, Jared Bruce, Bradley Cherry, Laura Martin, Ann Davis, et al., "Brain Responses to Food Logos in Obese and Healthy Weight Children," *Journal of Pediatrics*, vol. 162, issue 4, 2013.

[5] Dawn C. Chmielewski, "Disney Bans Junk-Food Advertising on Programs for Children," *Los Angeles Times*, June 6, 2012.

[6] South Carolina Department of Mental Health, "Eating Disorder Statistics," 2011.

[7] Galia Slayen, "The Scary Reality of a Real-Life Barbie Doll," *Huffington Post*, April 8, 2011.

CHAPTER 9

[1] John G. Rodwan Jr., "Bottled Water 2011: The Recovery Continues," www.bottledwater.org.

[2] Jared Blumenfeld and Susan Leal, "The High Costs of Bottled Water," *San Francisco Chronicle*, February 18, 2007.

[3] Andrew Pollack, "Monsato Wins Big Award in a Biotech Patent Case," *New York Times*, August 1, 2012.

[4] Kaayla Daniels, *The Whole Soy Story: The Dark Side of America's Favorite Health Food* (Newtrends Publishing, Inc., 2005).5 P. Fort, N. Moses, M. Fasano, T. Goldberg, and F. Lifshitz, "Breast and Soy-Formula Feedings in Early Infancy and the Prevalence of Autoimmune Thyroid Disease in Children," *Journal of the American College of Nutrition*, vol. 9, issue 2, 1990.

CHAPTER 10

[1] Alice G. Walton. "How Much Sugar Are Americans Eating?" Forbes.com, August 30, 2012.

[2] "Broccoli profile," USDA Economic Research Service, 2011.

[3] Walton, "How Much Sugar Are Americans Eating?"4 Clif Bar & Company, www.clifbar.com.

[5.] "Coffee Frappuccino® Blended Beverage," Starbucks Corporation, www.starbucks.com.

[6] "The Global Burden," International Diabetes Federation, *Diabetes Atlas*, fifth edition.

[7] Basu, et al., "Relationship of Sugar to Population-Level Diabetes Prevalence."

[8] Magalie Lenoir, Fuschia Serre, Lauriane Cantin, and Serge H. Ahmed, "Intense Sweetness Surpasses Cocaine Reward," *PLOS ONE*, vol. 2, no. 8, 2007.

[9] Qing Yang, "Gain Weight by 'Going Diet'? Artificial Sweeteners and the Neurobiology of Sugar Cravings," *Yale Journal of Biology and Medicine*, vol. 82, no. 2, 2010.

[10] David Barbano, "BST Fact Sheet," FDA Connection.

[11] "Quality Low Impact Food," Danish Institute of Agricultural Sciences and University of Newcastle.

[12] B. J. Abelow, T. R. Holford, and K. L. Insogna, "Cross-Cultural Association Between Dietary Animal Protein and Hip Fractures: A Hypothesis," *Calcified Tissue International* (Yale, 1992).

[13] "The Consumers Union Guide to Environmental Labels," www.eco-labels.org.

[14] Coffee Statistic Report 2012 Edition.

[15] "Coffee: Health Food or Simply Not a Risk?" American Institute for Cancer Research, December 11, 2006.

[16] "WHO Issues New Guidance on Dietary Salt and Potassium," World Health Organization, http://www.who.int/mediacentre/news/notes/2013/salt_potassium_20130131/en/.

[17] Michael Jacobson, *Salt: The Forgotten Killer*, Center for Science in the Public Interest, February 2005.

[18] "World Salt Awareness Week," Centers for Disease Control and Prevention, 2013.

[19] "Raised Blood Pressure," World Health Organization, Global Health Observatory, 2013.

[20] Jacobson, *Salt*.

[21] "Who Consumes the Most Chocolate?" CNN Freedom Project, January 17, 2012.

CHAPTER 11

[1] FairShare CSA Coalition, www.csacoalition.org.

[2] Ibid.

References

The 3-Season Diet: Eat the Way Nature Intended: Lose Weight, Beat Food Cravings, Get Fit by John Douillard, Ph.D. Three Rivers Press, 2000.

The Art of Listening by Harvey Jackins. Rational Island Publishers, 1981.

The Book of Macrobiotics: The Universal Way of Health and Happiness by Michio Kushi. Japan Publications, Inc., 1977.

Can't Buy My Love: How Advertising Changes the Way We Think and Feel by Jean Kilbourne. Touchstone, 1999.

Diet for a Small Planet by Frances Moore Lappé. Ballantine Books, 1972.

Eat, Drink and Be Healthy: The Harvard Medical School Guide to Healthy Eating by Walter Willett, M.D. Free Press, 2001.

Eat More, Weigh Less by Dean Ornish, M.D. HarperCollins Publishers, 1993.

Eat Right for Your Type: The Individualized Diet Solution to Staying Healthy, Living Healthy & Achieving Your Ideal Weight by Peter D'Adamo, N.D.G.P. Putnam's Sons, 1996.

Energetics of Food: Encounters with Your Most Intimate Relationship by Steve Gagné. Spiral Sciences, 1990.

Enter the Zone: The Dietary Road Map to Lose Weight & More by Barry Sears, Ph.D. and Bill Lawren. HarperCollins Publishers, 1995.

Food and Our Bones: The Natural Way to Prevent Osteoporosis by Annemarie Colbin, Ph.D. The Penguin Group, 1998.

Food Politics: How the Food Industry Influences Nutrition and Health by Marion Nestle, Ph.D., M.P.H. University of California Press, 2002.

Get the Sugar Out: 501 Simple Ways to Cut the Sugar out of Any Diet by Ann Louise Gittleman, Ph.D., C.N.S. Three Rivers Press, 1996.

The Glucose Revolution Life Plan by Jennie Brand-Miller. Avalon Publishing Group, 2001.

Grub: Ideas for an Urban Organic Kitchen by Anna Lappé and Bryant Terry. Jeremy P. Tarcher/Penguin, 2006.

Healing with Whole Foods: Asian Traditions and Modern Nutrition by Paul Pitchford. North Atlantic Books, 1993.

The Longevity Diet: Discover Calorie Restriction—The Only Proven Way to Slow the Aging Process and Maintain Peak Vitality, by Brian M. Delaney and Lisa Walford. Marlowe & Company, 2005.

The Master Cleanser: With Special Needs and Problems by Stanley Burroughs. Burroughs Books, 1976.

The Mood Cure: The 4 Step Program to Rebalance Your Emotional Chemistry and Rediscover Your Natural Sense of Well-Being, by Julia Ross. M.A. Viking Penguin, 2002.

Nature's First Law: The Raw-Food Diet by Stephen Arllin, Fouad Dini and David Wolfe. Maul Brothers Publishing, 1996.

Nourishing Traditions: The Cookbook That Challenges Politically Correct Nutrition and the Diet Dictocrats by Sally Fallon with Mary Enig, Ph.D. NewTrends Publishing, 1999.

Nourishing Wisdom: A Mind-Body Approach to Nutrition and Well-Being by Marc David, with Patrick McGrady, Jr. Bell Tower, 1991.

Pritikin Program for Diet and Exercise by Nathan Pritikin, M.D. Grosset and Dunlap, 1980.

The Self-Healing Cookbook: A Macrobiotic Primer for Healing Body, Mind and Moods with Whole, Natural Foods by Kristina Turner. Earthtones Press, 1987.

Soul Work: Finding the Work You Love, Loving the Work You Find by Deborah Bloch and Lee Richmond. Davies-Black Publishing, 1998.

The South Beach Diet: The Delicious, Doctor Designed, Foolproof Plan for Fast and Healthy Weight Loss by Arthur Agatston, M.D. Rodale, Inc, 2003.

Staying Healthy with the Seasons by Elson M. Haas, MD. Celestial Arts, 1981.

Sugar Shock!: How Sweets and Simple Carbs Can Derail Your Life—and How You Can Get Back on Track by Connie Bennett, C.H.H.C. and Stephen T. Sinatra, M.D. Berkley Trade, 2006.

The Truth about Drug Companies: How They Deceive Us and What to Do about It by Marcia Angell, M.D. Random House Publishing Group, 2004.

Your Body's Many Cries For Water: You Are Not Sick, You Are Thirsty! by Fereydoon Batmanghelidj, M.D. Global Health Solutions, 1992.

Index

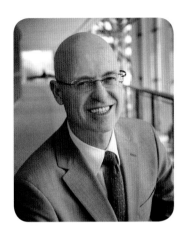

About the Author

Joshua Rosenthal is the founder, director and primary instructor of the Institute for Integrative Nutrition®, the world's largest online nutrition school, based in New York City. He is a highly trained leader with a Master's of Science degree in Education, specializing in counseling. With 30 years of experience in the fields of whole foods, personal coaching, curriculum development, teaching and nutritional counseling, Joshua has pioneered Integrative Nutrition®, a whole body approach to holistic nutrition and living. His simple methods allow people to quickly and successfully reach new levels of health and happiness.

About Integrative Nutrition

Since 1992, the Institute for Integrative Nutrition® has led the field of holistic nutrition education. Our proprietary online learning course allows students from all over the world to experience our cutting-edge Health Coach Training Program.

We are the only school in the world integrating all the different dietary theories—combining the knowledge of traditional philosophies like Ayurveda, macrobiotics and Chinese medicine with modern concepts like the USDA food guides, the glycemic index, The Zone, the South Beach Diet and raw foods. We teach more than 100 different dietary theories and address the fundamental concepts, issues and ethics of eating in a modern world.

In addition, the curriculum bridges the gap between nutrition and personal growth and development by addressing what other dietary theories don't talk about—a concept called primary food. Healthy relationships, regular physical activity, fulfilling careers and a spiritual practice feed your soul and satisfy your hunger for living. When primary food is balanced, the fun, excitement, love and passion of your daily life nourish you on a deeper level than the food you eat.

The school is a place of profound learning, with guest teachers, who are the world's greatest nutrition and personal development experts, including Dr. Andrew Weil, Dr. Barry Sears, Deepak Chopra, Paul Pitchford, and Geneen Roth.

Our mission is to play a crucial role in improving health and happiness, and through that process create a ripple effect that transforms the world. Students learn about healthy nutrition and lifestyle choices and receive business training to help them work with the public around these crucial matters.

Graduates who are Integrative Nutrition® certified partner with physicians, chiropractors, fitness facilities, spas, schools, restaurants, retail stores, publishers, websites and corporations and work in private practice.

For more information about Integrative Nutrition, go to our website:
www.integrativenutrition.com